AIDS AWARENESS THROUGH COMMUNITY PARTICIPATION

AIDS
Awareness Through Community Participation
An Action Research

Meenu Sharma

Publications

KALPAZ PUBLICATIONS

Delhi-110052

AIDS Awareness Through Community Participation
An Action Research

ISBN: 81-7835-471-3

Reprinted in 2012 in India by
Kalpaz Publications,
C-30, Satyawati Nagar, Delhi-110 052
E-mail: kalpaz@hotmail.com

Printed at: G. Print Process, Delhi

Contents

List of Tables

List of Figures

List of Pictures

List of Appendices

List of Annexures

List of Acronyms Commonly Used in the Research

AIDS	–	Acquired Immuno Deficiency Syndrome
CDC	–	Centre for Disease Control and Prevention
CSW/s	–	Commercial Sex Worker/s
DBT	–	Department of Bio-technology
EMS	–	Extramarital Sex
Ft. Pd	–	Field-testing Period
GIPA	–	Greater Involvement of People Living with or Affected by HIV/AIDS
HAART	–	Highly Active Anti Retroviral Therapy
HIV -	–	HIV Negative
HIV +	–	HIV Positive
HIV	–	Human Immuno Deficiency Virus
ICMR	–	Indian Council of Medical Research
IDU	–	Injecting Drug User/s
IEC	–	Information Education & Communication
ILO	–	International Labour Organization
Int. Pd	–	Intervention Period
KABP	–	Knowledge, Attitude, Behaviour & Practices
MTCT	–	Mother to Child Transmission
NACO	–	National AIDS Control Organization
NACP/s	–	National AIDS Control Programme/s
NGO/s	–	Non-government Organization/s
ORG	–	Operations Research Group
ORG CSR	–	Operations Research Group, Center for Social Research
%	–	Percentage
PMS	–	Premarital Sex
PWHA	–	People Living with or Affected by HIV/AIDS
SPPC	–	Strategic Plan for Prevention and Control
STD	–	Sexually Transmitted Disease/s
STI	–	Sexually Transmitted Infection/s
T.V.	–	Television
UCMS	–	University College of Medical Sciences
UN	–	United Nations
UNAIDS	–	Joint United Nations Programme on HIV/AIDS
UNDCP	–	United Nations International Drug Control Programme
UNDP	–	United Nations Development Fund
UNESCO	–	United Nations Educational, Scientific and Cultural Organization

UNFPA	–	United Nations Population Fund
UNICEF	–	United Nations Children's Fund
USAID	–	United States Agency for International Development
UTA	–	Universities Talk AIDS
UTs	–	Union Territories
WBC	–	White Blood Cells
WHO	–	World Health Organization

Preface

World is a beautiful place and so is the experience of living in it. It would be tragic if this beautiful experience of living life is shortened by HIV/AIDS, when its prevention is within one's control, though not the cure. The Acquired Immune Deficiency Syndrome commonly known as AIDS is caused by the Human Immuno Deficiency Virus (HIV), which completely breaks down the immune system of a body to combat infections, even the commonest ones. The infection in a HIV positive person remains dormant for about 5-10 years before the onset of full blown AIDS, which is terminal.

Globally, the number of people living with HIV/AIDS at the end of the year 2004 stood at nearly 40 million, while the epidemic is estimated to have claimed more than 3 million lives the same year according to the recent UNAIDS/WHO (2004) estimates. The statistics are raising grave concern since the infection is rapidly spilling over to the general population from those with high-risk behaviour like the commercial sex workers, truck drivers and migrant populations with known vulnerability to the HIV. In India, the first case of HIV was reported in 1986 and since then the country has been experiencing an exponential rise in the number of new HIV infections each year. According to the National AIDS Control Organization (NACO) estimates, 5.1 million people in India were HIV infected by the end of the year 2004. The HIV has taken the form of an epidemic and is also one of the leading causes of life threatening diseases such as tuberculosis, cancer, dementia and eventually death amongst the most productive and reproductive sections of the population.

The problem is aggravated by the fact that there is a lack of overall awareness about the disease among majority of the masses. Continuing myths and misconceptions regarding the cause and transmission of the disease are causing "AIDS phobia" where in people living with or affected by HIV/AIDS are being strongly discriminated by the general population while at the same time it is also leading to "physicians bias" that poses a major deterrent to treatment and care of HIV/AIDS infected people. Further, the stigma attached to certain populations practicing high-risk behaviour extends the marginalization of the most vulnerable sections.

Efforts are underway in almost all parts of the country to implement large-scale information and education programmes for HIV/AIDS prevention. However, the increasing number of HIV infections strongly suggests that there is an urgent need to increase the coverage area of such interventions.

The present study was undertaken with a broad objective to create awareness about AIDS amongst the most vulnerable sections of the society using community participation approach. The sample for the study comprised of the commercial sex workers, the truck drivers and the rickshaw pullers each thirty in number. These groups have been reported to be most vulnerable to the HIV infection due to their indulgence in high-risk behaviour. The situation is further aggravated because of lack of awareness about the disease and the general apathy.

The specific objectives of the present study were to have an insight into the respondents' myths, misconceptions relating to HIV/AIDS, their living and work environment followed by development of a set of communication material for AIDS awareness. The thread running through these objectives was the intervention aimed at enhancing awareness about the disease. The main thrust of the study was to involve the community for achieving sustainability of this action research.

The study was done in three distinct but related phases. The first step in the process of bringing about HIV/AIDS awareness was to make an initial assessment of the knowledge level, types of attitudes and forms of behaviour and practices of the sample groups with regards to HIV/AIDS. To achieve this, regular visits were made to the three sites selected on the basis of a pilot study, located in Delhi and information was gathered with the help of interview, focus group discussion and observation methods of data collection. The process aimed at identification of "gray areas" in the form of myths and misconceptions, negative attitudes, high-risk behaviour and practices of the sample groups. This marked the first phase "the pre-intervention period" of the study.

Since the knowledge, attitude, behaviour and practices (KABP) scores of the sample in context to HIV/AIDS were found to be abysmally low (as assessed by the KABP scale developed for the study on the basis of core indicators used by the WHO and Operations Research Group – Center for Social Research) a suitable intervention based on the needs of the communities was planned and carried out accordingly. The need assessment of the sample took into consideration their living and work environment, substance use patterns, day-to-day behaviour and practices, the value system upheld by them along with recognition of other vulnerability factors hindering their ability to protect themselves from HIV. This marked the second phase of the study denoted by the actual conduction of the intervention.

Community participation was ensured at various stages of the intervention such as development of the audio-visual aids, training of few members of the sample communities as peer educators as well as conducting of HIV/AIDS related out-reach activities within their respective communities by the peer educators. This period termed as the "intervention" represented the transition phase in which the sample was seen moving ahead from ignorance to a state of factual knowledge and awareness regarding HIV/AIDS and its ramifications. Rapport building and gaining their trust were crucial for such community-involved action.

In the third and final phase of the study "the post-intervention period", KABP of the sample were re-assessed using the same scale as was used at the time of the pre-intervention. A comparative analysis was done for specific contents/areas to see changes in the knowledge, attitude, behaviour and practices of the sample as a result of the intervention.

The study depicted findings of a wider significance in terms of recognition of not merely superficial but core factors enhancing samples' vulnerability to HIV/AIDS. For instance, the sample's tendency to practice sex with non-regular partner/s without using a condom was not merely viewed as conducting of unsafe sex but the underlying reasons for this practice were analyzed in detail. Lack of condom use negotiation skills, not carrying a condom (non-accessibility) during the time of sexual transaction, treating condoms as a hindrance to pleasure, as well as wrongly treating many sexual partners as steady partners with whom condom usage was not considered necessary, were seen as some of the reasons for their unsafe behaviour. These vital issues were subsequently addressed through the intervention, which empowered the sample with related skills.

The results of the study portrayed a significant change brought about as a result of the intervention in KABP of the sample with regards to HIV/AIDS. For instance, the awareness regarding crucial aspects of the disease like its transmission modes and symptoms, concept of fatality of the disease and most importantly of HIV preventive methods showed a significant rise. Few case studies were also conducted to explore trends in human behaviour with regards to HIV/AIDS. These studies while highlighting the HIV vulnerability factors also effectively documented the impact of the intervention on the sample by way of desirable changes.

Based on the prior need assessment, a set of communication material in the form of audio-visual aids, which included a photo-script, a poster and a pamphlet were designed for the sample groups. These audio-visual aids aimed at generating HIV/AIDS awareness along with emphasis on certain subtle human values to improve their behaviour in context of HIV vulnerability. These aids were field-tested both within as well as across the three sample groups. The results indicated significant changes in the overall KABP of the sample.

The study showed that the sample appreciated the efforts of the researcher in seeking community participation thereby removing several inhibitions. The interactive mode of communication used in these aids seemed to be a viable solution as the sample was able to dispel its doubts, myths and misconceptions regarding the disease.

The study concluded with the crucial theme that awareness, care and empowerment of the communities (ACE strategy) can lead them to a positive beginning directed towards safe behaviour.

Meenu Sharma

Acknowledgements

First and foremost, I am grateful to God for bestowing on me the courage to carry out this research work.

I take the opportunity to pay my deepest sense of gratitude to my revered supervisors Dr. Savitri Ramamurthy, Former Reader and Dr. Sarita Anand, Senior Lecturer, Lady Irwin College, University of Delhi, for their valuable guidance, keen interest and cooperation from initiation till culmination of the present research. I am thankful to them for leading me through this wonderful learning experience.

It is a matter of privilege to have worked under the able guidance of Dr. (Mrs.) K. Khanna, Head, Department of Home Science, University of Delhi. I am extremely thankful to her for the constant encouragement and support rendered throughout the course of this study.

Behind visible success, there are numerous invisible efforts. I must thank Mr. K. K. Arora, SPA, Lady Irwin College, Delhi, for making all such efforts and providing support throughout the course of my study. His gentle reminders encouraged me to keep the work going, even through phases that were not so easy.

My deep sense of indebtness is due to Mr. Anil Kumar, Senior Programmer, Indian Council of Social and Scientific Research (ICSSR), Delhi, for helping me to quantify the huge volume of data gathered for the study.

From the core of my heart, I thank all my study participants for allowing me to tread and many a times intrude into their personal lives. Without their complete and honest involvement, this endeavour would not have been possible. I am indeed, indebted to them.

I owe tremendous gratitude to my family; especially my mother for giving me unstinted love and support. My acknowledgement would not be complete without saying a "Big Thank You" to my lovely daughter Urvashi, who had to bear my absence for long period of time.

Heartfelt thanks to all my friends for their unforgettable cooperation and support at times when required the most.

Meenu Sharma

Introduction

As the twentieth century drew to a close and mankind entered into a new millennium, the world witnessed a lot of spectacular events celebrated with magnanimous enthusiasm and joy. Indeed, it was time to celebrate because we as mankind have achieved a lot in terms of growth and development. But for the families of a few million people, there were no celebrations at all because they had lost their dear ones to AIDS (Acquired Immune Deficiency Syndrome). Unfortunately, even today AIDS is still continuing to take it's toll of human lives rather very harshly necessitating the setting up of the millennium achievement goal to halt and reverse the epidemic by 2015.

AIDS cases were first reported in the U.S.A. in the year 1981. Today, twenty-four years later AIDS has engulfed the entire globe by transforming itself into a pandemic. According to the new estimates from the Joint United Nations Programme on HIV/AIDS (UNAIDS) and the World Health Organization (WHO) more than 70 million people have been infected with the virus out of which over 30 million have already died. At the end of the year 2004, an estimated 40 million people globally were living with the HIV (Human Immuno Deficiency Virus). The number of children now alive with HIV is 2.5 million and women represent nearly 43 per cent of all people living with HIV/AIDS. Global estimates indicate that more than 95 per cent of all HIV infected people live in the developing world that has likewise experienced 95 per cent of all AIDS deaths till date. As many as 11 men, women and children around the world were infected every minute during 1998 amounting to 16,000 infections per day. Further, tuberculosis, the second biggest infectious killer is also on the rise, driven in large part by the HIV epidemic. Around 30 per cent of all AIDS deaths result directly from tuberculosis (UNAIDS/WHO, Dec., 2003, 1998).

Need for Creating AIDS Awareness

The impact of AIDS is now being increasingly felt by many countries across the globe. The disease is tearing away the social and economic fabric of the global-community by killing people in the prime of their youth on whom the society relies for production and reproduction. The epidemic is eroding the hard-earned gains in development indicators by regressing life expectancy, rising child mortality rates and leading to a substantial fall in gross domestic product (GDP) growth rate in many countries. Huge number of farmers, teachers, doctors and other human resources are being claimed by the epidemic leading to widespread shortages of food and access to medical care (UNAIDS/WHO, Dec., 2001).

In India by the end of the year 2000, the overall cost on account of AIDS rose to US $ 11 billion (WHO, 1999). AIDS is seen not just as a health problem; but a potential threat to human welfare, development as well as social and economic stability. *The challenge to contain the spread of HIV and to convert this commitment into a sustained strategy is the need of the hour.* Identifying people with propensity to acquire and transmit the HIV infection and addressing factors that make individuals vulnerable to the disease become crucial.

Statistics from various countries including India show that behaviours that cause the highest risk of acquiring HIV infection are unprotected sexual contact with multiple partners and sharing of needle and syringe. This in turn implies that the most vulnerable groups include commercial sex workers, truck drivers, migrant workers, injecting drug users and other youth groups. While men and women, both are vulnerable to HIV, the latter are more so because of their sexual and economic subordination to men.

Although, there has been a growing awareness to identify factors that make individuals particularly vulnerable to HIV infection, there is paucity of systematic analysis (UNAIDS/WHO, Dec., 2001). The social, economic and cultural situations that create vulnerability to HIV infection have not been adequately studied or explained. Surprisingly, there is virtually no information in many countries on the basic sexual and drug taking behaviours and patterns of sexual networking that determine how the virus spreads amongst a population (www.unaids.org. June, 1998). Although various parts of the world have witnessed the epidemic among the diverse populations - poverty, lack of skills, violence and harmful social norms are some of the manifestations (UNAIDS, 1999). The problem is further aggravated by illiteracy. Since many of the populations most affected by the disease are among the world's least educated, there has been a temptation to say, "AIDS is a disease of ignorance" (www.unaids.org. June, 1998). More than twenty years into the epidemic, millions of young people know little about HIV/AIDS. According to UNICEF, over 50 per cent of the young people (aged 15-24 years) in more than a dozen countries have never heard of AIDS or harbour serious misconceptions about how HIV is transmitted (UNAIDS/WHO, 2001). Although there is no single solution to these closely interlinked problems, still since HIV is primarily associated with high-risk behaviour, changes in individual behaviour would go long way to prevent this dreaded disease. But building awareness regarding HIV/AIDS would be a prerequisite. Gaining awareness and knowledge is the first stage in the process of acceptance of new ideas, practices and change of behaviour (Seth and Capila cited in Vasuja, 1999).

Worldwide, studies have shown that well designed and carefully focused HIV prevention campaigns that rely on increasing knowledge of HIV and how to avoid it; creating an environment where safer sexual or drug taking behaviours can be discussed and acted upon; providing services such as treatment for sexually transmitted diseases (which if left untreated greatly augment the risk for HIV transmission), access to cheap condoms and clean injection equipment and lastly but most importantly helping people to acquire the skills they need to protect themselves have managed to arrest or even reverse HIV trends. Thailand's 100 per cent condom usage programme enforcing a policy of 100 per cent condom usage in brothels by the commercial sex workers and in Nepal, a vigorous campaign to inform truck drivers and sex workers of the risk of unprotected sex have helped substantially in raising awareness about HIV/AIDS, subsequently, leading to a significant decline in HIV infection rates due to cutting down of risk behaviour among such populations. Thus, what seems evident is that awareness works and it does lead to prevention. At present, since prospects for a HIV cure or vaccine seem remote, HIV prevention efforts take on even greater role in containing the spread of the epidemic and minimizing its future impact.

The Joint United Nations Programme on HIV/AIDS (UNAIDS) is leading the global response to HIV/AIDS along with a host of other UN agencies, countries and partner organizations in developing and advocating the use of "best-practices" which strive to reduce the impact of HIV/AIDS. Some of the key areas in which efforts are being massively scaled up include – rationalizing measures and providing facilities for HIV testing, providing counselling, care and support to people infected with HIV, countering stigma and discrimination against PWHA (people living with HIV/AIDS) in order to recognize the important contribution they can make within the society, and most crucially helping countries gain an access to anti-retroviral therapy at affordable prices. The WHO and UNAIDS have taken what is termed as the 3 by 5 initiative which aims at providing anti-retroviral treatment to 3 million people in areas of most need, by the end of the year 2005 (UNAIDS/WHO, Dec., 2003).

Large-scale information, education and communication (IEC) programmes continue to be implemented, essentially to contain the spread of HIV/AIDS. It is, however, important that the messages that are seen or sent out must be sensitive to cultures, traditions, the literacy levels and the environment of the people (WHO, 1999). While designing/implementing HIV/AIDS awareness programmes many factors need to be taken into account. A "*client-centred model*" can help service providers to work more effectively with populations resistant to behvioural change. In such model, interactions are tailored to assess the clients' needs, including behavioural risks and contextual issues (social, psychological and economic factors etc.). Further, the use of a "harm-reduction approach" (i.e., gradual minimization of risk behaviour over time) as the basis for interventions encourages the clients and the service providers to select specific behavioural changes, which realistically reflect the clients' circumstances and willingness to change (Brookman, 1996).

Prevention initiatives that rely on community-participation in terms of energy, commitment and spirit of the targeted communities are emerging to be a credible and cost-effective solution in combating AIDS. The grass-root participation of community members is vital in developing a culturally appropriate programme (Sin, 1996) and in ensuring community acceptance of the same (Ayala, et al., 1996). Thus, peer educators are being encouraged and trained to disseminate HIV information. The importance of peer educators to bring about behvioural change and to help keep HIV infection at a low level has been effectively demonstrated by the Sonagachi initiative in which groups of sex workers were mobilized as peer educators and trained to disseminate HIV/AIDS information. Further, peer educators can crucially help in sustaining HIV/AIDS prevention efforts due to the fact that they can draw upon from their existing social networks and identify shared problems and experiences thus, building the solidarity necessary for a truly community-based programme (Skinner, et al., 1996).

Another area requiring mounted focus is empowerment of communities with skills required to practice safe behaviour. There is a critical need to integrate life-skills education into HIV prevention programmes. WHO defines life-skills as "abilities for adaptive and positive behaviour to enable individuals to deal with the demands and challenges of everyday life" (UNFPA, Sept., 2000). It has been realized that people cannot transform HIV awareness information into safe behaviour and practices until they have the required skills to do so. Promoting condom usage messages cannot be of much help till people know the skill to use a condom correctly. Based on the rising HIV incidence, massive efforts are needed to equip young people with life-skills training such as correct condom usage and disposal, negotiation skills, disinfecting needle and syringe etc., that is essential to protect them from the virus.

Although, concerted efforts backed by strong political leadership and high level of public commitment are being stepped up yet, behavioural data mapping knowledge, attitude, behaviour and practices (KABP) related to HIV/AIDS reflects an overall lack of awareness coupled with widespread complacency amongst vast populations across the globe. This is also evident from the extensive spread of the epidemic.

Hence, a successful response to the AIDS epidemic calls for a dynamic action in the form of programmes, which are need-based, foster community-participation, include mobilization of peer educators, empower targeted communities and are sustainable in the long term.

State of the HIV Epidemic in India

At the end of the year 2004, an estimated 5.1 million Indians were living with HIV/AIDS. Presently in the six states which are Maharashtra, Tamil Nadu, Andhra Pradesh, Karnataka, Manipur and Nagaland, the HIV prevalence in the general population is more than one per cent indicating the presence of generalized epidemic (UNAIDS/WHO, Dec., 2004). Out of all the reported AIDS cases nearly 75 per cent are represented by men while transmission through sexual mode accounts for 83 per cent of all the HIV infections (NACO, 2002). Although there are significant variations among and within the states yet, the emergence of a common pattern nationwide is causing great concern, which depicts that the HIV is rapidly shifting from populations with high-risk behaviours to the general population. The virus is logging itself fast and firmly in the general population, which was earlier supposed to be safe from the epidemic. In the national capital Delhi, the threat of HIV prevalence is looming large over several residential colonies. A recent survey has indicated that all the nine districts of the capital have at least one or more high-density areas of the virus. Further, the number of people living with HIV in the city is estimated to be more than 25,000 with several areas turning fast into hubs of HIV positives (Chabbra, 2003).

Given the current evidence, a much larger and generalized epidemic cannot be ruled out. Some of the factors propelling the epidemic are high prevalence of STDs, presence of red light areas and commercial sex workers and large-scale migration from rural to urban areas in search of work (NACO, 2002). Besides, populations such as those of injecting drug users, men having sex with men, and people with high mobility (e.g., truck drivers) are also known to boost the transmission of HIV by indulging in high-risk behaviour. The situation is further worsened by lack of awareness about the disease and its preventive aspects. To combat the epidemic, the National AIDS Control Programme (NACP) in India established the National AIDS Control Organization (NACO) in 1992 with the aim of leading and catalyzing an expanded response to the HIV/AIDS epidemic. NACO in collaboration with UN and bilateral agencies, NGOs, educational and research organizations and government as well as private sector is continuously accelerating a broad-based effective response to contain the spread of the HIV. Some of the major issues being addressed on a priority basis are – awareness generation among the masses through various programmes including suitable IEC strategies, implementing targeted interventions for specific populations, and encouraging health-seeking behaviour among the masses. Integrating HIV/AIDS and STD control within the existing health-care system, ensuring blood safety measures, establishing voluntary counselling and testing centers, providing care and support to those infected with HIV and most importantly propelling the participation of NGOs and other voluntary groups in the NACP are some of the efforts in the prevention and control of the HIV, a notoriously dreaded disease of the century.

Recently, there has been a growing focus on the decentralization of prevention efforts and services including financial and administrative powers from the national to the state level. Efforts are also being marshaled to counter discrimination against PWHA, which is proving to be a major hurdle in prevention efforts in India. Although, progress is being made on many fronts still there is not yet persuasive evidence to show that the epidemic is being curbed (UNAIDS/WHO, Dec., 2003). The appropriateness, reach, efficacy and sustainability of the programmes need to be reviewed in view of the troubling rise in HIV prevalence. Various KABP assessment surveys (Balaganesh, et al., 1994; Ghosh, et al., 1997; Roy & Chowdhury, 1997) show an overall lack of awareness among the masses including medical practitioners regarding vital aspects of HIV/AIDS, leading to increased vulnerability. *The solution to this problem largely lies in generating HIV/AIDS awareness amongst populations through need-based programmes.*

Vulnerability of Commercial Sex Workers, Truck Drivers and Rickshaw Pullers to HIV/AIDS

Commercial sex workers, truck drivers and rickshaw pullers (representing the migrant population) have been recognized by the National AIDS Control Organization as populations with high-risk behaviour leading to their remarkably increased vulnerability to HIV/AIDS (NACO, 2002). Statistics depict that level of infections among sex workers and their clients (the bulk mostly constituted by transport workers and the migrant population) are rising at alarming levels (UNAIDS/WHO, June 1998 & Dec., 2001). The HIV infection rate among commercial sex workers in Mumbai was 52 per cent in 1996 (WHO, 1999), which has lately risen to 60 per cent primarily due to ignorance and lack of information (UNFPA, Sept., 2000). Similarly, in Delhi HIV testing conducted on 30 sex workers from the G.B. Road revealed that as many as seven of them (23 per cent) were HIV positive (Chabbra, 2003). Further, a number of studies with truck drivers and migrant workers also continue to ascertain their vulnerability to HIV/AIDS by reflecting rising HIV prevalence amongst them. HIV prevalence rates as high as 8.33 per cent (Roy, et al., 1997) and 1 per cent (Ramakrishnaiah, et al., 1997) have been recorded among truck drivers and migrant workers respectively.

Many inter-related factors in their lives such as poverty, low literacy levels, lack of employment opportunities, mobility, migration and exploitation often force them into a vicious cycle of poverty to high-risk behaviour to increased probability of acquiring HIV infection; deprivation and death. The problem is aggravated due to lack of awareness and apathy about the disease.

Concerted efforts are being made to reduce the onset of HIV infection through the targeted interventions. A comprehensive intervention propagates best practices regarding general health, well-being and safety against contracting HIV, culminating in full blown AIDS. At present 554-targeted intervention projects are being implemented in the country out of which 132 are for commercial sex workers, 127 for truckers and 185 for migrant workers (NACO, 2002).

Because of the scattered nature of these programmes and interventions, many such high-risk communities still remain untouched. For instance, a recent survey by the Delhi State AIDS Control Society (DSACS) has identified as many as 276 new sites in the capital where 20 or more commercial sex workers are operating, 117 sites which have men having sex with men in large numbers and 171 sites where many eunuchs are selling sex. Further, the number of sex workers in Delhi is estimated to be over 35,000 out of which 30,000 have been identified for the first time, pointing to a staggering rise in the sex-trade (Chauhan, 2003). Another study mapping the most vulnerable populations in the capital estimates the number of migrant workers to be around 8,88,000 while 35,000 truckers are known to transact in the city each day (*Indian Express*, 9 Dec., 2003). A survey puts the number of people to 10 lac in Delhi with propensity to acquire HIV/AIDS (Chauhan, 2003).

The increasing prevalence of HIV/AIDS in India highlights the urgency to expand targeted interventions to cover the entire HIV/AIDS vulnerable population in the country. This need has also been acutely felt by NACO, which plans to expand the coverage area for its targeted interventions. Recent reports by NACO stress on the need to develop peer-based approach; which enables and sustains behavioural change among the high-risk populations in the country. "Targeting such high-risk groups can make prevention a concerted effort instead of individual struggle for existence" (NACO, 1996).

Further, involving the community in awareness building would strengthen the information inputs, make them more convincing and thus, would sustain the overall interest of people without outside intervention. Keeping this in mind and also a sense of social responsibility, the present study entitled "AIDS Awareness Through Community Participation - An Action Research" was proposed.

Significance of the Study

The objectives of the study are in line with the Global AIDS Strategy of creating an enabling environment, addressing critical poverty related issues and the HIV/AIDS vulnerability. While most of the countries have developed strategic frameworks for effective HIV prevention yet, only a fraction of people at risk of HIV infection have access to basic prevention services (UNAIDS, 2003). Thus, there lies an urgent need to reach the most vulnerable populations with a comprehensive package of HIV prevention services. In the present study, efforts have been made to reach few such communities (comprising of commercial sex workers, truck drivers and rickshaw pullers) identified to be having an increased vulnerability to HIV/AIDS.

Further, as has been experienced till recently, surveillance systems were concentrated only on tracking the HIV prevalence and AIDS cases in the country. But such process only documented the damage wrought on the communities and the country. This did "not help in identifying factors like current behaviour which fuels the HIV pandemic. Documenting such behaviour and documenting behavioural change which predisposes to the spread of HIV/AIDS is of crucial importance for prevention of HIV/AIDS" (NACO, 2001). Therefore, a new framework for HIV surveillance called the Second Generation Surveillance system has been developed which is based on tracking behavioural changes in the country (NACO, 2001).

Keeping this new and upgraded aspect in mind, the present study too focuses on documenting high-risk behaviour as well as in delineating factors fueling them among certain communities. A concerted effort has been made to understand various factors that can effect desirable behavioural changes in context to HIV/AIDS. Critical 'gray areas' in the form of lack of awareness, myths and misconceptions relating to HIV/AIDS, negative attitudes towards people living or affected with the disease and practicing unsafe behaviour that need urgent attention have been delved into, as these can help in evidence-based planning of strategic interventions for the control of HIV/AIDS.

Further, the study envisages to demonstrate how community participation can be effectively used in raising HIV/AIDS awareness as well as in achieving sustainability of the programme with the help of peer educators. The endeavour applied efforts to lead to the development of a set of need-based audio-visual aids, which can be further used with similar populations at various sites to generate HIV/AIDS awareness. In essence, in the present research efforts have been made to document desirable behavioural changes among the sample communities brought about as a result of creating HIV/AIDS awareness amongst them with the help of community participation.

Objectives of the Study

The present study was undertaken with the following main objectives–

1. To have an insight into the respondents:
    (i) Awareness, myths and misconceptions relating to HIV/ AIDS, its manifestations, prevention and control.
    (ii) Living and work environment with special reference to socio-cultural ethos and health care.
2. To review the above, identify areas of action and carry out a suitable intervention for AIDS awareness through community participation.
3. To develop a set of communication material for AIDS awareness through community participation and field-test the same.

The research entailed not merely data collection, but a well-meaning action research involving the communities using their holistic participation. Community participation formed a vital component of the study design and the same was ensured at the following levels:

(i) Development of need-based audio-visual aids with the help of the community.

(ii) Community members trained as peer educators to strengthen HIV/AIDS awareness in the community.

(iii) Community participation reflected by way of innovative interventions like drama/role play, fictional stories and sharing of experiences.

Operational Definitions

Some operational definitions conceptualized for the study are as follows:

Myths	:	Traditional narrative usually involving supernatural or imaginary persons and embodying popular ideas on natural and social phenomena.
Misconceptions	:	Wrong ideas, badly arranged/organized information and the knowledge base.
Community	:	People living in a specific locality doing similar jobs/professions; alternatively specific locality and its inhabitants forming a group, being addressed as a community.
Participation	:	To take part/getting involved/become an integral part of the programme.
Awareness	:	Well informed/conscious, not ignorant but having knowledge.
Knowledge	:	Understanding, familiarity, person's range of information (of subject).
Attitude	:	Opinion, way of thinking.
Behaviour	:	Manner, conduct, way of behaving.
Practice	:	Habitual action/procedure.
Action Research	:	Doing something/getting things done after some ground work and investigation for identifying the need and suitable areas of action.
Intervention	:	Targeting specific communities with the aim of creating HIV/AIDS awareness as well as promoting safe behaviour amongst them.

1
Review of Literature

With the increasing number of HIV infections and AIDS related deaths running into thousands each day, the need for prevention of this epidemic has become imperative. To achieve this, the importance of creating AIDS awareness as one of the best and cost-effective method of prevention has been unanimously accepted world wide. It has been shown time and again, that awareness regarding HIV/AIDS can vitally help in bringing down the number of HIV infections by cutting down high-risk behaviour and practices. Presently, research is increasingly being focused on ensuring community participation while planning interventions for the same, with the goal of achieving sustainability of the programmes. To get a comprehensive insight into the magnitude of the AIDS epidemic and various related aspects accelerating its fast spread, the available literature was reviewed. It is presented in this section under the following heads:

- (i) Spread of the HIV - A Regional Overview.
- (i.) AIDS Threatening the Global Development.
- (iii) Factors Driving the AIDS Epidemic.
- (iv) How HIV Spreads.
- (v) HIV - The Dangerous and Fast Mutating Virus (including counselling, support, ART and Vaccine Development).
- (vi) Global Response to the AIDS Epidemic.
- (vii) AIDS in India.
- (viii) Discrimination of PWHA.
- (ix) Community Participation.
- (x) Use of IEC in creating HIV/AIDS Awareness.
- (xi) Limited Success of HIV Prevention Programmes.

Spread of the HIV — A Regional Overview

In the summer of 1981, the Center for Disease Control and Prevention (CDC), in the USA reported that five homosexual men were suffering from an unusual type of pneumonia caused by a parasite - Pneumocystis carinii. CDC also confirmed that 26 homosexual men in New York and Los Angeles had developed a rare type of skin cancer called Kaposi's sarcoma (WHO, 1997). These were the first reported cases that announced the arrival of AIDS. Today, AIDS pandemic (global epidemic) has become one of the biggest public health problems worldwide.

Africa, the global epicenter, continues to dwarf the rest of the world on the AIDS balance sheet. Since the start of the epidemic, 83 per cent of all AIDS deaths so far have been reported from this region and at least 95 per cent of all AIDS orphans have been African. The bulk of new infections continue to be concentrated in East and Southern Africa (UNAIDS/WHO, Dec., 1998). According to recent estimates, Southern Africa is home to about 30 per cent of people living with HIV/AIDS world wide, while the region has less than 2 per cent of the world's population. By the end of the year 2003, nearly 27 million people in Sub-Saharan Africa were living with HIV while another 2.3 million succumbed to the disease the same year (UNAIDS/WHO, Dec., 2003).

Further, new trends project that HIV incidence (i.c., the annual number of new infections) now seems to be stabilizing in Sub-Saharan Africa. This fall in HIV incidence is attributed to two basic factors – firstly, the epidemic has already affected so many people that there is only a small pool of people left to acquire the infection. Moreover, although high levels of new HIV infection are still persisting in the region but ironically, they are now being matched by equally high levels of AIDS mortality. Secondly, in contrast to this, few countries like Uganda and Senegal have been able to demonstrate that sustained prevention efforts can reduce national HIV infection rates as in their own countries (UNAIDS/WHO, Dec., 2003, 2000). Recent estimates by UNAIDS/WHO (Dec., 2003) for various other continents are as follows:

The Caribbean records the second highest HIV infection rates worldwide after Africa. More than 2 million people are now living with HIV in Latin America and the Caribbean, with the region experiencing the highest death toll after Sub-Saharan Africa and Asia. Heterosexual transmission predominates in the Caribbean while in the bulk of South American countries, all modes of transmission co-exist.

In Eastern Europe and Central Asia the number of people living with HIV/AIDS is estimated to be nearly 1.5 million. Injecting drug use and unsafe sex account for bulk of new infections in these regions along with the possibility of hidden epidemic brewing among men having sex with men.

Similarly, North Africa and Middle East are also experiencing a rise in new HIV infections. The number of people living with HIV/AIDS had reached 600,000 by end 2003. Heterosexual contact, men having sex with men and injecting drug use were found to be mounting the HIV epidemic.

North America, Western Europe, Australia and Canada represent the high-income regions of the world and together have nearly 1.6 million people living with HIV/AIDS. Homosexuality is the leading cause for majority of new HIV infections over here followed by injecting drug use. Yet, in these regions AIDS deaths continue to reduce significantly because of access to anti-retroviral (HIV) therapy. However, unfortunately, the wide access to anti-retroviral therapy is also encouraging widespread public complacency and giving rise to misperceptions that there is a cure for AIDS (UNAIDS/WHO, Dec., 2000).

In Asia over 7.4 million people are already infected and HIV is clearly spreading fast in the vast populations of India and China. Commercial sex and injecting drug use remain the predominant modes of viral transmission in the region with India providing an interesting example of the shifting trends of the HIV. According to UNAIDS/WHO (Dec., 1998) HIV infection is exhibiting the following significant patterns in India:

1. Until recently, it was commonly assumed that HIV infection in India was concentrated mostly in urban sex workers, their clients and in drug injectors. But the last round of sentinel surveillance has shown that in a few states, more than 1 per cent of the pregnant women in urban areas are now HIV infected.
2. India's rural areas, which are home to 73 per cent of the country's population, were thought to be relatively spared by the epidemic. Again new studies show that HIV is becoming worryingly common in villages too. For example, in Tamil Nadu, a survey of randomly selected households revealed that 2.1 per cent of the adult population living in rural areas had HIV, as compared to 0.7 per cent of the urban population.
3. The virus is firmly embedded in the general population, especially among women whose only risk behaviour is having sex with their own husbands. In a study of nearly 400 women attending STD clinics in Pune, 91 per cent had never had sex with anyone but their husband and yet, 13.6 per cent of them tested positive for HIV.

All these trends are acting as warning signs, showing the massive transcend of the HIV from high-risk behaviour populations to the general population.

AIDS Threatening Global Development

The epidemic constitutes an urgent and massive threat to the development in many ways such as:

1. **Life expectancy regressed -** Life expectancy at birth is used as an indicator to measure human development. According to UNAIDS/WHO (Dec., 1998) AIDS is wiping out the gains of development by reducing life expectancy. Taking countries like Kenya, South Africa, Zambia and Zimbabwe which have an adult HIV prevalence rate of 10 per cent or more, calculations predict that AIDS on an average will cost them 17 years of life expectancy. Instead of rising and reaching 64 years by 2010-2015, life expectancy due to AIDS will be cut down on an average to 47 years.
2. **Rising child mortality rates** – HIV/AIDS is by and large threatening child survival rates. According to UNAIDS/WHO (Dec., 1998) by the year 2005-2010, 61 out of every 1000 infants born in South Africa are expected to die before their first birthday. Infant mortality, otherwise in the absence of AIDS would have been only 38 per 1000 births.
3. **Pushing children into orphanhood** – The number of children being orphaned and thus, in need of care is rising with each passing day as AIDS is cutting into their families. A study in Zimbabwe showed that many households are being headed by adolescents and children (some as young as 11 years), as majority of them had lost both parents to AIDS (UNAIDS/WHO, Dec., 1998). The study further revealed that majority of such children on being interviewed, said that they would become delinquent and drift into prostitution and onto the streets if their needs were not met. They were also worried about exploitation and abuse by their relatives.

   India too, faces a grim situation in view of the fact that the country reportedly has the second largest number of HIV infections in the world (Shreedhar, 2002). In the absence of any cure, these infections are likely to turn into fatalities in the near future thus, rendering many children into orphanhood. Although, globally the number of children orphaned by AIDS is projected to rise at least 25 million by 2010 yet, 39 per cent of countries with generalized HIV epidemic (i.e., HIV prevalence exceeding 1 per cent) have not been able to place a national policy to provide essential support to such children (UNAIDS, 2003).

4. **Businesses beginning to suffer** – Many businesses are suffering heavily as AIDS is decimating the pool of skilled workers and eating away the economy too. The epidemic is exacerbating the severe shortage of skilled labour in many sectors of the economy. As a result, Botswana is being forced to import white-collar workers from the neighbouring countries. Zambia is facing an acute shortage of teachers as many of them are increasingly dying of AIDS. Similarly, Swaziland will have to train twice the number of teachers than usual over the next 17 years and is expected to spend around US $233 million towards extra hiring and training costs of new teachers by the year 2016 (UNAIDS/WHO, Dec., 2000). Similarly, another UNAIDS/WHO (Dec., 2001) report estimates that in some countries, health care systems are losing up to a quarter of their personnel to the epidemic.

In the Indian capital Delhi, a study conducted by the Operations Research Group revealed that a majority of those infected with HIV/AIDS were in their most productive age group. For instance, out of 646 confirmed cases of AIDS in the city till Nov. 2001, as many as 534 belonged to the age group of 15-49 years (*Indian Express,* April 4, 2002). If the present trend continues, productivity in many businesses is expected to fall significantly giving a major set back to the economic development.

Further, various reports suggest that a widespread and destabilizing Indian AIDS epidemic is not inevitable (Gates, 2002). Gates (2002) while stressing on the challenges faced by India due to HIV/AIDS observes, "India's ability to realize its extraordinary potential is at risk...If India follows the tragic path of countries hard hit earlier by HIV/AIDS, the countries lifeblood – its teachers, scientists and business professionals – could be in jeopardy."

The Macro Economic Impact of the AIDS Epidemic

The impact of HIV/AIDS on individuals, families, communities and nations is terribly huge. As people across the globe continue to become affected by AIDS, there is a growing need to look at the pandemic from a macro perspective. Many countries have started exhibiting a significantly inverse relationship between their HIV prevalence rate and gross domestic product (GDP) growth rate. Gross domestic product growth rate of a country is measured in terms of total national income as well as the growth in the national income. Growing evidence suggests that as HIV prevalence rate of a country rises, its economic growth and thereby GDP fall substantially. For instance, in South Africa, AIDS epidemic is predicted to reduce the economic growth rate by 0.3- 0.4 per cent per year, resulting in a GDP 17 per cent lower by the year 2010. This implies that South African economy will be poorer by US $22 billion by 2010 (UNAIDS/WHO, Dec., 2000).

UNAIDS/WHO report (Dec., 2000) also estimates that majority of households will be forced to spend more on care of AIDS patients and orphans and the disposable income/person will be less by 13 per cent on an average. In the hard-hit areas, households are trying to cope by cutting their food consumption and other basic expenditures and also by selling their assets to cover the costs of health-care and funerals (UNAIDS/WHO, Dec., 2001). The government is in need to direct more money to health care services, which could otherwise be used to build economy. Calculations predict that many countries in Sub-Saharan Africa would need at least US $1.5 billion per year to prevent new HIV infections from taking place among their population and another US $1.5 billion per year is needed to look after people already affected by AIDS. Treatment with anti-retroviral therapy (ART) would cost another few billion dollars annually (UNAIDS/WHO, Dec., 2000).

In India, the epidemic is estimated to have costed $11 billion as direct and indirect costs of AIDS by the end of year 2000 (WHO, 1998). The cost is by no means small and these resources could have been utilized for development/welfare purposes such as providing food, shelter and health care facilities to the poor people in the absence of the AIDS epidemic.

According to a United Nations Food and Agricultural Organization (FAO) report, 7 million farm workers have died because of AIDS since 1985 and another 16 million are expected to die in the coming 20 years. FAO predicts that agricultural output especially of staple crops cannot be sustained under such conditions and chances of widespread food shortages and hunger threaten us in the near future (UNAIDS/WHO, Dec., 2001).

Children are being increasingly removed from schools to look after family members ill from HIV and also to help in regaining the income lost due to death of earning member/s from AIDS. UNAIDS/WHO (Dec., 2001) report reveals that almost everywhere across the globe, the extra burden of care and work is being deflected onto women. Families are removing girls from school to take care of sick members and assume other family responsibilities, hampering girls' education and future prospects. The report also estimates that in Swaziland, school enrolment has fallen by 36 per cent due to AIDS, with girls being most affected.

Companies facing a dilemma – HIV epidemic is forcing many organizations and companies to radically change their policies regarding recruitment and payment of death benefits to staff members. Many companies because of the fear of HIV/AIDS fatalities are now hiring employees on casual basis, thereby escaping the responsibility of paying death and other benefits. In Botswana, many companies are taking "key man insurance" (for people in critical positions) in case they die of AIDS (UNAIDS/WHO, Dec., 1999).

The challenge of meeting needs of people living with HIV/AIDS has led some insurance firms in South Africa to provide benefits of up to US $ 4000/person/year which is substantial to cover a good share of the cost of anti-retroviral therapy. Similarly, some benefit schemes have agreed to pay death benefits to employees certified as terminally ill with AIDS before they die, so that they are able to spend their final days at home with peace (UNAIDS/WHO, Dec., 1999).

In India, such initiatives are unfortunately profoundly lacking. On the contrary, majority of insurance companies have excluded HIV/AIDS condition from their benefit plans making the disease more devastating. There lies an urgent need to include HIV/AIDS illness in the benefit plans offered by various insurance companies in order to reduce the burden of the disease. In the long run, this could substantially help people to enhance their coping ability to the fatal infection.

Factors Driving the AIDS Epidemic

In the recent years, there has been a growing awareness of the complex biological, socio-cultural, economic, political and psychosocial forces shaping the face of the AIDS pandemic. Meaningful strategies to reduce HIV related risks among populations are not possible without a thorough understanding of these factors. Some of the major factors fueling the AIDS epidemic have been summarized in Table 1.1.

Table 1.1. Factors Shaping the AIDS Epidemic

I.	**Biological Factors**	(*a*) *Age at the time of initial HIV infection*
		(*b*) *Sexual vulnerability*
		(*c*) *Presence of STD*
II.	**Socio-cultural Factors**	(*a*) *Sex and Sexuality - A Taboo*
		(*b*) *Machismo Behaviour*
		(*c*) *Violence Against Women*
		(*d*) *Norms and Practices*
		(*e*) *Education and HIV*
		(*f*) *Myths and Misconceptions*

III. Economic Factors	(*a*) *Migration* (*b*) *Prostitution*
IV. Political Factors	(*a*) *War* (*b*) *Ethnic Conflict*
V. Psychosocial Factors	(*a*) *Physical and Sexual Abuse* (*b*) *Substance Abuse* (*c*) *Stigma and Shame* (*d*) *Gender role expectations*

The above-mentioned factors have been elaborately discussed as follows:

I. Biological Factors. Studies conducted in nine different African countries suggest that for every ten HIV infected African men, there are around 12 to 13 women infected with the HIV (UNAIDS/WHO, Dec., 1999). Why more women than men are being infected with HIV can be explained by the following basic factors, which are:

(a) Age. Women across the globe tend to become HIV infected at younger age than men due to prevalent biological and cultural factors. Recent studies in Africa show that girls aged 15 to 19 years are about 5 to 6 times more likely to become HIV positive than boys in the same age group (UNAIDS, 1999).

The increased vulnerability of women can be attributed to cultural norms in many countries, which require women to be younger than their husbands. This in turn implies that if a husband is subsequently infected with HIV, he would be infecting his wife at a far younger age. Research in many industrialized countries has shown that the length of survival of HIV positive individual depends on the age at initial infection. The younger the person at the time of initial HIV infection, the longer the survival time.

Thus, women who become infected at younger age as compared to their male counterparts are expected to live longer and be counted for a longer time as female population living with HIV/AIDS.

(b) Sexual Vulnerability, Currently, almost half of all new HIV infections are taking place among women. Eighty-four per cent of these HIV infected women are in the reproductive age group, i.e., 15 to 45 years and 9 out of 10 infected women are living in a developing country. In India, around 230,000 women are getting HIV infected each year and more than four-fifth of all these infections are accounted by unprotected heterosexual contact (NACO, 2000).

HIV transmission from male to female is more efficient than vice versa because females have a larger mucosal surface area exposed to their partner's sexual secretions during sex. The risk of acquiring HIV for females is reported to be higher by 2 to 17 times by different studies (Nicolosi, et al.; Padian, et al. cited in NACO, 2000).

(c) Sexually Transmitted Diseases (STD) Facilitate HIV Transmission. The World Health Organization (WHO) estimates that about 333 million people worldwide suffer from STD every year and about one million new infections are taking place every day globally (NACO, 2000).

The term sexually transmitted diseases is used for all infections that are transmitted through vaginal, anal or oral sexual contact. STD can also be transmitted from mother to child before or during birth, through contaminated blood, blood products, donated organs or tissues and by contaminated needles. Sexually transmitted infections (STI) is the new term that is now being commonly used to cover asymptomatic cases (i.e., symptom free cases) of STD.

India, also has a high incidence rate of STD with 40 million new infections each year and an annual incidence rate of 5 per cent (NACO, 2000). There exists a strong association between the presence of STD and the occurrence of HIV infection. STD are confirmed to facilitate HIV transmission by damaging the inner lining of the genital tract. Thus, HIV can freely pass from the infected partner to the uninfected one by exchange of body fluids through these broken linings. The risk of acquiring HIV infection is enhanced 4 to 6 times by the presence of STD (WHO, 1997).

II. Socio-cultural Factors. HIV is certainly a behavioural epidemic that is driven by individual behaviours. Individual behaviours are in turn largely influenced by social, cultural and religious factors that leave people with little or no control over their exposure to HIV. According to Betancourt, Lopez and Cole (cited in Bee, 1995) culture in essence "describes some system of meanings and customs including values, attitudes, goals, laws, beliefs, morals as well as physical artifacts of various kinds - tools, forms of dwellings, and the like. Further more to be called a culture, this system of meanings and customs must be shared by some identifiable group...and transmitted from one generation of that group to the next."

Extensive studies have been carried out which, show that meaningful strategies to reduce HIV related risk behaviour cannot be realized without understanding the dynamics of family history, cultural norms, feelings of self-power and self-sufficiency as well as gender role expectations (Lewis et al., 1996; Sikos, 1996; Oetomo, 1996). The need to determine the salient factors in socio-economic structure and culture, which contribute to the spread of AIDS and also have implications on HIV prevention efforts, has been stressed by various researchers (Dlamini – Kapanda, et al., 1996;

Coll–Seck, et al., 1996). Similarly, the role of social environment in promoting behavioural changes related to HIV risks has also been well documented by various studies (Metsch, et al., 1996). For instance, sustaining behavioural change among rural women was found to be influenced by social, cultural and gender related factors (Nankunda, 1996).

Although tremendous progress and advancement in fields of education, science and technology have led to radical changes in primitive norms and practices yet, in many parts of the world certain socio-cultural practices have been recognized as hindering factors to HIV prevention efforts. Some of the socio-cultural factors impeding HIV prevention efforts are:

(a) Sex and Sexuality: A Taboo. Talking about sex and sexuality is still a taboo in many parts of the world. Cultural norms, societal practices and family values by and large dictate sex to be a private and prohibited issue, which is not to be discussed openly in public. The sense of secrecy surrounding sexual talks has led to a major lack of sex education especially among young people who are making an early sexual debut. A study conducted by Pan American Health Organization (PAHO) in 1998 in 100 schools showed, more than 40 per cent of the sexually active adolescents had made their sexual debut before the age of 10 (UNAIDS, 1999).

Similarly, in Zambia though people under 18 can not choose to be tested for HIV without their parent's consent yet, nearly half of women have had sex by the time they were 16 and many teenagers are infected with HIV (www.unaids.org., June1998).

In India, relevant data assessing knowledge, attitudes and beliefs regarding HIV/AIDS among school/college going adolescents indicate a lack of AIDS awareness. A study conducted among secondary school students in rural areas surrounding Delhi showed that although 25 per cent of them were sexually active yet, majority of them were not aware about HIV prevention methods (Sharma, et al. cited in Mathai, et al., 1997).

(b) Machismo behaviour. Machismo, a Spanish word is often used for predatory behaviours, which young men practice to prove their masculinity. It is a commonly practiced and accepted social norm in many parts of the world (UNAIDS, 1999). Young men are socialized to be aggressive and virile whereas women are expected to be passive and sexually subordinating. Machismo is leading young men to have early and frequent sex with multiple partners. A study by Reproductive Health Surveys in Latin America showed that premarital sex is much more common among 15-24 year old males than females (www.unaids.org., 1999). Following the same trend in Mexico City, 15 per cent of boys as compared to 4.5 per cent of girls have first intercourse before the age of 15 (UNAIDS, 1999).

(c) Violence Against Women. Women subjected to violence at the hands of their husband or partners are at a greater risk of acquiring HIV. The UNAIDS (1999) report reads "Even when the violence is not sexual, however, the mere threat of it makes women wary of challenging their partner's extra-marital relations or afraid to demand condom use". One out of every three women worldwide has been abused, beaten or coerced into sex according to the recent global data (NACO, April, 2000). Forced sex is known to transmit HIV more readily because of the greater probability of genital injury and because of no condom use in such situations (UNAIDS, 1999). Surveys in the USA indicate that 4 per cent to 30 per cent of women who have been raped acquire a sexually transmitted disease as a result (UNAIDS, 1999). The report also reveals that contrary to the belief, sexual abuse and rape are most often perpetrated not by strangers but by relatives, friends and husbands of young women (although rape in marriage is seldom punishable by law).

In India, the incidence of adolescent rape (10-16 years) had increased by 26 per cent between 1991 and 1995. According to government's statistics, of all sexual assaults reported 35 per cent are against minors. Further, dowry killing has also been acknowledged as a particular form of violence against women in India (UNFPA, Sept., 2000).

(d) Norms and Practices. Adverse societal norms and practices also challenge women's ability to protect themselves from HIV. For instance, certain communities in India like the Bedias and Bancharas have a history of practicing community-based prostitution. Likewise, in some South Indian states religious-based prostitution (Devdasi system) and exploitation of girls is routine and part of the ritual of "growing up" (UNFPA, Sept., 2000). Such practices coupled with a lack of negotiating power make young girls more vulnerable to HIV/AIDS.

Globally, there exists an imbalance of power between men and women based on gender lines. Women's ability to make decisions about sex/safe sex and subsequently to protect themselves from HIV infection is impeded by poverty, illiteracy, lack of economic independence and high levels of sexual subordination. In many societies across the globe, differentiation based on gender is fundamental. The virginity myth is a necessary condition for women to marry (Castaneda, et al., 1996) whereas no such prerequisite exists for men. Similarly, the responsibility of practicing safe behaviour usually lies on women, as worrying about condoms is considered unmanly by men (NACO, April, 2000).

(e) Education and HIV. AIDS is a disease fuelled by poverty and ignorance. Globally, it is certainly the poor and the less educated who are

reeling under the impact of the HIV epidemic. Since better-educated people have better-paid jobs, they can afford goods and services that allow them to protect themselves from HIV. The global HIV/AIDS epidemic report shows that countries with high levels of literacy have low levels of HIV. The data comparison of 161 countries across the globe confirms a pattern of this kind (UNAIDS/WHO, June, 1998). Further, analysis of studies focusing on 15-19 year old teenagers show that teenagers with higher education are more likely to use condoms than their counterparts with lower levels of education (UNAIDS/WHO, Dec., 2000).

Similarly, in Western Uganda survey reports of child-bearing women aged 15 to 24 years showed that HIV infection rates of educated women had dropped by half in 1995-97 (UNAIDS/WHO, Dec., 2000).

(f) Myths and Misconceptions. Myths and misconceptions regarding HIV/AIDS are in abundance and deeply ingrained in almost all communities worldwide. Today no community seems to be immune to commonly held beliefs that have no scientific validity. Although myths and misconceptions are largely associated with low levels of education yet, studies continue to indicate that even medical professionals have their own share of such beliefs.

A study conducted in Delhi on 100 general medical practitioners (GMPs) registered with the Delhi Medical Association, revealed many of them to be believing that HIV could be transmitted by sharing soap, drinking glass or cup, telephone and swimming pool with a HIV infected person (Roy and Chowdhury, 1997). Similarly, while assessing HIV/AIDS awareness among Indian communities it was observed that 56.7 per cent of the rural and 37.5 per cent of the urban respondents were of the opinion that AIDS could be acquired through kissing, hugging, shaking hands and sharing clothes and utensils with a HIV infected person (Balaganesh, et al., 1997).

Myths such as HIV infected people should be totally isolated from the society (Sehgal and Singh, 1997), HIV infected children should not be allowed to attend a school (Sehgal, 1997), eating hot things and urinating at bad places causes sexually transmitted diseases (Mittal, et al., 1997) and that AIDS is a God's way of punishing people for their evils (Wadhwa, et al., 1997) have been found to be prevalent among the masses.

Besides, myths like getting cured of STD/AIDS after having sexual contact with minors is leading to an alarming trend of infant girls (some as young as 8 to 9 months old) being sexually abused (www.excite.com, 26 Nov., 2001).

III. Economic Factors. Migration and prostitution, which are often a result of economic compulsions, are making people vulnerable to HIV.

(a) Migration. Today migration is one of the leading factors exposing people to HIV. People around the world are experiencing an unprecedented mobility. They are moving for very many reasons but the most common reason is to seek employment. Economic compulsions very often force these people to leave behind their homes as well as their families. UNAIDS/WHO (Dec., 1998) estimates that Carltonville, the heart of South Africa's gold mining industry is a home to 88,000 mineworkers, out of which 60 per cent are migrants. Around US $18 million are paid to these miners every month as wages. Wages bring along with them the purchasing power to buy sex and drugs. About 500 sex workers cater to the needs of these miners. HIV prevalence rates are all time high with 22 per cent of adults being infected. Periodically, these migrants return home and transmit the virus to their wives and communities. Similarly, a recent report by Delhi State AIDS Control Society has also recognized migration to be one of the major factors contributing to the increasing risk of HIV transmission (*Indian Express*, April 4, 2002).

Migration is leading people into extra-marital sex and in many communities this trend is being increasingly accepted as a societal norm. A study conducted in a rural district of Natal with about 60 per cent households having one or more male migrants found that sex outside marriage is accepted as inevitable in separated families for both men and women (UNAIDS/WHO, Dec., 1998).

(b) Prostitution. Poverty manifests itself in the form of sexual abuse, sexual exploitation and prostitution. Economic pressures are forcing an ever-increasing number of people into flesh trade. The induction of minors is now being recognized as a key factor in keeping sex trade at flourishing levels. As sex tourism expands so does the pandemic of AIDS. Costa Rica, the Dominican Republic, Brazil, Haiti and several other countries have become a hot spot for sex tourism with minors (www.unaids.org., 1999).

In India, there are about 9 lac sex workers involved in the flesh trade (UNFPA, Sept., 2000). Although prostitution is illegal in India yet, it flourishes and more so in metropolitan cities of the country. In Delhi, Mumbai and Kolkata there are well-demarcated areas commonly known as the "red light areas" where prostitution is openly practiced as a profession. Young girls including many minors are kidnapped/lured on the pretext of employment or marriage and sold to brothel owners for money. These women generally live in hostile conditions and are most often subjected to abuse and exploitation by the brothel owners as well as clients. Sex industry faces an increased vulnerability to HIV/STD because of low levels of education, lack of assertive skills regarding safe sex and poor access to health care services. In Mumbai, 70 per cent of the commercial sex workers are now HIV positive (Span, Sept./Oct., 2001) while in Tamil Nadu HIV prevalence among sex workers in the year 1996 was estimated to be around 30 per cent (WHO, 1998).

IV. Political Factors. Political turmoil and civil war in many countries have also been instrumental in the rapid spread of the HIV. For example., Cambodian soldiers who have been battling Khmer Rouge Rebels in the northwest of their country perceive risk as a way of life. For many of them sex is a source of comfort and not of any special danger. Behavioural studies have shown that over a third of Cambodian soldiers visited a brothel and HIV prevalence in the military was around 7 per cent in 1998 (UNAIDS/WHO, Dec., 1998).

Similarly, epidemiological estimates by the Indian army indicated that there were at least six thousand armed forces personnel who were HIV positive by the end of the year 1998. According to a report, since these personnel are subjected to immense physical as well as mental stress and they have to stay separated from their families under inhospitable conditions for long periods; the desire to seek sexual satisfaction often leads them to sex workers. Thus, perceiving the enormity of the AIDS threat, the Director General of Medical Services (Army) brought out a handbook on AIDS with the aim of promoting safe sex among the armed personnel (Kumar, 1998).

In Rwanda too, widespread conflict has created fertile conditions for the spread of the HIV. For instance, HIV prevalence among people who had spent the years of conflict in refugee camps was 8.5 per cent. These people had fled from rural areas where HIV prevalence was only 1.3 per cent. The rise in HIV infection among refugees in the camps was due to overcrowding, violence, rape and despair (UNAIDS/WHO, Dec., 1998). Recently, Djibouti and the Sudan have also been facing growing epidemics due to political instability (UNAIDS/WHO, Dec., 2001).

V. Psychosocial Factors. The word psycho is derived from the Greek word "Psyche" which relates to the mind, spirit and soul (Bee, 1995). Thus, psychosocial factors refer to those social issues, which have a lasting impact on an individual's mind. Many a times societal oppression in the form of neglect, abuse and exploitation especially during childhood, leaves a deep impact on the psychology of an individual. People who have been abused and exploited at the hands of society are more vulnerable to HIV. Their abuse has been known to lead them to a feeling of loss of self-esteem and control over their lives. They are also known to become more prone to drug taking and commercial sex.

For instance, a study in a country showed that 80 per cent of children entering the sex trade had been sexually abused (UNAIDS, 1999). According to Morill and Ickovics (1996) women who are physically and sexually abused contribute to risky heterosexual behaviour by virtue of their association with substance abuse and depression. Substance abuse in the form of alcohol or drugs is known to increase aggression, diminish inhibitions and impair the capacity to make decisions about HIV protection (UNAIDS/WHO, Dec., 1998).

A study by Weinrich et al. (1996) showed that family environment of an individual also predicts his preferences for safe and unsafe behaviour. The study found that familial factors such as childhood physical abuse, neglect and parental alcoholism were associated with submissive sexual behaviour in adulthood for homosexual and heterosexual men.

As a part of European Union concerted action on HIV risks, social scientists from different European countries are trying to study the psychosocial determinants of sexual behaviour and attitudes to HIV risk. They are focussing on different theories such as social learning theory, social system theory and health belief model and their impact on psychology of an individual to practice safe/unsafe behaviour. Effectiveness of HIV prevention efforts can be greatly increased by an understanding of why people prefer the acts they do.

In the Indian context, Mane and Maitra (cited in Mathai, et al., 1997) observed that there is a tendency to be psychologically oriented towards morality rather than towards real life issues related to sex. Women are brought up to be psychologically passive in talking about sex, sexuality and condom use with their partners. Female sexuality to them means being sexually subordinating to men and fulfilling roles of reproduction as well as motherhood.

Even the needs of people living with HIV/AIDS (PWHA) have been found to differ in accordance to their gender roles. For instance, in a study in Mumbai (India), it was found that the needs of HIV infected men were more self-centred relating to their own health condition and personal image in society. On the contrary, the needs of HIV infected women were more family oriented including concerns for jobs, shelter, sustenance of self and children and ensuring the future of their children (Bharat, 1996).

Stigma and shame attached to HIV/AIDS are also proving to be major psychosocial issues that place hurdles in HIV prevention and care efforts. As HIV/AIDS is largely believed to be a disease associated with infidelity, people are ashamed of accepting their HIV positive status due to the fear of stigma and societal rejection. In a study conducted in South Africa, several HIV positive people confided that they had not disclosed their HIV positivity to any one including those who were caring for them (UNAIDS/WHO, Dec., 1998).

Similarly, in a survey conducted by Kenya's Population Council in the year 2001, more than half of the women who knew they were HIV positive said they had not disclosed their HIV status to their partners for the fear of exposure to violence or abandonment (UNAIDS/WHO, Dec., 2001). In India, upcoming reports keep conforming the fact that majority of women with HIV/AIDS have acquired the infection from their husbands/ partners who chose to remain silent about their HIV positivity (*The Week*, Dec., 2000).

Thus, various factors contributing to the spread of the HIV epidemic need to be urgently as well as seriously explored in order to contain the spread of the fatal disease. The solution to the problem largely lies in adequately addressing these core issues on one hand, while simultaneously empowering people by creating HIV/AIDS awareness on the other hand.

How HIV Spreads

HIV is found in body fluids such as blood, semen, vaginal secretions, breast milk, tears, and saliva. However, HIV transmission is known to be possible only through blood, vaginal fluids and breast milk. For other body fluids, it would require enormous quantities to be exchanged to transmit HIV.

Presently, there are only three well-defined routes by which HIV is known to spread –

(i) ***Sexual Intercourse.*** HIV can spread through heterosexual as well as homosexual intercourse when one of the partners is already infected. Though the probability of HIV transmission by sex is only one in a hundred to one in a thousand, (WHO, 1997) the sheer number of heterosexual activity taking place across the world makes it the single largest factor in spreading HIV.

(ii) ***Blood and Blood Products.*** HIV infected blood, blood products, transplanted organs, tissues and contaminated needles and syringes can effectively transmit HIV. This is the most efficient transmission mode with a probability of more than 90 per cent (WHO, 1997). Although universal precautions (adopted in the healthcare set up) and blood screening have greatly reduced the risks of HIV transmission in health care settings yet, in some countries HIV transmission risk

through blood and blood products remains potentially high (UNAIDS/WHO, Dec., 2003).

(iii) ***Mother to Child Transmission (MTCT).*** A pregnant women with HIV has approximately 30 per cent chances of passing the infection to her child during pregnancy, at birth or shortly after birth, i.e., through breast-feeding. 5, 90,000 children are infected with HIV each year by vertical transmission, i.e., mother to child transmission (USAID cited in NACO, 2000). Evidence shows that vertical infection can occur as early as 12-15 weeks of gestation (NACO, 2000).

The gap between the rich and poor countries in terms of vertical transmission is growing. For instance, in France and the USA less than 5 per cent of the children born to HIV infected women in 1997 were HIV positive whereas in the developing countries, the transmission rates were between 25 per cent to 35 per cent (UNAIDS/WHO, June, 1998). There are primarily two reasons accounting for this wide gap namely - breast-feeding practices and access to anti-retroviral therapy (drugs for HIV infection).

(a) Breast-feeding practices. In industrialized countries, breast-feeding by HIV positive mothers is not recommended. Some governments such as Thailand's have taken the initiative of distributing free/subsidized artificial milk to such women (UNAIDS/WHO, June, 1998). But in most developing countries there are no such subsidized programmes and even if a women chooses to bottle-feed, she may be exposing her newborn to deadly infections if the drinking water supply is unsafe. Therefore WHO/UNICEF recommend continuation of breast-feeding by all women including HIV positive women in the developing world (NACO, 2000).

(b) Access to anti-retroviral therapy (ART). In 1994, studies showed that giving anti-retroviral drugs to HIV infected women during pregnancy, childbirth and to their infants after birth could cut down HIV transmission rates by two-thirds (UNAIDS/WHO, June 1998). Soon this became a common practice in the developed countries. But this regimen is long-term and costs around US $1000 per pregnancy (UNAIDS/WHO, June, 1998). Thus, many developing countries are not able to afford to provide this costly therapy to HIV infected women.

A major breakthrough has been reported in Uganda that proved the efficacy of drug Nevirapine as a single dose treatment in reducing vertical transmission. The study showed that a single dose of Nevirapine given to a HIV infected mother during labour and to her infant during the first 72 hours after birth cut down the HIV transmission rate by 50 per cent. This single dose regimen is 30 times cheaper than short-term treatment in Thailand and 70 times cheaper than long-term treatment in the USA. The cost of single dose of Nevirapine is only US $3-4 (WHO, Jan.-April, 2000).

The National AIDS Control Programme in India too, has initiated a feasibility study with the aim of preventing MTCT by Azidothymidine (AZT) prophylaxis. The prophylactic measures are being provided to HIV positive pregnant women in five high prevalence states which are Maharashtra, Tamil Nadu, Karnataka, Andhra Pradesh and Manipur (NACO, Dec., 2000). However, a note of caution is required here to stress the fact that seeing the exponential spread of the HIV in many other states of India, it may not be easy in the near future to provide such regimen to all HIV infected pregnant women. Thus, prenatal prevention from the deadly disease by creating AIDS awareness seems to be the most viable solution.

HIV and Drug Abuse – On the basis of global 1992 data, WHO estimated that more than 5 million people injected drugs and around 200,000 drug injectors died every year with half of these dying due to HIV/AIDS (UNAIDS/WHO, June, 1998). HIV is undoubtedly spreading rapidly among injecting drug users (IDUs) because many of them share injecting equipment viz. needle and syringe. When drugs are injected, some blood is usually sucked back and remains in the syringe. In the eventuality of this blood being HIV infected, the subsequent user of the same contaminated needle/syringe is very likely to become HIV infected too.

In Eastern Europe and Vietnam, many drug users go to "shooting galleries" for their injections. In these galleries, which are usually small rooms/shacks, the drug dealer mixes heroin or opium solution and puts it in a communal pot. Clients pay for a shot of solution drawn from this pot and administered by the dealer to the drug user. One such communal pot is usually shared by 50 clients, all using the same needle and syringe with no cleaning in between (UNAIDS/WHO, June, 1998). The report further revealed that in Vietnam, until 1997 more than 70 per cent of HIV infections were in drug injectors.

Studies also indicate that due to unavailability/non-affordability of needles and syringes many injecting drug users in developing countries like Myanmar and India are using home-made equipment consisting of a needle attached to an eyedropper or a polythene tube (UNAIDS/WHO, June, 1998; Sehgal and Singh, 1997). The use of a polythene tube makes it virtually impossible to sterilize the equipment. To make matters worse, the practice of sharing such home-made injecting equipment was found to be very high among drug users. For instance, a study conducted in Manipur revealed that 63.9 per cent of the IDU were using home-made injecting equipment and that 42.6 per cent of IDU did not clean their injecting equipment. Further, 50.2 per cent of the drug users washed the equipment with any available water (Sehgal and Singh, 1997). In Manipur, HIV prevalence among IDUs in the year 1996 was reported to be 73.26 per cent (NACO, 2000). Ironically, HIV spread is aggravated by the fact that majority of drug users virtually have no access to HIV/AIDS information and prevention services due to social stigma or legal complexities attached with drug use. For instance, fewer than 5 per cent of injecting drug users receive the recommended prevention services in countries where injecting drug use is an established mode of HIV transmission (UNAIDS/WHO, Dec., 2003).

Casual Contact does not Transmit HIV

HIV cannot spread by casual contact such as hugging, kissing, sitting next to an HIV positive individual, sharing water, food, clothing and utensils. It is also confirmed that lice, mosquitoes, flies, bedbugs, fleas and other insects and pests do not spread HIV (WHO, 1997). Ironically, myths and misconceptions linking these modes to the transmission of HIV/AIDS are widely prevalent among the masses. This in turn is giving rise to an attitude of discrimination against people living with or affected by HIV/AIDS. Hence, there is an urgent need to demystify the disease as well as the fears and apprehension of people related to it.

HIV - The Dangerous and Fast Mutating Virus

In order to understand various aspects of the HIV that have made it resilient to all present day treatments as well as vaccines, it is important to have some knowledge regarding certain crucial aspects of the virus. Some of these aspects have been touched upon in the proceeding sections to provide clarity regarding certain characteristics of the virus that make HIV/AIDS a fatal condition.

Acquired Immuno Deficiency Syndrome is not a single disease but a set of diseases. Hence, it is named as a "syndrome". With a view to understand the reason for fatality of this syndrome, it is important to understand the immune system of a human body.

The functioning of the immune system in our body is shown in Fig. 1.1.

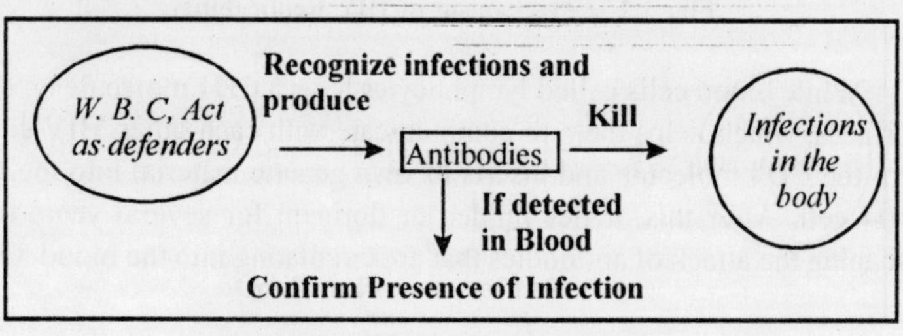

Fig. 1.1 : Immune System of the Body.

In a healthy individual, infections are kept at bay by white blood cells (WBC) that act as defenders of our body. The WBC recognize foreign bodies (infections) and in response produce specific chemicals called antibodies, which neutralize the invaders. Each disease results in the production of specific antibodies. The detection of these antibodies in blood is used to determine the presence of various infections including HIV (WHO, 1997).

Now, HIV is unique in its action as it targets the WBC that are vital in protecting our body from all the infections as shown in Fig. 1.2.

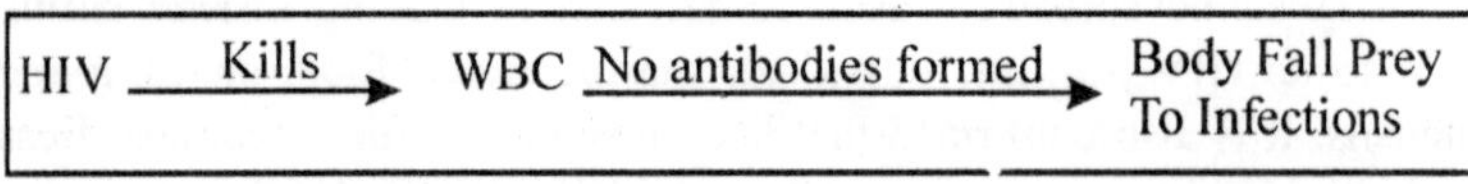

Fig. 1.2: HIV Targets the Immune System (WBC).

In other words, HIV directly attacks the protective cells (immune system), of our body. Once the protection giving cells are destroyed, each and every infection (called opportunistic infections) can prove to be fatal.

Mechanism of HIV replicability – The crucial process which helps the HIV in escaping the attack of antibodies and also in its fast and undetected replication in a human body, is shown in Fig. 1.3.

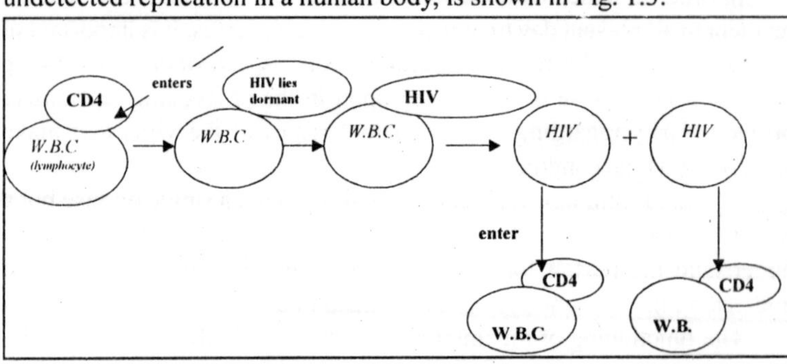

Fig. 1.3 : Mechanism of HIV Replicability.

White blood cells called lymphocytes have a CD4 molecule on their surfaces, which helps them to communicate with each other. HIV enters into the CD4 molecule and inserts its own genetic material into the host CD4 cell. After this, it lies hidden or dormant for several years thus, escaping the attack of antibodies that are circulating into the blood. Once this dormancy period is over, the HIV starts replicating and produces several new copies of itself. These newly multiplied HIV destroy the host CD4 cell, come out in the blood stream and start infecting new CD4 cells (WHO, 1997). Once majority of the white blood cells has been destroyed, the body starts falling prey to opportunistic infections.

Discovery of the HIV – In 1983, Professor Luc Montagnier and his team in Paris discovered a new virus from the lymph glands of a male homosexual suffering from persistent generalized lymphadenompathy (PGL), i.e., enlargement of the lymph glands. They called the virus as lymphadenopathy associated virus (LAV). Shortly afterwards, a team led by Dr. Robert Gallo in USA, also isolated a new virus from patients with AIDS. The virus was called human T-lymphocytic virus III (HTLV, III). A general consensus was reached by the international committee on taxonomy of viruses to name the virus as human immuno-deficiency virus (HIV) (WHO, 1997). The microscopic structure of the HIV is shown in Fig. 1.4.

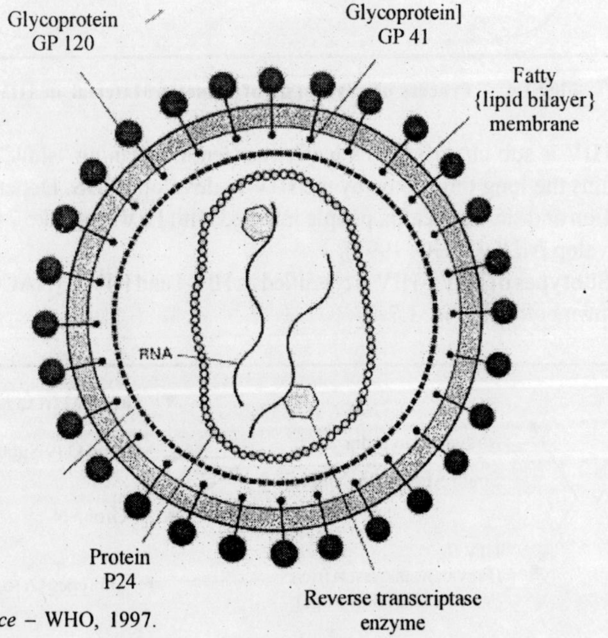

Source – WHO, 1997.

Fig. 1.4 : Structure of the HIV.

HIV: A retro-lentivirus – HIV belongs to a family of viruses called retroviruses. Retroviruses defy the general biological rule whereby deoxy-ribose nucleic acid (DNA) leads to the synthesis of ribose nucleic acid (RNA) in most living organisms as shown in Fig.1.5.

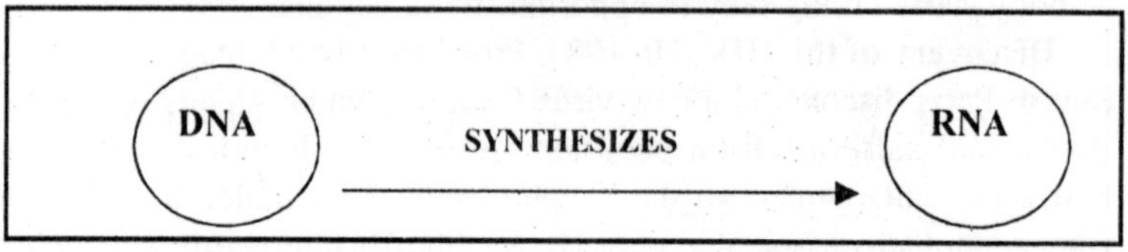

Fig. 1.5 : Process of Synthesis of Genetic Material in Most Organisms.

But in HIV, RNA leads to the synthesis of DNA due to the presence of an enzyme called reverse transcriptase (Fig. 1.6).

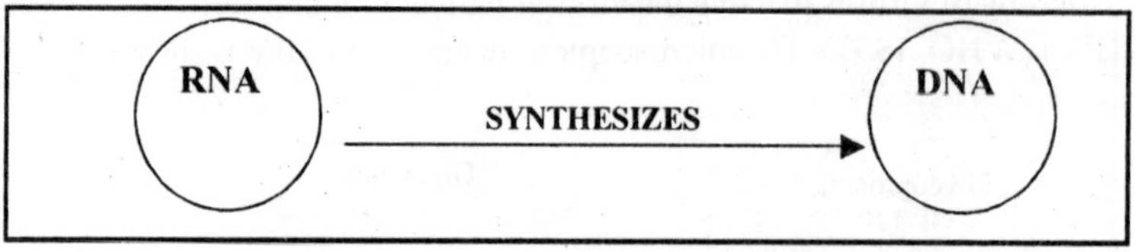

Fig. 1.6 : Process of Synthesis of Genetic Material in HIV.

HIV is sub classified as a lentivirus (lentus meaning "slow"), which explains the long time taken by the HIV to develop AIDS. Depending on nutrition and state of health, people infected with HIV may take 7-10 years to develop AIDS (WHO, 1997).

Subtypes of HIV – HIV is classified as HIV-I and HIV-II (NACO, 2000) as shown below in Fig. 1.7.

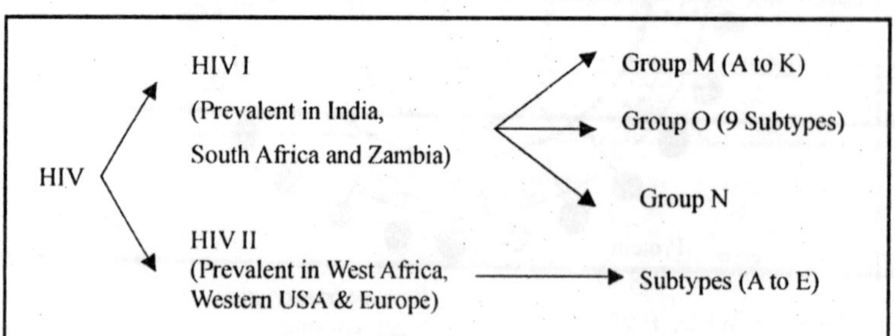

Fig. 1.7 : HIV Classification.

HIV I is predominant and further subdivided into three groups –

1. Group M (consisting of 11 subtypes from A to K)
2. Group O (consisting of 9 Subtypes)
3. Group N

India, South Africa and Zambia have HIV I subtype C as the dominant mode of infection. HIV II has 5 subtypes (A to E) and is principally found in West Africa, Western US and Europe. Further, recent reports are confirming the fast emergence of drug resistant strains of HIV not just from the US and the Europe but also from Mumbai and Chennai in India (Jain, 2001).

Life span of the HIV Virus – The virus itself cannot survive for a significant length of time outside the human body. Studies at the Center for Disease Control and Prevention (USA) have shown that drying causes 90-99 per cent reduction in HIV concentration in human body within several hours (NACO, 2000). According to ICMR (cited in NACO, 1997) the life span of HIV producing cells is only about two days. The daily rate of HIV production in an infected individual is shown to be around 10^8-10^9/day. Roughly an equal number of virions are also being destroyed in the earlier stages of the HIV infection. But after the initial infection, the rate of virus replication stabilizes at a "set point" in each HIV positive individual as shown in Fig. 1.8.

HIV Levels in Asymptomatic Individual
= $10^2 - 10^6$ HIV/ml of Plasma

HIV Levels in AIDS Patient
= More Than 10^8 HIV/ml of Plasma

Fig. 1.8 : Levels of HIV.

The HIV level in an asymptomatic individual remains stable at 10^2 to 10^6 HIV RNA/ml of plasma. Over a few years in an AIDS patient this level rises to more than 10^8 virions/ml of plasma.

Progression of the HIV infection to AIDS - The Center for Disease Control and Prevention (USA) has used CD4 count in blood as an indicator to mark the progression of HIV infection to AIDS. According to NACO (2000) the progressive stages of the HIV infection are as follows:

1. ***Primary Infection** (Seroconversion) Stage* – Begins at 2-6 weeks after primary infection and the individual may show symptoms like fever and pharyngitis. The initial illness usually lasts 2 weeks or less.
2. ***Asymptomatic disease** (CD4 Count > 500/mm^3)* – This stage may last for 8-10 years and is usually marked by dermatitis (skin disease), PGL and various opportunistic infections such as diarrhoea and fever.
3. ***Intermediate HIV infection** (CD4 count 200-500/mm^3)* – Marked by worsening of opportunistic infections like Tuberculosis. Lasts for 18 to 28 months.
4. ***Late stage of HIV disease** (CD4 Count is 50-200/mm^3)* – Marked by neurological manifestations such as dementia, meningitis and visual impairment.
5. ***Advanced HIV disease** (CD4 Count $<50/mm^3$)* - Person dies of opportunistic infections usually within 2 years of diagnosis of this stage.

Clinical Confirmation of AIDS - According to the WHO (1997) AIDS is confirmed in an individual by the presence of the following three conditions-

(a) ***Opportunistic infections*** – Like pneumocystis carinii, chronic diarrhoea, weight loss more than 10 per cent of body weight, skin cancer (Kaposi's sarcoma), prolonged fever and infection of the nervous system (dementia).

(b) ***CD4 cell count less than 200/ml of blood*** – Number of CD4 cells drops below 200/ml of blood whereas the normal count is between 800 to 1200/ml of blood.

(c) ***ELISA positive test*** – ELISA (enzyme linked immuno sorbent assay) is a sensitive blood test, which is used to detect the presence of HIV antibodies in our body.

However, it is important to note that antibodies against HIV start appearing in blood in significant amounts only 6-12 weeks after a person has been infected with the HIV. This time period, i.e., time from initial infection till 12 weeks is called the "window period" as shown in Fig. 1.9.

Time From Initial Infection	TILL → "WINDOW PERIOD"	12 Weeks After HIV infection

Fig. 1.9: Window Period.

A blood test to detect HIV antibodies during the window period will give false negative results due to the absence of significant amount of antibodies even when the person is HIV infected.

Objectives of HIV Testing – In 1992, the World Health Assembly adopted a resolution endorsing that there is no public health rationale for any measures like mandatory HIV screening, which limit the rights of the individual (WHO, 1997). In fact, mandatory testing measures have proved to be counter-productive as they tend to drive the most vulnerable sections of the society "underground". Once underground, these people may not have an access to HIV education and prevention as well as other health care services. WHO emphasizes and recommends voluntary HIV testing (wherein an individual volunteers to undergo a HIV test) as the best measure for HIV control.

Some of the worst hit states in India like Manipur and Tamil Nadu have taken the initiative of encouraging people to go in for pre-marital voluntary HIV testing. Similarly, in a significant move the government of India has changed its policy of not revealing the HIV status of blood donors. Effective from December 2002, all blood banks have been instructed to reveal the HIV status of blood donors who would like to know it, after careful counselling (Jain, 2002). The government has taken this stand in view of the fact that an early detection of the virus can help prolong the life of an individual by teaching the person how to live with it.

Measures like motivating people to go in for voluntary premarital HIV testing as well as revealing the HIV status to consenting blood donors need to be effectively promoted. Such strategies can help a long way not only in checking the further spread of the HIV but also in helping HIV positive individuals to cope up with the disease in an effective manner.

Globally, WHO (1997) recommends HIV testing only for following purposes –

(a) *Surveillance* - to monitor trends of the HIV infection using unlinked anonymous testing (i.e., the identity of the person tested is not known).

(b) *Transfusion safety* – to test blood, organs or tissues for ensuring safety of the recipients.

(c) *Diagnosis of symptomatic infection* – among those clinically suspected of having AIDS (with informed consent).

(d) *Early diagnosis of HIV infection* – among asymptomatic persons who would like to know their HIV status (with informed consent).

Counselling and Support – HIV/AIDS counselling helps people to assess their risk of HIV infection and also provides them information so that they are able to reduce the risk of passing HIV to others. Counselling is essential to reinforce safe behaviour and is a cost-effective way of supporting prevention efforts. Studies show that people who have received counselling are more likely to adopt or maintain safe behaviours. For instance, patients in an urban primary health care clinic receiving AIDS education, skills-training and peer support reported a 40 per cent increase in condom use (Kelly, et al. cited in JAMA, 1996). Similarly, studies of discordant couples (i.e., where one is HIV infected and the other is not) have shown that discordant couples who received repeated HIV testing and post-test counselling showed increased condom use from 3 per cent to 57 per cent (Allen, et al. cited in JAMA, 1996).

It is important to note that people diagnosed with HIV/AIDS require not only clinical care but also need profound social, emotional and behavioural adjustments in family life, sexual and social relations, at work place as well as an understanding of spiritual needs and legal and civil rights. Counselling helps infected people make decisions about their life, to cope effectively with stress and to improve family and community relationships as well as quality of life. It also provides support to the families as well as loved ones of HIV positive people so that they are able to look after HIV positive members in a more supportive manner.

In order to be effective, counselling needs to be undertaken at various levels, which are –

(a) *Pre-test counselling* – Counselling before the HIV test is done to provide the individual being tested with information on personal, medical, social and psychological implications of being tested positive or negative.

(b) *Post-test counselling* – This is done to provide support and hope for problems that may result if the person tests positive. The client is informed about the resources that are available and possible treatment for symptoms of the HIV infection.

(c) *Preventive counselling* – This counselling helps individuals to change their behaviour irrespective of their HIV status. It is not restricted to HIV infected people and their families but is also available to all people who are at risk of HIV infection.

Hence, preventive-counselling needs to be vigorously pursued as a HIV prevention strategy among the masses especially those practicing high-risk behaviours. Seeing the huge cost incurred on the treatment of the HIV infection in terms of human and material resources, preventive counselling can prove to be a cost-effective method of checking the further spread of the virus.

Anti-Retroviral Therapy (ART) – Anti-retroviral drugs introduced in 1996 are being used to delay the progression from HIV infection to AIDS and to prolong the life of an infected individual. There are various drugs like Azidothymidine (AZT), Saquinavir, Ritonavir, ddc and 3TC that are currently available. But recent studies show that combination therapy (i.e., using three drugs together) is more effective than single drug therapy. This is because HIV rapidly develops resistance to single drug use. Highly Active Anti-Retroviral Therapy (HAART) is the term commonly used for combination therapy (i.e., AZT + 3TC + Protease Inhibitors). However this regimen should only be started when the immune cell count of the infected person falls sufficiently low (NACO, 2000).

Till recent years, HAART in India costed around Rs. 15,000-20,000 per month thus, rendering it inaccessible to majority of people living with HIV/AIDS (NACO, 2000). In fact, the high cost of HAART has forced an HIV positive prisoner lodged in Tihar Jail to resist his release from the jail since last 15 months despite being granted bail. He wants to remain jailed because as long as he is a prisoner he is entitled to get free drugs and treatment for AIDS according to jail rules. The jail authorities are spending Rs. 2000 every week on his treatment. Once out of the jail this man knows that he will not be able to afford his treatment and will eventually die at an early stage (Sharma, 2001). Similarly, reports of many HIV positive patients mainly from low-income groups being forced to stop life-sustaining antiretroviral therapy because of high costs are becoming common phenomena day by day (*Times of India*, Dec. 2, 2003).

Although an Indian pharmaceutical company has come up with a generic triple drug cocktail priced at less than $ 1 a day yet, the price is by no means affordable for poor people who live on day-to-day basis. Ironically, it has also been reported that majority of those who need these drugs in India do not get them due to the fact that the Indian company exports its anti-retrovirals to some African countries (Shreedhar, 2002).

The United Nations through its accelerating access initiative (AAI) is collaborating with pharmaceutical corporations to help drive anti-retroviral drug prices down. Backed by a strong social commitment, few countries like Brazil, Argentina, Uruguay and Botswana are providing HIV/AIDS patients free anti-retroviral drugs (UNAIDS/WHO, Dec., 2001). Presently in the Indian scenario, providing free regime of anti-retrovirals to a huge population of HIV positive people seems to be a distant possibility. However, the government has taken the initiative of providing free HIV/AIDS control drugs to all HIV positive children less than 15 years of age as well as all HIV positive mothers (Sharma, 2003).

Further, studies to determine the efficacy of natural and cheaper therapies for HIV/AIDS are continuing in various countries. The French Ministry of Health has classified SPV-30 (a natural boxwood evergreen extract) as a natural anti-retroviral drug (Stokes and Mestman, 1996). In

India too, the Indian Council of Medical Research (ICMR) is coordinating research into Indian systems of medicine and Homeopathy to look for natural and cheaper alternatives, which may be easily available to PWHA. However, till such alternatives become available, the only option for PWHA remains the anti-retroviral therapy. Unfortunately the latest UNAIDS/WHO (Dec., 2003) report showed that many countries and more so in the Asia-Pacific region, have not yet, been able to adopt policies to promote access to HIV related medications, including anti-retroviral drugs.

Vaccine for HIV – Scientists around the world are working hard to develop an effective HIV/AIDS vaccine. Globally, around $ 300 million is being spent annually for the development of AIDS vaccine and more than 60 HIV vaccine trials have taken place all over the world (*Span*, Sept./Oct., 2001). The Rockfellar foundation launched a programme in 1994, which is now known as the International AIDS Vaccine Initiative (IAVI). The major donors of this social venture are the governments of U.K., USA, Canada, Netherlands, World Bank and Bill and Melinda Gates Foundation. The goal of this initiative is to develop, manufacture and distribute AIDS vaccine at affordable prices.

Clinical trials to test IAVI's first vaccine began in Kenya in January 2001. IAVI has also signed an agreement in March 2001 with ICMR (India) to develop and evaluate HIV/AIDS vaccines in India. The Department of Bio-technology (India) and Chiron (a US Company) are also working out on a collaboration to develop AIDS vaccine (*Span*, Sept./Oct., 2001). On the same hand, care is also being taken to address ethical issues relating to clinical trials of AIDS vaccine. For this purpose, ethical guidelines for research involving human beings have been prepared by the ICMR (India). An effective HIV vaccine in the near future is being hopefully awaited, which can put a stop on the spread of the epidemic.

India makes Indigenous HIV Testing Kits – Until the mid 90's India was totally dependent on imported HIV testing kits, which proved to be expensive by Indian standards. With the aim of becoming self-reliant and providing cheaper HIV testing kits, the Department of Bio-technology (DBT) took the initiative to develop indigenous kits in 1993-94. The kits developed indigenously and sponsored by the DBT are:-

- NEVA HIV (naked eye visible agglutination assay) kit.
- X Cyton's HIV Chex.
- HIV TRI-DOT and Microlisa HIV kit.

All these kits have been assessed by the WHO, National AIDS Research Institute (NARI), Pune and National Institute of Communicable Diseases (NICD), Delhi. The cost of HIV testing with these kits varies from

Rs. 40 to Rs. 100 per test. The Tata Memorial Center (Mumbai) has also developed an indigenous Western Blot kit (used for confirmatory HIV test). This confirmatory test costs anywhere between Rs. 700 to Rs. 1500 (*Span*, Sept./Oct., 2001).

Global Response to the AIDS Epidemic

The massive devastation inflicted by the AIDS pandemic has led many nations to unite and jointly wage a war to combat the HIV. Some of the efforts that are being jointly implemented by the United Nations at the global level are –

The Global AIDS Strategy - The different phases of evolution of the present day global AIDS strategy are shown in Fig. 1.10.

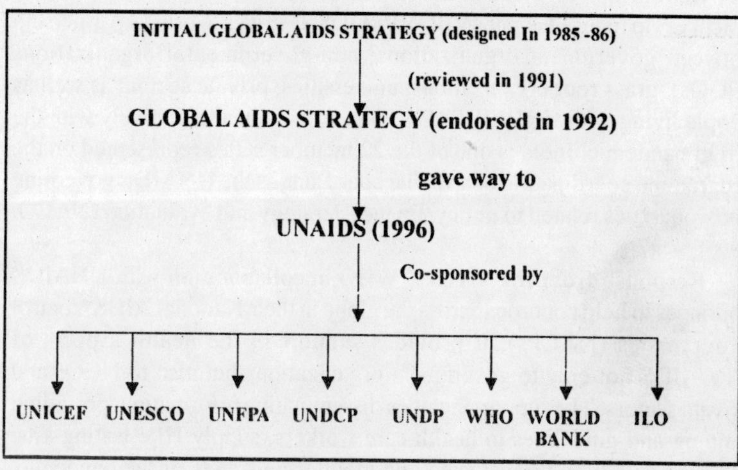

Fig. 1.10 : Evolution of the Global AIDS Strategy.

The initial global AIDS strategy was designed in 1985-86. It was reviewed in 1991 and endorsed in 1992 by the World Health Assembly and the United Nation's Social Council (NACO, 1996). The strategy was designed with the following three main objectives: -

1. To prevent infection with HIV.
2. To reduce the personal and social impact of HIV infection.
3. To mobilize and unify national and international efforts against AIDS.

UNAIDS - The global AIDS strategy was replaced in 1996 by a new Joint United Nations Programme on HIV/AIDS (UNAIDS) whose secretariat is based in Geneva, Switzerland. UNAIDS is co-sponsored by eight organizations which are the United Nations Children's Fund (UNICEF), the United Nations Development Fund (UNDP), the United Nations Population Fund (UNFPA), the United Nations Educational, Scientific and Cultural Organization (UNESCO), the United Nations International Drug Control Program (UNDCP), the World Health Organization (WHO), the World Bank and the new eighth entrant in 2001, i.e., International Labour Organization (ILO).

The goal of UNAIDS is to lead and assist in an expansion of the international response to HIV/AIDS on all fronts: medical, social, economic, political and human rights.

It gathers, analyses and disseminates information about the epidemic. UNAIDS is also involved in developing and advocating the use of "best practices" to reduce the impact of HIV/AIDS. It strives to bring a partnership between government organizations, non-governmental organizations (NGOs), grass root organizations, universities, private sectors as well as people living with HIV/AIDS (PWHA), so as to deal effectively with the AIDS pandemic. India is one of the 22 member states represented on the programme coordinating board. The board acts as the UNAIDS governing body on issues related to policy, finance, strategy and evaluation (NACO, 1996).

Response from the WHO – WHO in collaboration with UNAIDS continues to help countries across the globe in their National AIDS Control Programmes (NACPs). It provides support in the health aspects of HIV/AIDS not only to government organizations but also to NGOs and private sectors. The support includes disseminating information, providing training and guidelines to health-care workers, supply HIV testing kits, ensuring safe blood transfusion and monitoring trends of the pandemic. WHO is also promoting the concept of continuum of care for people living with HIV/AIDS at various levels and proposes that HIV/AIDS care should be integrated with primary health care.

United Nation's (UN) General Assembly Responds to AIDS - The United Nations General Assembly Special Session (UNGASS) on HIV/AIDS was held in New York in June 2001. The Assembly recognized that HIV/AIDS is not just a medical problem but an economic, social and human rights issue. Women represent 52 per cent of adults who have died of AIDS since the epidemic started. Thus, the pandemic can be averted if women are protected against exploitation and from being forced into unsafe sex. UN Secretary General Kofi Annan said, "If there is one idea that stands out in this declaration, it is that women are in the forefront of this battle." The meet unanimously agreed to a global agenda of reversing the epidemic by 2015. Kofi Annan also proposed for the establishment of a global HIV/AIDS fund to finance programmes in the developing nations (*Times of India*, June, 2001).

The assembly pledged to pursue a series of targets relating to HIV/AIDS prevention, care and support. Some of the important targets are as follows:-

1. To reduce HIV infections among 15-24 year olds by 25 per cent by 2005-2010.
2. To reduce the proportion of infants infected with HIV by 50 per cent by 2010.
3. To strengthen health care systems and provide ART at affordable prices by 2003.
4. To provide supportive environment for orphans and children infected and affected by HIV/AIDS by 2005.
5. To address the factors that make individuals particularly vulnerable to HIV by 2003.
6. To develop multi-sectoral strategies to combat HIV/AIDS epidemic at family, community and national levels by 2003 (UNAIDS/WHO, Dec., 2001).

The 189 members General Assembly adopted the "Declaration of Commitment on HIV/AIDS" and this marked the end of an unprecedented special session of General Assembly on a health issue.

Political Response to AIDS – Experience across the globe shows that prospects for success of AIDS prevention programmes are brightest when a country has a top level committee or body often reporting to the president or prime minister responsible for planning and managing the AIDS prevention programme (UNAIDS/WHO, Dec., 2000). Such a high level body can collaborate with many sectors such as the education, health, defence, agriculture, industrial as well as the private sectors. A large number of countries have set up a top level AIDS coordination committee in their respective nations. The global community is also coming closer by forging International Partnership against AIDS. Formed in 1999, the International Partnership against AIDS in Africa is working to find and mobilize new partners inside and outside the continent in the fight against AIDS (UNAIDS/WHO, Dec., 2000).

Similarly, prime ministers and finance ministers of the Caribbean group of countries at a meeting in June 2000 recognized AIDS as a major development challenge. The Caribbean community (CARICOM) pledged a strong political commitment to combat the epidemic at a massive scale. Growing political commitment has also led countries of the Commonwealth of Independent States to develop a special declaration on AIDS. Similarly, the president of Ukraine set a positive example by declaring 2002, the year of the fight against AIDS (UNAIDS/WHO, Dec., 2001).

US President Bill Clinton during his historic visit to India in March 2000, addressed both the Houses of the Parliament and stressed on the need of scaling up AIDS prevention programmes as well as putting an end to stigma attached to the disease. The address led to an agreement between India and the USA to jointly wage a war against HIV/ AIDS (NACO, April, 2000).

Similarly, while urging to the masses to practice safe behaviour, Indian Prime Minister Atal Bihari Vajpayee during his Independence Day speech from the Red Fort on August 15th, 2000 said, "Recently, the rapidly spreading disease of HIV/AIDS has become a grave challenge to our nation. I appeal to all sections of society to fully participate in building awareness about the epidemic. They should also make necessary changes in their behaviour so that this dreaded disease can be controlled" (NACO, July-Sept. 2000). The prime minister's meeting with business leaders and industrialists on 1st December, 2000 led to the development of a government-business partnership to control further spread of HIV/AIDS in the country (NACO, Oct. - Dec. 2000). Further, the year 2002, marked the beginning of the initiative "Delhi Declaration" which vows to achieve liberation from AIDS (*India Abroad*, June- July, 2002). Under this Declaration, India has confirmed its pledge to make concerted, sustained and effective action in the struggle against HIV/AIDS.

Although, the political response to the AIDS epidemic has been phenomenal in our country yet, the growing number of HIV infections indicates that such responses need to be transformed into effective policies, which in turn should be stringently implemented. The National Convention on HIV/AIDS held in Delhi made deliberate efforts to make political leaders take a public stand regarding HIV/AIDS management for which they could be accountable (*Times of India*, July 28, 2003).

Religious Impact - Helping in AIDS Awareness

In most continents across the globe, the daily lives of people are strongly influenced by spiritual beliefs about God, supernatural powers and life after death. Religious institutions and preachers form an integral part of many communities in these continents especially in rural areas. They have been known to be powerful influencers and are being currently trained to create AIDS awareness in the communities. For instance, religious leaders and volunteers in countries like Kenya, Zimbabwe and USA are actively persuading communities to understand and participate in providing care and support to PWHA (Dortzbach, et al., 1996; Drew, 1996). Similarly, female minstrels in Burkina are spreading AIDS prevention messages during ceremonies such as marriages and baptism (Yameogo, et al., 1996).

The tremendous impact of religion and the vast outreach potential of various festivals in India have also been used for creating AIDS awareness. For example, Indian Health Organization (IHO) has organised various AIDS awareness exhibitions during major festivals such Kumbh mela (in Nasik), Ganpati immersion (in Mumbai) and during Navratri at various places (Bora and Gilada, 1997). In Mysore (Karnataka), a local community has erected a shrine for what they call as AIDS goddess- "AIDS Amma" (*Span* Sept./Oct., 2001).

Prime Minister Vajpayee while addressing a meeting on HIV/AIDS stressed on the need to involve religious institutes in our fight against AIDS. In his words, "We should also actively involve religious establishments who can have a strong positive influence over large sections of society" in combating AIDS.

World AIDS day - Reinforcing the Response

December 1 is being observed as the World AIDS Day every year since 1988. The day emerged from a call given by the world summit of ministers of health in January 1988 to promote and coordinate international efforts against AIDS. The World Health Assembly, the UN organizations, the governments and communities across the globe support the World AIDS day. In 1997, the first *World AIDS Campaign* took place to stress on the need of sustaining HIV prevention efforts all through the year and not just observing 1st December every year as the World AIDS Day. Since then a particular theme focusing on a priority issue is chosen for the World AIDS Day and the same is observed through the year.

For AIDS awareness, a red ribbon logo (shown in Fig. 1.11) was conceived in 1991 by a group of US artists who wanted to draw attention to AIDS (www.unaids.org. Sept., 1998). Since then it has become an international symbol of AIDS awareness.

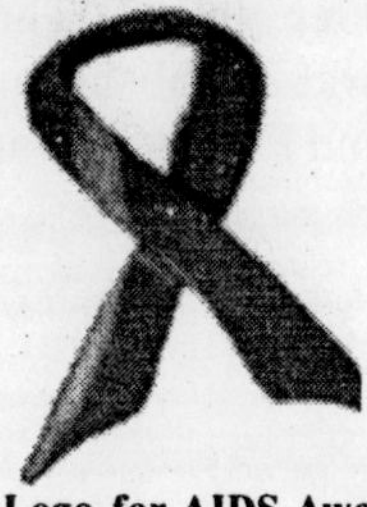

Fig. 1.11 : Logo for AIDS Awareness.

AIDS in India

India has the highest number of people in Asia living with HIV/AIDS according to the latest UNAIDS/WHO (Dec., 2004) report. Recent estimates suggest that about 5.1 million people in the country are infected with HIV and that children comprise 10 per cent of the infected population (*UNAIDS/ WHO*, Dec. 2004, *Times of India*, Dec. 2, 2003). In the six states of Maharashtra, Tamil Nadu, Andhra Pradesh, Karnataka, Manipur and Nagaland the HIV prevalence in the general population is more than 1 per cent, making it a generalized epidemic with Maharashtra alone accounting for nearly 50 per cent of all reported HIV/AIDS cases in India (NACO, 2000). NACO admits that these numbers do not reflect the true situation in India, as there is significant under reporting. According to the recent WHO estimates half of all HIV infections in Asia come from India (NACO, 2000). Commercial sex and injecting drug use remain a dominant feature in the spread of the HIV.

Epidemiological trends in India as observed by NACO (2000) show that:

1. By January 1999, a sero-positivity rate (i.e., number of infections/ 1000 of population) of 24.22 per thousand was estimated.
2. 89 per cent of all the people infected by HIV are in the age group of 15-44 years.
3. The predominant mode of HIV infection in India is through heterosexual contact (74.17 per cent), followed by blood transfusion (8.15 per cent) and injectable drug use (7.05 per cent).
4. Men account for 78.77 per cent of AIDS cases whereas women represent 21.23 per cent. The ratio of HIV infection between men and women is 3:1.

National AIDS Control Programme in India - The first case of HIV in India was detected in 1986 by the Christian Medical College (CMC), (Vellore), in the blood sample of a commercial sex worker (CSW) from Chennai. Soon after, a National AIDS Committee was set up under the chairmanship of Minister of Health and Family Welfare. In 1987, the government launched the National AIDS Control Programme (NACP) with the goal of increasing AIDS awareness and also to keep a check on the spread of the epidemic. The National AIDS Control Organization (NACO) was established in May 1992 in New Delhi by the Ministry of Health and Family Welfare to manage the activities of the NACP.

Fig. 1.12 depicts the functioning of the NACP.

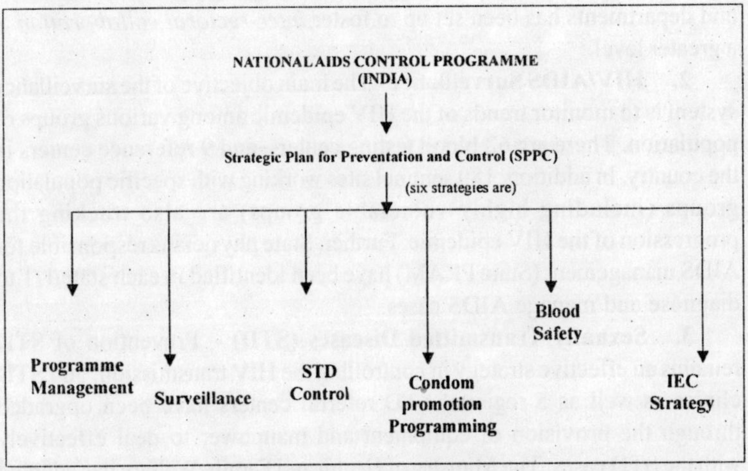

Fig. 1.12: Functioning of the NACP.

The National AIDS Control Programme implemented its Strategic Plan for Prevention and Control **(SPPC)** in 1992. As per the updates from NACO (2000), the six strategies identified to achieve the goals of the SPPC are:

1. Programme Management - The NACP is managed at the national level by National AIDS Committee (NAC), National AIDS Control Board (NACB) and NACO. NACO co-ordinates, monitors and evaluates the programme in various states with the support of the National AIDS Control Board. The board exercises all financial and administrative powers. In order to strengthen the programme management at the state level, all the states/UTs have established their own State AIDS Control Societies.

Intersectional collaboration is much needed as the challenges posed by HIV/AIDS stretch beyond the health sector to many other sectors. Therefore, NACO encourages the involvement of every possible sector in the fight against AIDS. It is collaborating with various multi-lateral/bilateral agencies, government ministries and NGOs. Effective collaborations with the private sector represented by TATA Iron and Steel Company and the Bengal Chamber of Commerce are successfully ongoing. The private sector has also formed a Business Coalition to respond to HIV/AIDS. NACO is working closely with ministries like Defence, Railways, Labour, Steel and Social sector ministries such as Youth Affairs, Social Justice and Empowerment of Women and Child Development. A *multi-sectoral committee*, which has representatives from major government ministries and departments has been set up to foster *inter-sectoral collaboration* at a greater level.

2. HIV/AIDS Surveillance - The main objective of the surveillance system is to monitor trends of the HIV epidemic among various groups of population. There are 62 blood testing centers, and 9 reference centers in the country. In addition, 180 sentinel sites working with specific population groups (including highly vulnerable groups) are also tracking the progression of the HIV epidemic. Further, State physicians responsible for AIDS management (State PRAM) have been identified in each state/UT to diagnose and manage AIDS cases.

3. Sexually Transmitted Diseases (STD) – Prevention of STD remains an effective strategy in controlling the HIV transmission. 504 STD clinics as well as 5 regional STD referral centers have been upgraded through the provision of equipment and manpower to deal effectively with the STD cases. The Ministry of Health and Family Welfare has adopted a policy to integrate STD control in the ongoing family welfare services.

4. Condom Programming – NACO has initiated a programme to ensure that good quality and affordable condoms are easily accessible to people especially the vulnerable groups. Condom quality specifications as described by the WHO have been adhered to through the revision of schedule "R" of the Drugs and Cosmetics Act. Condom vending machines are being installed at strategic sites to make condoms easily available. Social marketing of condoms whereby the user pays a subsidized price for the product is also being initiated to increase condom use.

5. Blood Safety - Blood safety is an integral part of the NACP. 154 zonal blood-testing centers have been established for HIV screening. Mandatory measures such as licensing of all blood banks and testing every unit of blood for HIV are being enforced stringently. 815 blood banks have been upgraded and 40 blood component separation facilities have been established. The Supreme Court of India passed a judgement on 4th January, 1996, which led to the formation of National and State Blood Transfusion Councils that ensure the availability of safe blood. Professional blood donation has also been banned w.e.f. 1st January, 1998 in order to curb the selling of blood especially by vulnerable sections of the society.

6. Public Awareness through Information, Education and Communication (IEC) – Efforts are under way in all parts of the country to educate people about HIV/AIDS. A comprehensive Information, Education and Communication (IEC) strategy was prepared by NACO in 1994 and is operational at two levels. At the national level, political and media advocacy is being enhanced to create a supportive environment whereas at the state level, State AIDS Control Societies are undertaking IEC activities in accordance to their social and cultural context. The wide spectrum of IEC strategy includes the following components:

(a) ***Generic material*** – It is developed by NACO and disseminated to all the states, Union Territories and NGOs for further use.

(b) ***Mass Media Approach*** – Multimedia campaigns using talk shows, music programmes, TV spots, cinema, press advertisements, cinema slides, posters, and pamphlets etc., are being used to mobilize community efforts against AIDS.

(c) ***Reaching Rural Youth*** – NACO is supporting about 700 Yuva Kendras in rural areas with the objective of spreading HIV/AIDS/STD awareness among the rural youth.

(d) ***Outreach Projects*** – The Department of Youth Affairs and Sports has been using rural art forms like puppetry, folk dance and music in disseminating HIV/AIDS information messages.

(e) ***AIDS education in Schools*** – In consultation with the National Council of Educational Research and Training (NCERT), NACO has prepared training packages for imparting AIDS education in schools.

(f) ***Universities Talk AIDS (UTA)*** – The UTA programme was launched in 1991 by the Department of Youth Affairs and Sports with technical assistance from the WHO. The programme continues to sensitize the college going youth on causes, consequences and prevention of HIV/AIDS. It is operational in all universities in India and has more than 1.35 million student volunteers who act as peer educators. The UTA is a low cost programme, which aims to train 10 new peer educators/college/year (WHO, Nov., 1998).

(g) ***Mobilizing Women Organizations*** – Keeping women's vulnerability to HIV infection in mind, NACO has held workshops with grass root level women's organizations to specifically address issues related to women and HIV.

(h) ***Targeted Interventions*** – Targeting groups practicing high risk behaviour makes prevention a concerted effort in reducing HIV transmission. At present, 570 targeted interventions are being implemented throughout the country (NACO, Dec.1, 2001). These interventions are being implemented for the vulnerable and marginalized groups such as migrant workers, sex workers, truck drivers, street children, injecting drug users, prison inmates and men having sex with men. Some of the successful interventions which have resulted in increased condom usage and decrease in STD rates have been for — the commercial sex workers (CSWs) in Sonagachi area (Kolkata) and in Khetwadi area (Mumbai), men who have sex with men (Chennai), truck drivers (Rajasthan) and intravenous drug users (Manipur).

Most of these projects are operating on an integrated approach and are providing a host of services like information, education, communication, health-care, and condom programming services. The integrated approach ensures maximum impact of the programme. IEC print material targeting specific groups like commercial sex workers, intravenous drug users, slum dwellers and street children has also been developed by NACO with a goal of creating HIV/AIDS awareness among these vulnerable sections of the society.

Continuum of Care – Providing care and support to people living with HIV/AIDS (PWHA) is an integral component in NACP—Phase-II. People living with HIV/AIDS require care and support at various levels such as – home, community, clinics, and hospitals thus, necessitating a continuum of care. Apart from the therapeutic measures, which treat opportunistic infections, supportive measures are also essential to combat stress and stigma. NACO plans to train family members, community volunteers, health care workers and doctors so as to reduce the social and psychological impact of AIDS and to improve the quality of life of PWHA. In Manipur, a "continuum of care" project initiated jointly by NACO, WHO and Oxfam has been a success (NACO, 1996). The project provides care and support to PWHA through a network of home, community and health care services as shown in Fig. 1.13.

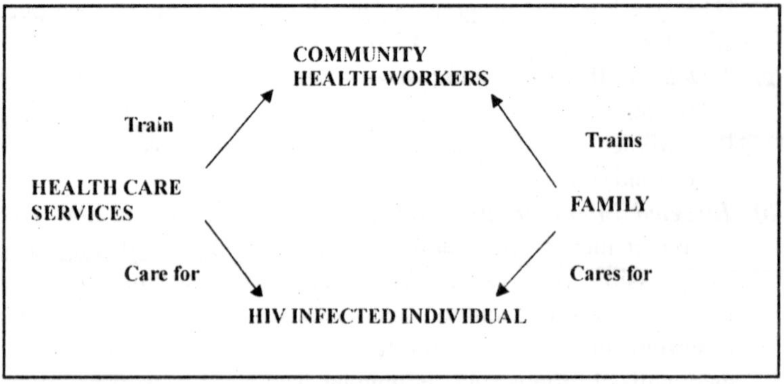

Fig. 1.13 : Continuum of Care.

Similar projects have also been taken up in Tamil Nadu and Maharashtra since they represent the worst affected areas. At present twelve care and support centers which aim to provide low cost community based care for people living with HIV/AIDS and their families are operating in different states (NACO, Dec. 1, 2002).

Research Programmes - Studies regarding knowledge, attitudes, behaviour and practices (KABP) with regards to HIV/AIDS are being taken up by various organizations with the aim of providing guidance and direction to policy-makers.

Counselling - Recognizing the vital importance of counselling as a supportive and cost-effective measure, NACO has established 145 Voluntary Counselling Centers all over the country. A counselling training module for training apex level, intermediate level and grass-root level counsellors has also been developed by NACO.

Online Discussion Forum - NACO in association with UNAIDS has launched an online discussion forum, i.e., www.youandaids.org. The forum is operational on every Wednesday between 2 to 3 p.m. and shares knowledge and experiences on the web.

Telephone Hotline - A National AIDS Telephone Helpline (no.1097) has been initiated in most of the states which offers free HIV/AIDS information and counselling to the masses. The helpline is presently operational in 77 cities and towns.

Second Phase of NACP (1999-2004) – On 15th December 1999, India launched its second five year National AIDS Control Programme (NACP) with a budget of US $ 230 million including $ 191 million assistance from the World Bank and $39 million from the government of India and the state governments. The programme emphasizes on decentralization of service's delivery at the state level, protection of human rights of PWHA and encourages ownership of the NACP by the implementing agencies (NACO, Dec., 2001).

To evaluate the NACP, WHO has developed a set of *ten prevention indicators*, which measure achievements in knowledge level, use of condom and reduction in the incidence of sexually transmitted diseases. This evaluation is called the Prevention Indicator (PI) Survey (NACO, 1996).

Non-Governmental Organizations (NGOs) - Complementing NACP- In India, a number of NGOs have responded very positively to the HIV/AIDS epidemic. The role of NGOs in reaching the marginalized groups is vital, as they are better acquainted and have close interpersonal interaction with the communities they work with (Narain and Jha, 1997). Many NGOs continue to help in preventing new HIV infections through awareness generating activities. They are also instrumental in reducing the personal and social impact through their support and counselling programmes.

Some of the NGOs recognized for their efforts in combating HIV/AIDS epidemic are:

1. AIDS Awareness Group (Delhi) – working with commercial sex workers.
2. Calcutta Samaritans (Kolkata) – working with street children.
3. CINI-Asha (Children in Need Institute, Calcutta)–working with street children.
4. Community Health and Education Society (Chennai) – working with children.
5. Kripa Foundation (Manipur) – working with street children for community-based rehabilitation.
6. Naaz foundation (Delhi) – working with men who have sex with men (MSM) and also runs a care-home in Saket (Delhi), where HIV infected patients are taken care of both physically and spiritually.
7. Prayas and Prachi (Delhi) - working with different communities.
8. Prerana (Mumbai) - working with children.
9. Salaam Balak Trust (New Delhi) - working with street children and children affected by HIV/AIDS.
10. Sharan (Delhi) - working with intravenous drug users (IDUs).
11. Society for Promotion of Youth and Masses (SPYM) (Delhi) – working with truck drivers.

Although NGOs are bridging the gap between NACP and the communities yet, it has often been observed that most NGOs remain passive in exchanging information and reluctant in coming together in a coalition format (Gardner, et al., 1996). The coalition form can promote greater programme coverage and increase the accessibility of different services in an integrated manner. Narain and Jha (1997) while describing the role of NGOs state, "Whereas the number of NGOs working on AIDS related issues has increased quite appreciably over the years, the technical and managerial capacity of many NGOs needs strengthening."

WHO Policy for NGO – WHO collaborates with different NGOs on the basis of World Health Assembly Resolution (WHA 42.34), which calls for governments, NGOs and the WHO secretariat to work together by complementing each other's activities (Narain and Jha, 1997). WHO has recommended that 15 per cent of the fund it provides should be allocated to NGOs for AIDS activities. In 1994, WHO developed guidelines for NACPs, which stress that besides providing technical and material support to NGOs, NACPs should also collaborate closely with them. Assistance and guidance to various NGOs is provided by support organizations such as Asia-Pacific Council of AIDS Service Organizations (APCASO), the Global Network of People living with AIDS (GNP+) and the International HIV/AIDS Alliance (Narain and Jha, 1997).

Discrimination Against People Living with or Affected by HIV/AIDS (PWHA)

Discrimination against persons living with/affected by HIV/AIDS is socially, economically and legally detrimental. Under the UN Convention people living with HIV/AIDS have the same fundamental rights as uninfected people to education, employment, health, travel, marriage, procreation, privacy, social security, scientific benefits, asylum etc., (Honigsbaum and Neil, 1996).

Yet, growing evidence from many countries across the world suggests that many people with HIV/AIDS are being increasingly subjected to discrimination and rejection. For instance, many HIV-affected children in Europe do not have access to quality health and social services (Honigshaum and Neil, 1996). Similarly, in the USA claims of discrimination have been presented in a wide variety of contexts such as in employment, housing and health care establishments (JAMA, 1998).

HIV/AIDS is highly stigmatized in India too. The commonly held belief that HIV is associated with promiscuity has led many people to assume that HIV infected people have sinned and thus, deserve their fate (UNAIDS/WHO, Dec., 1999). Ironically, the discrimination against women is far greater than men. Women are frequently being blamed by their in-laws and husband for their spouse's HIV infection while on the contrary, majority of these women have themselves been infected by their husband. Many women have been turned out of their homes after their husbands died of AIDS and thus, made to lose their children (UNAIDS/WHO, Dec., 1999).

Exclusion, isolation and desertion of people living with HIV/AIDS have become usual responses of our society especially towards women. A study conducted in Mumbai (India), showed that responses towards people living with HIV/AIDS differed according to their gender and relationship in a family. For instance, men/sons/husbands with HIV/AIDS were given greater acceptance, care and support whereas the response towards women/daughters/wives infected with HIV/AIDS was not as supportive (Bharat, 1996).

Many hospitals and health care set-ups have also been reported to be turning away HIV positive patients due to the fear of contracting the disease (*Times of India*, Dec.1, 2001). "Physicians' bias" is strongly emerging as a major problem in HIV/AIDS management. For instance, many cases of HIV infected people being refused treatment at district hospitals because of AIDS phobia are being increasingly reported (Mishra, 2003). This attitude of medical professionals is resulting in non-accessibility of treatment to people suffering from HIV/AIDS related complications. With the situation taking a deteriorating turn, the Delhi government has planned to bring a legislation that will penalize doctors who refuse to treat those infected with HIV (Srivastava, 2003). Increasing levels of discriminatory attitudes towards people living with HIV/AIDS have also led NACO to work closely with International Labour Organization and the Ministry of Labour for formulating a code of conduct at work place. Similarly, many countries are increasingly enacting laws, which prohibit discrimination against PWHA in any context or form. A new international code of conduct on AIDS and the work place was ratified in the beginning of 2001 by the ILO with the aim of counteracting discrimination against PWHA at their work place (NACO, 2001). However, a recent UNAIDS/WHO (Dec., 2003) progress report on the global response to the HIV/AIDS epidemic indicates that 38 per cent of countries have yet to adopt legislation to prevent discrimination against people living with HIV/AIDS. It further needs to be emphasized that instead of having all these mandatory measures what actually is required, is a deep attitudinal change based on awareness regarding the disease and aspects related to it to put an end to discrimination against PWHA.

HIV/AIDS AND Human Rights – An international consensus stressing on equal rights for PWHA is gradually evolving. The need to protect and promote the human rights of HIV positive people has never been so acutely felt. Experience in many countries is reinforcing the opinion that non-discrimination of PWHA is an effective tool in preventing the further spread of the HIV. Many worst hit nations have started realizing that without adequate protection under law and a supportive social environment, PWHA are driven underground and do not come forward to avail information and prevention services even when they are freely available (WHO, 1997).

Protection and promotion of the rights of individuals living with HIV/AIDS, through legal and social environment has been one of the key policies of the "Declaration of the Paris AIDS Summit", held on 1st December, 1994. Forty-two countries including India signed the declaration and resolved to step up HIV prevention efforts. Keeping in line with the declaration, the Human Rights Programme in Zaire has used education and sensitization campaigns, which emphasize that women should use their rights for preserving their sexual relations against HIV (Musuamba and Mutombo, 1996).

Similarly, legal and social rights of children affected by HIV are being protected and promoted by the UN Convention on Rights of Children and the European forum on HIV/AIDS. AIDS activists in many countries are fighting for the rights of HIV infected people. Their efforts to empower PWHA have given rise to a new movement called AIDS Activism.

In India, a number of groups and organizations are striving for equal rights for PWHA. Maharashtra Network for Positive People (MNP +) (Mumbai), is one of such organizations which is formed by PWHA. The organization is committed to protect the basic human rights of PWHA including the rights to travel, to employment, to marry, to have children, job security, housing, education, access to medical care and to obtain an insurance cover. *Such efforts are at the initial stages in India and need to be evolved and implemented at a much wider scale.*

Greater Involvement of People Living with or Affected by HIV/AIDS (GIPA) – Philly Lutaaya, the Ugandan musician was the first African celebrity to disclose his HIV positive status. He stressed on the need to eliminate stigma and live positively. Lutaaya died in 1989 and is considered as one of the fathers of GIPA, the organization which stresses on the need to involve people living with or affected by AIDS in responding to the epidemic in an effective manner (UNAIDS, Sept., 1999).

The earlier term "people living with HIV/AIDS" has been widened by broad international consensus to the term "people living with or affected by HIV/AIDS (PWHA)". This includes individuals living with HIV/AIDS on the one hand to individuals such as HIV negative partners, family members and close friends of HIV positive persons on the other.

The 1994 Paris AIDS Summit declared that the principles of greater involvement of people living with or affected by HIV/AIDS (GIPA) is critical in forging ethical and effective national responses to the epidemic. GIPA basically means two important things, which are:

1. "Recognizing the important contribution people infected or affected by HIV/AIDS can make in the response to the epidemic.
2. Creating space within society for their involvement and active participation in all aspects of that response" (UNAIDS, Sept., 1999).

However, this principle has not been transformed into a reality so far. GIPA is not reflected or implemented in national policies and programmes of many countries on a large scale. Presently no major global, regional or national campaigns are being carried out to raise awareness and understanding of GIPA. High levels of fear, denial and stigmatization related to HIV/AIDS are further hampering the GIPA.

The importance of GIPA in reducing stigma and discrimination against PWHA has been globally acknowledged. PWHA can offer a lot to society in terms of their productive years and GIPA aims to give them an opportunity to realize this goal. Prominent examples of the successful GIPA related interventions are –

1. *The AIDS Service Organization (TASO)* which was created in Uganda in 1988 by a woman whose husband had died of AIDS. TASO has developed into one of the most innovative groups in the AIDS field.
2. *The United Nations Volunteers (UNV) Support to people living with HIV/AIDS project* – The UNV project recruits, trains and supports HIV positive people whom it places as UN volunteers in various host institutions.

In India, Delhi Network for Positive People (DNP+), Manipur Network of Positives and ACT- UP (AIDS Coalition to Unleash Power) are among the prominent organizations that are advocating the rights as well as greater involvement of people living with HIV/AIDS in all spheres of life. *Yet, such activities are in the initial stages and a lot remains to be done to recognize the needs and rights of people affected by HIV/AIDS as basic human rights.* Since India has the second largest population of HIV positive people in the world (Shreedhar, 2002) there is an urgent need to undertake in our national policies that all people living with or affected by HIV/AIDS are able to realize the full and equal enjoyment of their fundamental rights without any distinctions based on their HIV status.

Community Participation

In the recent years there has been a growing awareness about the crucial role played by different communities all over the world in shaping the course of the HIV epidemic. The recognition of community participation in facilitating or hampering HIV prevention efforts has led to the reformulation of both theoretical and practical efforts aimed at HIV/AIDS prevention and care. For instance, the focus of HIV/AIDS prevention efforts has been increasingly shifting from information based educational campaigns to intervention programmes aimed at enablement and empowerment of communities through their mobilization.

Community mobilization in essence is the process of sensitizing and motivating communities in bringing about a desired change. It has been earnestly recognized as a cost-effective way to control the spread of HIV. According to a recent UNAIDS/WHO report (Dec., 2001) "The axis of any effective response is prevention strategy that draws on the explicit and strong commitment of leaders at all levels, that is built on community mobilization, and that extends into every area of the country."

Many researchers are now increasingly stressing on the importance of community participation in planning, developing and implementing effective HIV/AIDS prevention and care efforts. According to O'Neill et al. (1996) "Current trends in HIV epidemic show an increasing need for access to and availability of comprehensive, community-based systems of care with linkages to research." A comprehensive strategy as described by Jayaseelan (1996) in her study is that which encompasses HIV/AIDS prevention and care, rights advocacy and networking with governmental bodies. The study also justifies the need of having small scale, people-centred prevention and care projects for communities such as commercial sex workers, injecting drug users and PWHA, which are usually excluded or antagonized from the mainstream HIV programmes.

Community participation approaches allow us to study and determine the salient features of the social structure, culture as well as the psychological factors of the community being studied. Gilliam et al. (1996) in their study have successfully used the participatory approach to assess the needs of the community under study and also for planning future strategies with key informants representing the cultural group. Similarly, participatory methodology has also been extensively used to develop culturally appropriate behavioural change programmes. Paula (1996) developed a cultural model for behavioural change, keeping in mind the cultural values of the sample being studied. Studies have also shown that participatory research methods allow communities to evaluate and track their programmes (Jayaseelan, 1996).

The Social Marketing Initiative (SMI) technique developed by the Center for Disease Control and Prevention (USA) represents an innovative example of the participatory approach. The initiative is based on community capacity to design sustainable HIV prevention programme using analytic case studies. Similarly, the Prevention Marketing Initiative (PMI) approach also developed by the CDC is actively engaged in involving, preparing and recruiting young people of the communities to effectively assist in HIV prevention efforts. Both initiatives recognize the fact that involving people in these approaches may be difficult yet, community participation must be ensured as it can enhance programme relevance, reach and credibility (Martin, et al., 1996).

Sehgal (1997) while describing ways to reduce the social and personal impact of the HIV infection observes that to reduce discrimination and marginalization of HIV positive/AIDS cases, family/community education and counselling services are necessary. Services of HIV positive individuals should be availed for peer group education. One of the finest examples of peer education and support system is provided by Self Help Therapy Groups formed by people living with HIV/AIDS in various countries, which are using self-help group techniques to give mutual support to each other. Similarly, Art Therapy Support Groups are trying to reinforce self-esteem of PWHA (Lelievre and Maison, 1996). The emergence of PWHA as a new social movement is significant as it reflects an increasing sense of bonding and unity among HIV positive people.

AIDS Europeer project is a collaborative venture working successfully in 14 European Union countries. It aims to provide HIV/AIDS knowledge through peer education process (Aids/europeer.htm). In India, Sonagachi project in Kolkatta qualifies as an exemplary peer education project that is running successfully among commercial sex workers of the Sonagachi slum area. Similarly, exemplary initiatives involving community participation are also exhibited by countries like Zimbabwe, Thailand and Kenya. In Zimbabwe, church groups are recruiting community members to visit AIDS orphans in their homes. The visitors know their communities well and pay weekly or fortnight visits to the neediest families, ensuring that carers and children get the material support such as clothing, blankets, school fees etc., as well as emotional support. Communities also contribute to activities such as farming communal fields and generating income to support the programme. Overall, the programme costs under US $ 10 per family supported, as against US$ 300-$500 a year for keeping an AIDS orphan in an orphanage. This community driven approach to support orphans is being reproduced all over Zimbabwe, Kenya, Malawi and Zambia (UNAIDS/WHO, Dec., 2000).

Similarly in Thailand, Home Based Care Model for supporting people living with HIV/AIDS is proving to be another success story. Teams of 2-3 community members visit homes of people living with or affected by AIDS and impart informal education on HIV/AIDS prevention and care (Guyer and Wooti, 1996). In Kenyan district, Thika, over a third of pregnant woman were found to be testing HIV positive. In response Ngethu, the district water processing plant's management has started training workers to educate their colleagues about HIV prevention and care. Kenya's government has also begun similar HIV prevention initiatives among workers in post offices, the national tax collection agency, the ports authority and the police force (UNAIDS/WHO, Dec., 2000).

In India, under National AIDS Control Organization's community care and support initiative, the first Community Care Center for PWHA was inaugurated in New Delhi on 6th April 2000. The center called Michael's care home is a collaborative effort by NACO and Sahara which houses HIV infected people with dignity and without stigmatization. The home makes efforts to train families to take care of their loved ones who are HIV positive, in an effective and supportive manner. Six similar projects are underway on a pilot basis (NACO, April, 2000).

Experience of various researchers has shown that reliance on energy, commitment and spirit of group members of various communities can be used to evolve an appropriate operational model for implementing a local initiative (Nowlan, et al., 1996)). Similarly, Chipo (1996) observed that community counselling could effectively help in facilitating the community to take the responsibility for change. Chipo, further states, "It is important to note the influence that change in one community can have in another community. The process is an indicator of behavioural change and sustainability".

Prostitute Outreach Workers project (POW) in UK justifies to be a role model representing sustainability of a programme. Launched in 1990, the research project shows that local women can create and sustain a community based STD/HIV/AIDS prevention programme (Gillies, et al., 1996). In the project, prostitute volunteers working in partnership with university colleagues were trained to assess local women's health needs. Using this data they designed a community outreach project that aimed at preventing other women from HIV.

Thus, what clearly emerges from such initiatives is the fact that since community participation can play a vital role in planning, implementing and sustaining HIV/AIDS prevention efforts; the same needs to be ensured for carrying out effective interventions.

Use of Information, Education and Communication (IEC) Material in Creating HIV/AIDS Awareness

IEC strategies are being extensively used in different ways across the globe to create HIV/AIDS awareness. The use of IEC material in the form of audio visual aids has been vitally helpful especially for people who are illiterate and can't be informed/educated by other means of IEC programmes such as written text in the form of brochures, booklets, pamphlets etc. For such communities, interpersonal communication channels such as talk shows, group discussions and street plays have proved to be best suited.

Various studies focusing on the development of IEC techniques show that the consideration of cultural background of the community, the message content, the type of media used for disseminating information and the theme conveyed by the IEC material have a large impact and direct relevance on the success of HIV/AIDS prevention efforts.

Mahler and Flanagan (1996) while reviewing contents of AIDS Community Action Programme (AIDSCAP), materials and messages stressed that instead of using fear-based prevention messages, programmes should emphasize on concrete action steps that can be taken to avoid negative consequences of HIV/AIDS. Similarly, Carneiro et al. (1996) state, "When a campaign uses positive approach connecting AIDS prevention to life and pleasure, individuals can engage more effectively in the practices the message proposes."

A study tapping the effectiveness of HIV prevention messages among women at high risk of HIV showed that messages using collectivist prevention themes (e.g., protect loved ones, avoid infecting a loved one/ family/friend) were far more effective in persuading women to use safe sexual practices then individualistic themes such as protect self and avoid death (Miller, et al., 1996).

Building on cost-effective theoretically based behavioural interventions and making them more relevant and culturally appropriate has been stressed by Jemmott (1996). Similarly, Castillo and Moreno (1996) have opined that HIV prevention services should be disseminated in an intelligible manner, which is sensitive to the personal and cultural needs of the clients. They further observe, "The use of culture, tradition and folklore to spread the information has been quiet helpful, especially when it comes to illiterates or people who can't read. To educate the population of rural areas it is necessary to communicate in their own terms."

Similarly, the need to emphasize on community cultural roots while planning HIV prevention campaigns has also been stressed in various studies (Fernandez, et al., 1996). The development of audio-visual aids based on a cultural model gives an explanation of the roots of attitudes and behaviours held by a community. Such models can also offer a range of directions targeting behavioural change (Paula, 1996).

Wide participation in programme development has been identified as the key to awareness and change in attitudes. Koo and Tang (1996) recruited community leaders to produce a poster involving a photo session of high profile individuals from a community along with a pamphlet on "Being gay and Asian". Similarly, studies have shown that AIDS awareness messages including personal testimonies are very effective in targeting high-risk populations (Grinard and Cato, 1996).

Innovative techniques such as provocative theatre and the use of fictional stories are being used to effectively reach the hard-to-reach groups. Provocative theatre was introduced in 1993, in the Dominican Republic. It allows the audience to play an active role in constructing solutions to problems encountered in their daily lives. This technique also allows the project educators to adapt their performance according to audience's spontaneous reactions and needs and provides them with useful information about the audience's level of knowledge, beliefs and attitudes about HIV/AIDS (Castillo and Moreno, 1996). Almeida et al. (1996) while emphasizing the need of theatre state, "Information and education activities aimed at HIV/AIDS prevention are not enough to provide incentive for behavioural change. Cultural activities such as theatre workshops can play an extremely important role in stimulating community attachment, affirming the value of safe sexual practices and providing a context for a positive collective response to the HIV/AIDS epidemic."

The role of fiction in supporting identification and social interaction has also proved to be an effective technique in imparting HIV awareness. A study in France showed that personal involvement and discussion on sexuality were more likely to be triggered when public campaigns were based on short film fictions and life stories presenting a diversity of everyday situation rather than directive messages (Rudelic-Fernandez, et al., 1996).

In the Indian context, the exponentially growing number of HIV infections across the nation compounded with low literacy rate demand an urgency of IEC implementation on a massive scale. According to Sehgal (1997) "IEC campaigns need to be intensified to increase knowledge and change attitudes so as to create behavioural changes that will prevent the spread of HIV/AIDS and STD."

Apart from assessing knowledge, beliefs and risk behaviours of the communities being studied, the factors associated with these risks behaviours also need to be thoroughly understood to design an effective IEC intervention. Whitt (cited in Mathai, et al., 1997) states, "Only recently have studies indicated that knowledge alone is insufficient. Also crucial are the attitudes and motivational factors which influence propensities to engage in risk behaviour, perceptions of personal vulnerability, behavioural intentions, competence to negotiate social situations and skills to implement prevention behaviours".

Besides, user-friendly documentation of audio-visual aids is a vital component that is required for their wider acceptance. An innovative IEC approach resulting in wide community acceptance has been tried by the Department of Preventive and Social Medicine, UCMS, Delhi. UCMS organized a AIDS Health Mela on 1st Dec., 1996 in Delhi. A large population especially from resettlement colonies visited the mela. Around 5000 people were estimated to have visited the mela in a short span of 7 hours. Apart from recreational facilities such as elephant ride, giant wheel, food counters etc., 21 stalls by different NGOs provided HIV/AIDS information and education to the people. (Aggarwal and Sharma, 1997).

Limited Success of HIV Prevention Programmes

Efforts of massive magnitude are being continuously put into HIV/AIDS prevention and care programmes and many have become success stories worldwide, in terms of their contribution in arresting the spread of HIV. Yet, some programmes have had limited success in containing the HIV epidemic. An understanding of the factors leading to partial success of HIV/AIDS prevention and care programmes can help in the reformulation of programmes that guarantee maximum impact and nearly 100 per cent success.

Ignorance, illiteracy, customs, attitudes and lack of both human and financial resources have been recognized as major factors responsible for the limited success of many programmes. Several constraints in implementing educational programmes effectively, which include the absence of standardized sex education programmes for the youth, the cultural stereotypes about gender appropriate sexual behaviour, the identification of indigenous skills in this area and the paucity of trained sex education experts have been identified (Mane and Maitra cited in Mathai, et al., 1997). Similarly, studies evaluating the role of AIDS awareness campaigns have concluded that many public service announcements (PSAs) have been ineffectual in addressing the needs of high-risk populations (Wolf and Dejong, 1996). The PSAs need to craft individual messages that address not only the needs of heterosexuals but also cater to the needs of homosexuals and bisexuals.

Extensive studies are increasingly showing that it is important to understand the behavioural epidemiology of HIV transmission within the social and cultural context. "Ignoring these complexities has resulted in the development of simplistic interventions which have not been effective in bringing about behavioural change" (Pachauri cited in Mathai, et al., 1997).

An evaluation study of IEC material prepared by NACO revealed that although 1/3rd of the NACO's budget is spent in developing IEC material yet, there are some major issues that need to be readdressed (Malhotra, 1996). The study in it's critical review of the IEC material developed by NACO showed that messages:

(a) are informative but do not address issues like AIDS and workplace and non-discrimination.
(b) cater only to literates.
(c) are ambiguous and rarely pre-tested.
(d) and, women are sidelined.

Similarly, Bharat (1996) in her study found that HIV/AIDS awareness advertisements were both a source of information as well as confusion. The study revealed that there was no way people could correct their misconceptions or seek clarifications. Community level efforts and visibility of NGOs were also found to be quiet poor in many communities. Thus, HIV prevention efforts based on interpersonal communication need to be evolved and implemented more vigorously to dispel the myths and misconceptions of communities.

Another hindrance making HIV/AIDS prevention and care efforts ineffectual is the total reliance on informational interventions. Studies have found that theoretical interventions integrating risk information along with motivation and prevention skills are more successful in changing high-risk behaviours than mere informational campaigns (DeWit, 1996). Equipping people with practical skills to implement their new knowledge is crucial for the success of HIV prevention programmes. Toppich et al. (1996) while describing efficacy factors of prevention strategies state, "The promotion and support of protective intentions and skills is essential".

Lack of sustainability is the biggest hurdle eluding success from HIV/AIDS prevention and care efforts. Effective management, monitoring and evaluation of the project along with skill building in the community can easily sustain prevention efforts. Further, understanding the value framework and the belief system of people of different social groups and their participation in all the initiatives of HIV/AIDS prevention and control can surely enhance programme effectiveness and its credibility. To summarize, building cost-effective, replicable and sustainable prevention programmes can go a long way in helping combat the HIV.

To conclude, prevention of the global community from HIV/AIDS has become an important research area. The epidemic is the underlying cause for reversal of hard earned progress on growth and development indicators. The devastation inflicted by the disease in terms of early and painful deaths, increasing number of orphans and depletion of human as well as material resources have all necessitated the compulsion of putting the virus under immediate control. Today prevention from HIV/AIDS has become our prime necessity. Further, few populations such as those of commercial sex workers, truck drivers, migrant workers, street children and injecting drug users are increasingly being recognized to be vulnerable to the disease because of their indulgence in high-risk behaviour and practices. To protect these populations from HIV/AIDS is a challenging yet, an urgently needed task since these groups are serving as bridges for HIV transmission from the high-risk behaviour populations to the general population.

India is known to have around 5.1 million HIV infected people (NACO, 2004), the second largest in the world (Shreedhar, 2002). Statistics continue to confirm that this number is rapidly growing and if preventive measures are not implemented at the earliest then the situation is very likely to become explosive. Thus, many programmes for the common masses as well as targeted interventions for the vulnerable groups are being implemented across the country with the aim of creating HIV/AIDS awareness amongst them. Similarly, efforts are underway to provide appropriate care and management for HIV/AIDS infected people. The ultimate goal is to prevent new infections from taking place while at the same time ensuring care for the infected ones. It is now being realized that prevention is possible only if people are aware about the disease as well as important aspects related to it.

Awareness for sure holds the key to success in containing the spread of the epidemic. People who are aware/educated are known to adopt measures to protect themselves from the virus as compared to those who are unaware about the disease (UNAIDS/WHO, June, 1998). Hence, their lies an urgent need to create awareness among the masses especially those who face increased vulnerability to the disease. Unfortunately in India, the task of creating AIDS awareness is complicated by various factors such as illiteracy (34.6 per cent - Census of India 2001), socio-cultural taboos and restrictions, adherence to gender inequalities as a norm as well as economic compulsions to name a few. Ironically, prevention from HIV/AIDS cannot take place in isolation. There is a need to review these factors while planning any intervention. Similarly, there also lies an equal necessity to base interventions on the needs of the communities as well as to ensure community participation for achieving sustainability in them. The coverage of the interventions also needs to be expanded to access the hard-to-reach groups whose number is phenomenally increasing.

2

Methodology

The study was conducted in Delhi among the commercial sex workers (CSWs), truck drivers and rickshaw pullers to assess their knowledge, attitudes, myths, misconceptions, behaviour and practices regarding HIV/AIDS. They have been identified as vulnerable groups to HIV by NACO due to their indulgence in high-risk behaviour. Studies continue to emphasize that the most effective and cost-efficient way to cause behavioural change is to target specific subgroups that have particular risks, existing affinities, indigenous communication channels and their own leadership structures (Velyvis, et al., 1996). The present study was undertaken with the goal of creating HIV/AIDS awareness amongst the sample communities. This chapter covers the sample selection, locale, variables and the study design inclusive of a few case studies.

The study was designed as a small-scale intervention and was conducted in three distinct but related phases, which have been briefly outlined in Fig. 2.1.

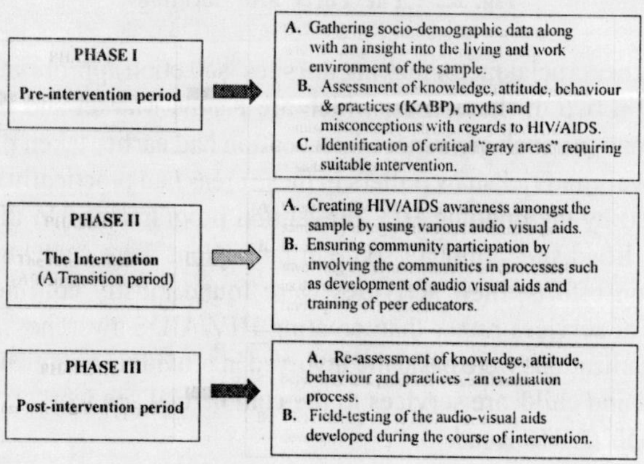

Fig. 2.1 : Conceptual Framework of the Study.

These phases have been elaborately discussed in the later part of this chapter.

Locale

The study was conducted in three areas of the National Capital Territory (NCT) of Delhi. These areas were selected on the basis of high concentration of commercial sex workers, truck drivers and rickshaw pullers found dwelling/floating here. The three site locations are shown in Fig. 2.2.

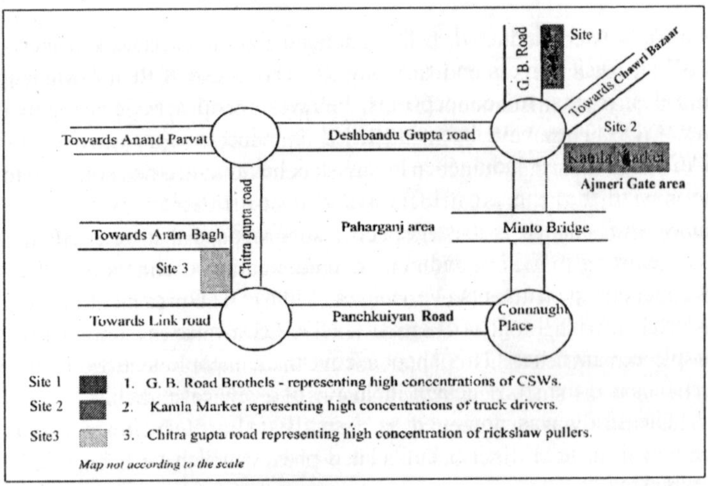

Fig. 2.2 : The Three Site Locations.

Another crucial factor making the sites' selection appropriate was the fact that in two of these sites, which are Kamla Market and the Chitra Gupta Road, no such awareness intervention had earlier taken place. The truck drivers and rickshaw pullers in these areas had practically remained untouched by the ongoing HIV prevention programmes. In the case of the G.B. Road site, although some organizations were carrying on HIV prevention efforts, their activities were found mostly confined to the delivery of services rather than creating HIV/AIDS awareness. Most of these organizations were basically involved in providing treatment of STD, condoms and childcare services to the commercial sex workers living in the brothels at G.B. Road.

Further, various studies continue to reveal the lack of HIV/AIDS awareness among the commercial sex workers over here and also stress on the need to expand HIV prevention efforts in this area (Ahmad, 1997; Khan & Sharma, 1997). A pilot study conducted in these three sites confirmed significantly low levels of HIV/AIDS awareness among the commercial sex workers, truck drivers and rickshaw pullers in these areas. Exploratory Nature of the Study - To begin with, no clear cut hypothesis or assumptions were made except recognition of the fact that the three sample communities have been identified by NACO (2003) to be at high-risk of acquiring and transmitting the HIV by virtue of their occupation (CSWs) as well as mobility and migration (truck drivers and rickshaw pullers). Thus, the study was designed to be exploratory in nature aiming to delve into various factors that were predisposing the sample to HIV/AIDS vulnerability with the aim of curbing the same. To achieve this, an assessment of the sample's knowledge, attitude, behaviour and practices and also an insight into the several myths and misconceptions held by them were looked into. The ultimate goal was to understand all the predisposing factors so that suitable control (intervention) for HIV/AIDS could be worked out.

The impact of the intervention carried out during the study was appraised using a null hypothesis stating that, "There is no change in knowledge, attitude, behaviour and practices of the sample due to the intervention."

Selection of the Sample

The study sample consisted of the commercial sex workers, truck drivers and rickshaw pullers. The sample was selected on the basis of the operational definitions conceptualized for the purpose of the study, which are as follows:

1. **Commercial sex workers.** Women living in the brothels of the G.B. Road and practicing sex work as a means to earn their livelihood. These women offer sex related services to their customers/clients.
2. **Truck drivers.** Interstate truckers plying on national highways and transacting (i.e., taking or delivering goods) at transport agencies in the Kamla Market area. The long interstate trips necessitate their staying away from homes. Moving goods from one state to another is their job.
3. **Rickshaw pullers.** Rickshaw pullers are primarily the migrant population who provide short distance mobility to commuters, usually near railway stations and market places. These migrants stay away from their families because of their work requirements.

The above mentioned three categories of the sample were selected on the basis of the updates by NACO which confirmed the vulnerability of commercial sex workers, truck drivers and rickshaw pullers because of their high-risk behaviour practices (NACO, 1996-2003). The choice of these three sample groups was also influenced by the fact that the research aimed at studying different types of communities on the basis of the specialized services provided by them. The commercial sex workers who render sexual services, the truck drivers who move goods from one state to another and the rickshaw pullers who provide cheap transport in congested locations, thus formed the three important communities for the above study. This type of study was considered to be more effective in the sense that inter-group problems of these communities that increased their vulnerability to HIV/AIDS could be studied realistically for a meaningful intervention. A pilot study showed that whereas the truckers and rickshaw pullers needed to be motivated to use condoms for safe sex, the sex workers were to be motivated to persuade their clients to use condoms when they visit brothels to experience sex.

Sample Size

Thirty subjects were chosen from each of the three communities as representative sample. These comprised of commercial sex workers, truck drivers and rickshaw pullers, the total final sample size being 90. A conscious effort was made to select equal number of respondents from each community to ensure equal representation of the three different sample groups. The sample size was limited to 30 subjects from each of the three communities keeping in mind the intimate and in-depth nature of the study. Efforts were focused on gathering relevant real life data depicting the true nature of the problem in a free atmosphere without any coercion. A few case studies were also conducted to have an in-depth insight into their life styles. The emphasis therefore was on building rapport, a confidence generating measure. It meant generous play of time without transacting any actual business but to build a relationship of friendship and trust.

The sample represented a cross section of the population with inherent attributes like age, sex, education, marital status, number of children, occupation, income and religion.

Sampling Strategy

The two communities comprising of the truck drivers and rickshaw pullers were approached purely on the basis of personal search and contact as there was no local NGO working with these groups at the time of the study. The truck drivers were contacted at their transport agencies in the

Kamla Market area, and the rickshaw pullers were contacted at the Chitra Gupta Road pavement area where they invariably throng.

The real challenge was faced in contacting the commercial sex workers in the brothels at the G.B Road, who were not interested to talk to the researcher. They feared that their profession would be jeopardized. The researcher's request during the initial visits made to these brothels, to contact commercial sex workers was turned down by the madams/pimps operating these brothels who gave some lame excuses. It was decided that initially it would be better to go through a local NGO operating a day care center nearby. The children of the sex workers were found to be attending this center. The NGO was subsequently approached and requested to facilitate entry of the researcher to these brothels purely for academic and social purposes.

The NGO too did not approve the idea of a research being conducted by an outsider in their premises and the request was subsequently rejected. The probable reasons for not allowing the research to be conducted in their center have been discussed in the chapter on Results and Discussion.

Lastly, efforts were made to contact some volunteers working for various social issues in the area. Two such volunteers came forward to help the researcher based on a mutual understanding. They enabled researcher's access to the brothels and the commercial sex workers; in turn the researcher was expected to help them impart non-formal education as well as in their campaign to bring some desirable changes among the sex workers. In brief, the researcher was seen as human resource, a channel for their ongoing activities. A doctor working in a nearby government clinic also joined in for furthering the cause. The researcher accompanied the doctor to the brothels to carry out the research, as planned. Thus, the initial resistance to enter these brothels was overcome with the help of these personnel. A few earlier visits were crucial for establishing rapport and gaining confidence of the community. Canvassing along with the team of Pulse Polio programme was also helpful in confidence building.

Soon the process of sample selection was started. The owners/madams operating two of the brothels were the first ones to be contacted, to gain a talking access to the sex workers. Sustained efforts went into convincing these owners/madams and the sex workers that the goal of the study was to help prevent the onset of HIV – the deadly infection. Most of them had to be constantly motivated and convinced to become a part of this prevention effort. Confidentiality was assured in all respects along with a genuine desire to fight the HIV/AIDS menace. Gradually, people showed eagerness to be a part of the ongoing research.

The communities of truck drivers and rickshaw pullers were also approached in a similar manner. The initial visits were utilized for steadily gaining confidence of these communities. Carrying out a few good-will gestures also formed a part of trust-building measures. For instance, talking to a local police constable who in spite of taking "*Hafta*" (i.e., weekly monetary favour) from the rickshaw pullers sometimes indulged in excesses towards them helped in bringing about a desirable shift in the attitude of this constable towards the pullers. This effort was crucial in winning over the trust of the rickshaw pullers. The concept of AIDS was deliberately not introduced in the earlier few visits, as it was seen as an encroachment to their privacy.

It was observed that most of the truck drivers and rickshaw pullers were eager to join the stir. There was a noticeable difference between these members and the sex workers; the former being more open to suggestions than the latter. Initially, there was some resistance from the owners of transport agencies in case of the truckers and the owners of rickshaws, as they feared waste of time and a threat to their meager survival. With the passage of time the resistance grew weaker and conviction grew stronger because of the social implications of HIV infection.

Since the study entailed information on the personal and intimate front, it was crucial to include as sample, only those who showed willingness and interest in the study. This was so essential to facilitate an open dialogue among participants. This kind of purposive sampling has been effectively used by various researchers for enrolling participants in various studies (Bharat, 1997; Warren, 1996; Kutikuppala, et al., 1996).

According to Jahoda et al. (1955) "The basic assumption behind purposive sampling is that with good judgment and an appropriate strategy one can select the cases to be included in the sample and thus develop samples that are satisfactory in relation to one's needs". In purposive sampling technique, a sample may be expressly chosen because in the light of available evidence, it mirrors some larger group with reference to a given characteristic.

Research Design

Keeping in mind the unanimous agreement that no single research method can take care of all aspects of an issue and that the best research design should include elements from both the cross sectional and longitudinal strategies (Clarke & Stewart, 1987) the present study is based on a "cohort sequential design" combining both cross sectional and longitudinal strategies. Different groups of people of different ages (cross sectional strategy) were studied over a reasonable period of time (longitudinal strategy) during the pre-and post-intervention periods, which altogether stretched for a time period of approximately 24 months for each community. This period was considered long enough for a transient nature of the sample.

The word "cohort" as used by Bee (1995) describes groups of individuals born within some fairly narrow band of years, who share the same cultural/historical experiences at the same time in their lives. Thus, the three categories of the sample may be classified as three cohorts since within each group (i.e., the CSWs, truck drivers and rickshaw pullers) individuals were fairly closer in age and shared the same cultural experiences.

Variables

The three different groups that comprised the sample formed the major independent variables with several intervening ones such as the social, cultural and economic factors. The dependent variables comprised of the awareness level, the myths and misconceptions relating to AIDS, the living and work environment and aspects related to health care of the three sample groups. The communication material developed during the course of study also formed a part of the dependent variable because of the inter-group needs/differences.

The time period for the study spanned between April 1998 till early 2004.

Tools for Data Collection

The research design employed both qualitative as well as quantitative techniques for data collection and analysis. Collecting accurate behavioural data has been recognized as the foundation of any AIDS prevention activity. Thus, many researchers are utilizing a variety of techniques to improve the accuracy of reported behavioural data.

Studies reveal that large-scale researches that rely solely on quantitative methods are often unable to detect the true effects of community level programme. "Scientific rigou is an important study design consideration but strict experimental designs have often shown disappointing results."(Westover, et al., 1996). It has been further suggested that assessing the impact of community level HIV prevention programmes requires the use of multiple methods comprising both qualitative and quantitative assessment.

Qualitative research methods such as focus group discussions, observations and key informant interviews have been extensively used by NACO to conduct HIV intervention studies in 65 Indian states (Sethi & Lal, 1996). Similarly, the AIDS risk reduction model developed by Shain et al. (1996) is based on qualitative data that assesses beliefs, values and existing behaviour of the population.

The present study too relied on a multi-pronged strategy to generate both qualitative and quantitative data. Qualitative techniques such as in-depth interviews, focus group discussions, participatory observations and case studies were used to collect comprehensive data. Knowledge, attitude, behaviour and practices of the sample, in short designated as "KABP" formed the core substance of the research. These tools have been described as follows:

1. Interview Schedules

Interview schedules were personally administered to study the sample demographics, socio-economic conditions and the KABP. Needless to say all information was relating to HIV/AIDS including myths and misconceptions shrouding the disease. Interviewing technique has been actively used to probe needs, ideas, thoughts and abilities of the subjects. Various researchers have deployed interviewing methodology to elicit information from respondents regarding sample demographics, behavioural patterns, history of STD, extra-marital sex and knowledge about HIV/AIDS (Bhave, et al., 1997; Pandey, et al., 1997; Manson, et al., 1996). Similarly, unstructured/semi-structured in-depth interviews have been conducted for mapping KABP of the subjects regarding HIV/AIDS (Halloran, et al., 1996).

In the present study the selection of interview schedules as a tool for data collection is justified by the fact that majority of the sample was found to be illiterate. The use of interview method allowed face-to-face interaction with the sample, building trust and emotional dialogue. The interview schedules were open-ended and hence amenable to free flow of information sharing. The atmosphere was made very friendly making room for clarifying and asking by the sample rather than passing on information, which is one-sided.

Three group specific interview schedules (Appendix I, II and III) were designed to elicit in-depth details about each sample group namely the commercial sex workers, truck drivers and rickshaw pullers. A separate interview format was used for each of the three groups due to the inherent differences in their work environment and life style. The common focus however remained on their vulnerability to HIV and its manifestations. The predisposing factors were keenly noted in each of the cases. Beside, the interview schedules which were common to all addressed specific information regarding sample's indulgence in pre/extra-marital sex (Appendix IV), assessment of physical/substance abuse patterns among the study groups (Appendix V), media exposure of the sample to find out the extent of accessibility and exposure to HIV/AIDS information (Appendix VI), and other information relating to STD (Appendix VII).

2. Focus Group Discussions

Focus group discussions form an important part of majority of HIV interventions. The basic idea of focus group discussions grew from the works of a sociologist - Robert Merton in 1956. The process has been described as "a method of getting information from a group of persons (usually 4 to 8 individuals) who have a common background and are brought together to discuss a particular topic of interest" (NACO, March, 1994). A deep reflection on quantitative assessment of knowledge and attitudes of participants can be evinced from focus group discussions (Warren, 1996).

This method of discussion is very helpful for issues like sex and sexuality (Warren, 1996), relationships and cultural/sexual orientation (Manson, et al., 1996). Various studies have applied focus group discussions to gather behavioural data (Koester, et al., 1996; Julia & Baume, 1996) and also as an effective HIV intervention strategy (Bhave, et al., 1997). Most importantly focus group discussions have proved to be an effective tool for behavioural change (Paula, 1996).

In the present study, focus group discussions were used as an effective communication tool to gather in-depth data regarding behaviour and practices of the sample groups. Their perceptions of personal vulnerability to HIV as well as factors impeding/promoting behavioural change were thoroughly studied with the help of these discussions. Social, cultural and psychological frameworks that explained patterns as well as tendencies to indulge in risky behaviour guided the discussions.

The focus group discussions in the study addressed the following issues/items:

- The needs of the target groups.
- Strategies for disseminating HIV/AIDS information.
- To help in skill building in the areas of self-care and HIV prevention.
- Training peer educators for creating further awareness regarding HIV prevention.

These discussions also paved the way for creation of culturally appropriate educational audio-visual aids for creating HIV/AIDS awareness.

3. Participant Observations

Real lives, typical activities and normal encounters of the sample groups were studied in their natural surroundings through participant observation method. The participant observation method helped greatly in data collection and also in bridging the gap between reported behaviour and actual behaviour. For example, many commercial sex workers reported that they knew and were practicing the right method of disposing the used condoms. This was verified by observing the condom disposal locations in the brothels.

The role of participant observation as a prominent tool in revealing actual behaviour/practices of the sample under study has been justified by various studies. According to Clarke & Stewart (1987) it is unlikely that people can or will disguise completely their usual ways of behaving just to put on a good show for the observer. Stratford & Ellerbrock (1996) have used participant observation to gather in-depth information about the full range and contexts of HIV related risk and protective behaviours used by men and women in different ethnic occupational groups. Similarly, the technique has been used to identify high-risk behaviours such as syringe sharing and injecting practices that place IDUs at risk of HIV (Koester, et al., 1996). Participant observation in conjunction with other techniques has also been used to develop a cultural model for behavioural change (Paula, 1996).

In the present research, participant observation methodology helped in focusing on the immediate environment of the sample groups and in determining its effect on their lives and behaviour. The process facilitated the study of the groups in great depth and to unearth the basic thought processes involved. A wide spectrum of components including verbal and non-verbal behaviour, peer relationships, child-care practices, norms and beliefs were observed through participant observation methodology.

Efforts were made by the researcher to record observations systematically and objectively, without projecting personal point of view or attitudes onto the sample. Inferences based on observations were kept to a minimum and for the ones that were made, due care was taken to confirm them with the sample through interviews/focus group discussions.

4. Case Studies

A few case studies have been conducted to have an insight into the real world of a few selected sample. The aim was to reach to the core of the matter for true understanding of the problems that underlie the issue of HIV vulnerability. Various researchers have used the case study method to increase an understanding of how community-based HIV prevention initiatives can be developed (Pinkney, et al., 1996). Further, this method has also been successfully used as a documentation process to quantify behavioural change (Martin, 1996).

In the present research too, case studies while highlighting the HIV vulnerability factors also documented the impact of the intervention on the sample by way of desirable changes.

Quantitative Techniques

Different researchers have used different tools/scales to assess components such as knowledge, attitudes, myths and misconceptions, norms, beliefs and behavioural practices regarding HIV/AIDS among different communities worldwide.

Large scale global variations in areas such as education, economic conditions, socio-cultural patterns, psychological frameworks and most importantly behavioural practices have hindered the standardization of knowledge, attitude, behaviour and practices (KABP) assessment scales which could be universally applied to all individuals of specific communities. For instance, AIDS awareness scales measuring components such as 'Patient Activism' (i.e., role of patients in making health care decisions), 'Patient Assertiveness' in health care interactions and potential for mindful non-adherence (Brashers, et al., 1996) are quite advanced measures and may not be applicable as valid assessment tools for majority of masses in a developing country like India because of high levels of illiteracy and lack of HIV/AIDS awareness.

Various researchers have stressed on the need to have HIV/AIDS intervention tools/techniques/scales that are designed on the basis of need assessment of the target group (Muncy, et al., 1996; Maticka, et al., 1996). Initial KABP surveys in specific sites and communities have given a baseline in doing various studies (Benjamin, 1996; Kagimu, et al., 1996). Martin et al. (1996) while describing strategies for actively involving youth in HIV prevention efforts have emphasized on the consideration of their developmental levels while evolving prevention strategies.

The general consensus that emerges from various studies is that tools/scales used to assess KABP should be largely based on the needs and background of the sample and that no rigid rules have been laid for designing these scales. For instance, a knowledge scale developed to assess knowledge regarding HIV/AIDS of school/college going students may not be suitable for assessing similar knowledge in the case of truck drivers or rickshaw pullers. Hence, the need to design and use tools and techniques that are based on the needs of the sample was fully justified.

In the present study the scales used to measure KABP of the sample were developed on the basis of a pilot study that gave an insight into the particular socio-cultural contexts and developmental needs. Additionally, scales developed by NACO (2001), Tikoo et al. (1997) and Wadhwa et al. (1997) were used for reference purposes. Each subject was separately assessed on these scales to avoid any reporting bias that could set in due to peer influence in case of group assessments. The assessment scales used in the study were jointly called as the "KABP scale" and are described as follows:

(i) Knowledge Assessment Scale

Knowledge assessment scales have been widely used to assess knowledge level of samples regarding HIV/AIDS as also to measure their reproductive knowledge (Tikoo, et al., 1997). Knowledge levels have been effectively quantified based on the use of the knowledge assessment scales in various studies (Campos, et al., 1996; Gray, et al., 1996).

The knowledge assessment scale (Appendix VIII) in the present study was developed to measure knowledge of the sample on HIV/AIDS, its etiology, transmission routes, serological aspects and methods of prevention. The items in the scale had both closed as well as open-ended questions. Each subject was first asked a simple question, i.e., "Have you heard anything about AIDS?" Only those who replied in affirmative were asked further questions on this scale. A score of one was awarded for every correct answer and for incorrect or no answers, a score of zero was given.

(ii) Attitude Assessment Scale

Various studies have emphasized the fact that in order to reduce discrimination and marginalization of people living with or affected by AIDS a radical change in attitudes of people is urgently needed (Sehgal & Singh, 1997; Dodds & Braidele, 1996). Therefore, attitudes of people towards HIV/AIDS have been assessed as being positive if they promote social support or being negative if they contribute to social stigma (Ruiz, et al., 1996; Campos, et al., 1996; Gray, et al., 1996).

In the present study the subjects' attitudes towards sex and sexuality, homosexuality, premarital, extra-marital relationships and gender related differences were studied on attitude assessment scale (Appendix IX). The scale also assessed values of the respondents and their attitude towards people living with HIV/AIDS (PWHA). Attitudes promoting social stigma and high-risk behaviour were rated as negative and the vice-versa.

(iii) Behaviour and Practices Assessment Scale

Behavioural change approaches are being vigorously pursued by majority of HIV prevention efforts. All of these emphasize on the importance of changing risk behaviours. Extensive studies have been carried out for mapping high-risk behaviours and practices with the goal of modifying them into safe behaviours. Studies assessing behaviours and practices such as practicing unprotected sexual behaviour including anal, oral and homosexual acts, indulging in premarital/extramarital sex and sharing of needles and syringes by injecting drug users have been taken up by various researchers (Mc Clure, et al., 1996; Bullock, et al., 1996; Shanmuganandan & Maniyosai, 1996).

Similarly behaviours and practices related to condom use are being extensively studied to have an in-depth knowledge about barriers to safe sex. Various researchers have examined issues such as why condoms are not used, the inability of people to negotiate condom use (Wolf & Cameron, 1996) and why people have negative attitude to condom use (Rosensvard & Campbell, 1996).

Commonly practiced behaviours and practices need to be assessed in order to bring about the desired changes. Condom use behaviour has been quantitatively assessed by various researchers through assessment scales based on numerical values (Fisherbein & Johnson, 1996; Ruiz, et al., 1996). Fisherbein & Johnson (1996) measured condom use behaviour on a five-point scale in which point 1 showed no intention to use a condom whereas point 5 showed consistent condom use for more than six months.

In the present study, patterns related to condom usage during sexual transactions as well as the general practices such as sharing of needles, blades and razors etc. as carried out by the respondents were assessed on the condom usage behaviour and practices assessment scale (Appendix X). Condom usage behaviour and practices were assessed on a single scale due to the fact that it is usually difficult to differentiate between behaviour and practices of an individual as the two seem to overlap each other. For instance, the practice of having unsafe sex at times by an individual can also be treated as non-consistent condom usage behaviour.

Similarly, the practice of sharing blades and razors can also be treated as conducting of unsafe behaviour. Thus, the line of demarcation between behaviour and practices at times is practically non-existent. Hence, condom usage behaviour and practices were assessed on the same scale.

The condom usage behaviour assessment consisted of 18 items found to be significant in indicating the condom use behaviour. Some items on the scale were further sub-categorized denoting various degrees of indulgence in certain behaviours. For instance, an individual's response regarding frequency of condom use with a commercial sex worker may range anywhere between "always, most of the times, sometimes or never."

Scoring – Pattern

Like a rating scale, higher scores were given for desirable behaviour and its consistency. For example, a score of 3 was given to a person who reported "always" for using a condom with a commercial sex worker, a score of 2 was given to a person who reported condom use "most of the times" but not always. A score of 1 was given to a person who reported the use of condom only "sometimes" and zero to those who reported having "never" used a condom with a sex worker. This question was addressed to both the sex workers and the sample who visited the brothels for sex gratification.

For assessing practices such as sharing of blades, razors, needles and syringes and indulging in premarital, extra-marital and homosexual relationships percentages were computed to quantify such data. Practices were not marked for scoring purposes due to the fact that most of the practices were descriptive in nature and could not be marked objectively. For example, the practice of having different types of sexual partners, the criteria for choosing different sexual partners and the different types of sexual practices that the sample indulged in, could be better explained in a descriptive manner rather than scoring these aspects in the form of numerical values.

The KABP scale developed for the study was critically evaluated by two experts* working with NACO, the apex body dealing with HIV/AIDS awareness generation. To ensure the validity of the scale these experts were requested to comment on the content of the statements and also the appropriateness of the response system. Necessary modifications were incorporated based on their suggestions prior to the use of this scale. The final scale was administered to six respondents, two from each of the three groups and the validity was determined through a pilot study.

---

* Dr. P. Salil (Joint Director) and Mr. Ninan Verghese CIEC (Consultant).

To test the reliability of the scale, test-retest method was used. Twelve respondents were administered the test on the scale; and retest on the same scale was administered after twenty days. The reliability was assessed using Karl Pearson's formula. The coefficient of the correlation was found to be .72, which shows that the scale was reliable to be used with the sample groups for eliciting their responses towards HIV/AIDS related aspects.

Pre-Testing of Tools /Techniques

Interview schedules and KABP assessment scale developed for the purpose of data collection were pre-tested on a sample of fifteen individuals (five subjects from each community under study) who were not included in the final sample. Modifications were made with regards to specificity of certain questions. Appropriate improvisations including restructuring of certain words as well as rephrasing of a few questions according to the socio-cultural and educational background of the sample were incorporated. For instance, the word HIV was replaced by the phrase *"Ek prakaar ka rogaanu"* meaning "a type of foreign body" for some individuals who were not able to comprehend the word HIV during the interview sessions. It was further observed that the time taken for rapport formation varied from one individual to another. Aspects related to personal and intimate behaviour were taken up only after gaining trust and confidence of the sample.

Methods of Data Collection

The data was collected in the natural surroundings of the sample with the aim of documenting their real lives in an unobtrusive manner. The interviews were conducted in the G.B. Road brothels, in the transport agencies located in Ajmeri Gate area and on the Chitra Gupta Road pavement for the sex workers, truckers and rickshaw pullers respectively. The visiting hours were as per the sample's convenience and accessibility. The periods when the subjects were not working were fully utilized for interviewing so as to get the needed time and space with the sample. Many visits were purposely scheduled during early morning and late evening hours (some extending till 9:00 p.m.) with the aim of capturing the real lives of the sample. Early morning visits were quite helpful in depicting how the truck drivers and rickshaw pullers were managing their day-to-day lives in the absence of basic amenities. Similarly, late evening visits were immensely helpful in portraying the living and work environment and the values of the CSWs. It was quite intriguing to see CSWs burning some stringent smelling substance (believed to possess magical powers) every evening. This ritual was practiced with the aim of attracting customers of another brothel to their own.

Interviews were conducted in small group settings during the initial visits to gather data regarding socio-economic demographics of the sample. During these interviews the investigator was careful not to dress or converse in a manner that could create social or economic distance between the researcher and the respondents. The interviews were conducted in Hindi in accordance with the local dialect of the sample. There was more of listening than talking.

In-depth information regarding personal lives and sexual behaviour was gradually accessed through sensitively crafted interviews conducted on one-to-one basis. Personal identifiers such as name and address were not insisted upon. The individual interviews in the case of rickshaw pullers were conducted in one of the vacant rickshaws/auto-rickshaws parked nearby. Similarly, truck drivers were usually interviewed either outside their travel agencies sitting near their trucks or at a tea stall nearby where most of them used to spend their time chatting and drinking tea with each other. Sharing a cup of tea with them became a routine activity.

Commercial sex workers were interviewed in their brothels and also at the stairs of the brothels where they used to sit and wait for their clients. The use of paper and pencil to record responses related to intimate behaviour was kept to a minimum. To avoid reporting biases on part of the sample, questions were worded in a manner that took into consideration the difficult situations faced by the study participants. For example, instead of asking CSWs a question like "Do you practice unprotected sex with your clients?", to which a majority of them would have said "No", they were asked "Are their times when your clients do not agree with your safe sex negotiations/proposals?" Questions like this helped the sample to realize that there was nothing wrong in admitting to the practice of having unprotected sex. Efforts were made to neither condemn nor condone samples' behaviour but to record it as reported.

The three different communities were studied simultaneously as this helped in the cross verification of data. For instance "all time availability of condoms to clients" was reported by CSWs to the researcher. This was verified from the truck drivers and rickshaw pullers who visited these brothels. More importantly certain improvisations in knowledge and attitudes of the respondents could be made as a result of these cross verifications. These improvisations have been elaborately discussed in the Results and Discussion chapter.

Implementation Stages of the HIV/AIDS Awareness Intervention in the Present Study

The present study was designed as a small-scale awareness intervention for three specific groups. The aim was to create awareness about HIV/AIDS among them and seek their participation at every step. The crucial stages followed during the study process are briefly described as follows:-

Phase I : The pre-intervention period – This entailed the following process :

A. Collecting baseline data. In-depth data regarding lives, needs, myths and misconceptions and KABP of the sample were collected and assessed prior to the intervention. This data primarily formed the background for the programme ahead. Key areas and issues that were not known to the sample were identified. This was an important step in building awareness in the areas where there was a need.

Phase II : The Intervention – (A transition period) - Moving from Ignorance to Awareness. This phase included the following steps :

A. Imparting AIDS Awareness - HIV/AIDS awareness was introduced among the sample. Their myths and misconceptions were thoroughly delved with the aim of dispelling them in a logical manner. Audio-visual aids developed by NACO and various NGOs (listed in Appendix XI) were extensively used for the study. Some changes that seemed pertinent were incorporated. These have been discussed in the chapter on Results and Discussion. Simple pictures, diagrams and charts as shown in picture 1 (a & b) for depicting the modes of HIV transmission and otherwise, symptoms of HIV infection and preventive methods were designed keeping in mind the needs of the sample. The very same pictures and diagrams were incorporated in the audio-visual aids (photo-script) prepared as a part of the intervention.

B. Community Participation Forms a Vital Part in Programme Development. In order to increase the acceptability and sustainability of the targeted intervention; community participation was ensured at various levels as follows:

I. Development of need-based audio-visual aids - Audio visual aids in the form of a photo- script, a pamphlet and a poster were designed and developed with the help of community participation. The development process of these aids has been briefly described as follows-

(i) Photo-Script- A photo-script titled *"AIDS Ka Gyan - Bachaye Jaan"* meaning AIDS Information - Saves Life was gradually evolved

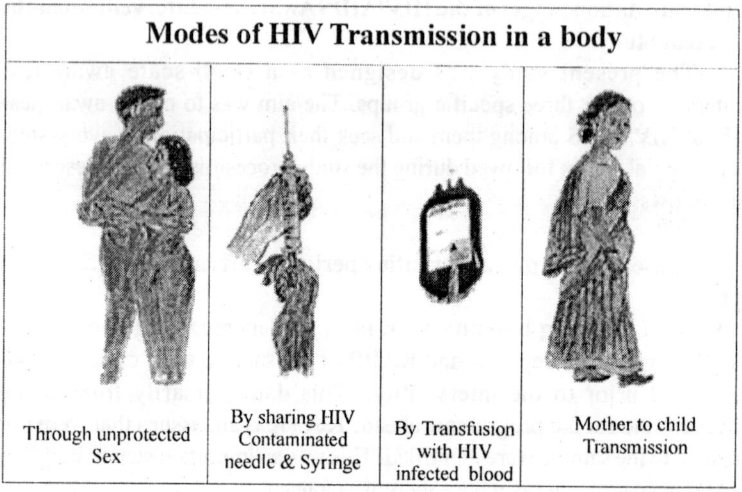

(a)

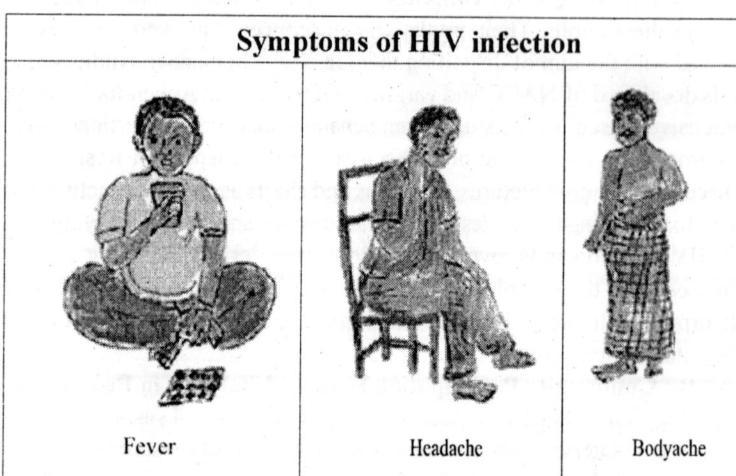

(b)

Picture 1 (a & b) : Set of Pictures Developed during the Study.

during the course of study. Short stories and skits containing different themes related to HIV/AIDS were presented in the form of provocative theatre before the respondents. The audience was asked to participate in constructing a solution to the problem narrated in the story or enacted in the skit. Such techniques have been successfully used with similar communities by various researchers like Castillo and Moreno (1996); Nordenberg & Bernstein (1996); Nickson & Kosch (1996). Following medical, social, legal and preventive themes were prominently emphasized in the story lines-

- HIV/AIDS -the disease and its symptoms.
- Modes of HIV transmission.
- Availability of HIV/AIDS testing facilities.
- Disclosure of HIV status to partner and family.
- HIV/AIDS preventive methods.
- Rights of PWHA with special emphasis on non discrimination.
- Rights of the sample as individual beings.
- Motivational appeals to the sample to promote safe behaviour in interest of spouse, children and family members.

The skills required to practice safe behaviour like asserting for safe sex and refusing to have unprotected sex were effectively staged to empower the audience with the same. The resolve to curb alcohol and substance abuse was effectively portrayed in the script.

The script content was designed in a way to give HIV prevention information in a generalized manner indicating that safe sex was in the public interest. Efforts were made to ensure that no specific community or behavioural patterns were stigmatized. The story content was designed to generate emotional and personal involvement for enhancing effectiveness of the programme. Collectivist messages emphasizing on protection of spouse and children were given preference over individualistic themes that were mainly limited to protection of self. Fathers and mothers were encouraged to consider the potential impact of their sexual behaviour on their partners, children and family members. Initially these skits were presented with the help of a group of students from District Institute of Educational Training (Delhi). They were given the story line and were trained by the researcher for enacting purposes.

In the later part of the study, few individuals from the sample groups were motivated and prepared to take up different roles and act in these skits. Emphasis was not laid on the respondents' ability to act or memorize specific dialogues of the script but on the willingness to stand up and speak in favour of safe behaviour. This strategy was very effective in creating a conducive atmosphere for dialogues and discussions.

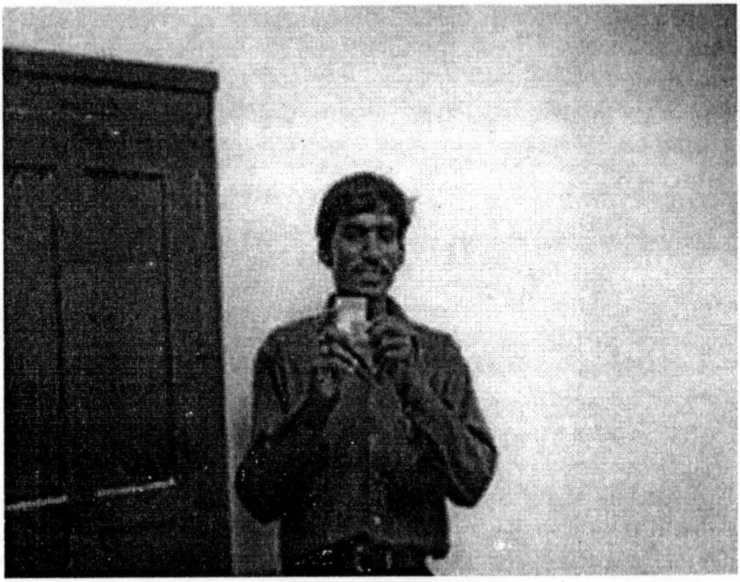

Picture 2 – A Rickshaw Puller Acting as Role Model in the Photo-script and Promoting Safe Sexual Behaviour.

Community participation helped to translate certain components of the audio-visual aids into language which was easy to understand and culturally acceptable to the sample. For instance, it was observed that the word "Nirodh" (brand name of a condom) was much more familiar than the English word "condom". Thus, the word condom was not used in isolation while developing the script for the audio-visual aids. The word "Nirodh" was used in conjunction with the word condom for easy understanding of the sample. Similarly, the word *"Sankraman"* commonly used to denote infection was substituted by words like *"Bimari/Rog"* which were easily understood by the participants.

The skits in which the rickshaw pullers played different roles were photographed in a sequential manner to form a set of flash cards. These flash cards were numbered in accordance with the events happening in the story. On the back of each flash card the script narrating the events seen in that particular flash card was written in a simple and lucid manner. The script was written in Hindi,* the language spoken and understood by the sample. These flash cards were later replicated and distributed to peer educators for further creating HIV/AIDS awareness in their own communities. The flash cards were bound together in the form of a photo-script (Annexure I) for easy handling.

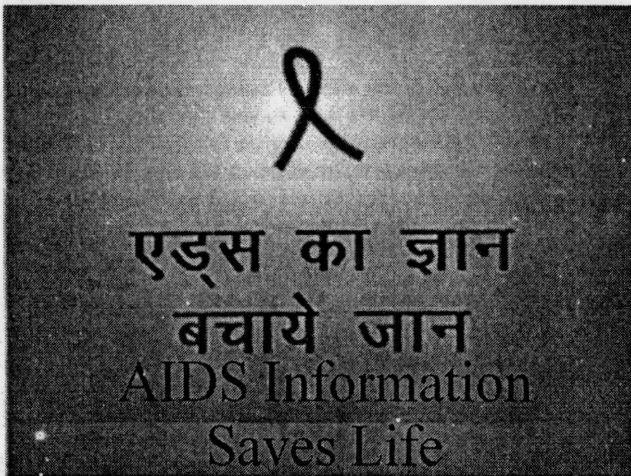

Picture 3 – The Photo-script: A Reflection of Whole-hearted Community Support and Participation.

(ii) Pamphlet. A pamphlet titled *"Mere Bhi Kuch Adhikar Hain"* meaning 'I too have some rights' was also developed during the study period. It featured first hand role model story of a commercial sex worker who as a result of this intervention had reduced her risk of acquiring HIV (Annexure II). Since, the CSWs were not willing to be photographed due to the stigma attached to their profession, hence, there was no coercion to take their pictures. Thus, the pamphlet was creatively designed as shown in picture 4.

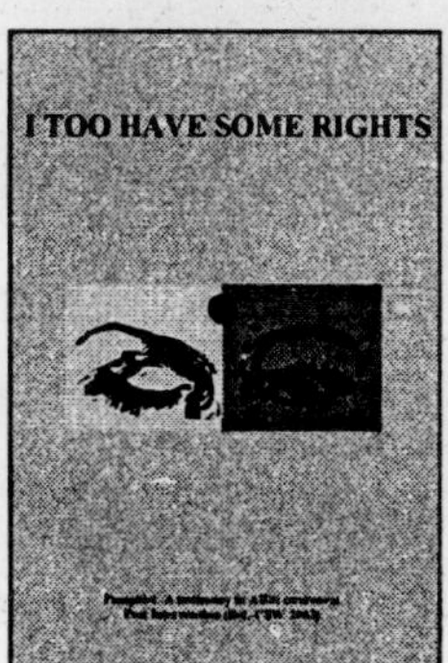

* To enable wide readership of the book, the audio-visual aids have been translated in English.

The pamphlet was thoughtfully crafted and symbolizes awakening of a woman from deep slumber as a result of AIDS awareness.

(iii) Poster. A photo session with the truck drivers was initiated and this led to the development of a poster advocating safe behaviour.

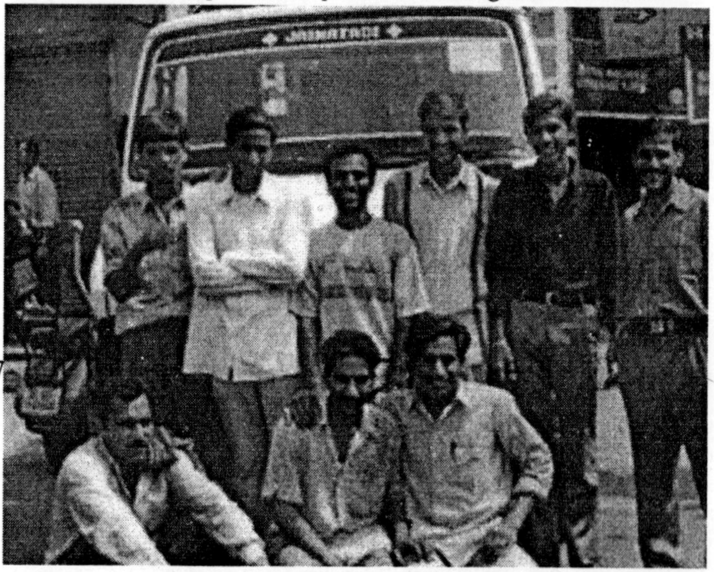

Picture 5 – Truck Drivers in a Photo-session.

The poster (Annexure III)* was appropriately titled *"Hum Khus Hain Kyon Ki Hum AIDS Se Surakshit Hain"* meaning "We are happy because we are safe from AIDS".

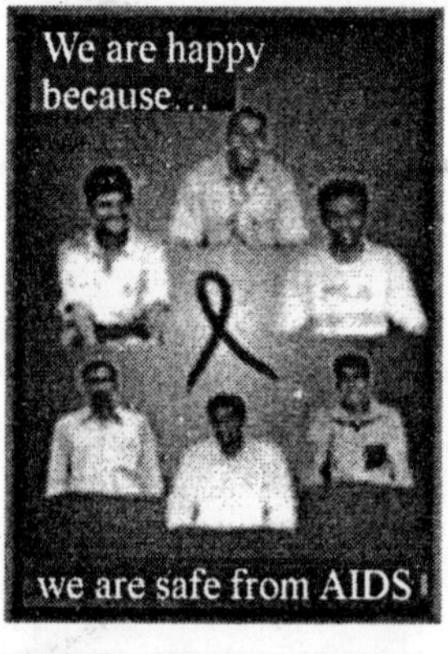

Picture 6 – The Poster: A Result of the Intervention among the Truck Drivers.

* The poster size has been reduced to scale for inserting it into the book. It can be enlarged as per requirement.

II. Peer educators trained to further create HIV/AIDS awareness among their colleagues. Many outreach prevention programmes have been heavily relying on peer educators to impart HIV/AIDS awareness among their communities. The role of peer educators has been significant especially among people hard to reach, conservative and unwilling to change. Many such 'hard to reach groups' like those of CSWs, IDUs and homosexuals continue to benefit by peer education system in which a few members of the particular group are trained to further train other peers. Realizing the effectiveness of the system many HIV prevention campaigns are now rapidly incorporating the peer education concept in their strategies. The need to train peer educators so as to create a supportive social environment especially for the vulnerable sections of the society has been stressed in various studies (Allen, 1996; Muncy, et al., 1996; & Chan, et al., 1996).

Keeping in mind the sensitive and intimate nature of the study it was felt that peer educators could play a crucial role in reporting as well as in modifying the sample's intimate behaviour by acting as role models. Therefore, few members from each of the three sample groups who had leadership/influencing qualities were motivated and trained to act as peer educators. Though it was time consuming to convince these people to act as peer educators but once they accepted this challenge, there was no looking back. They were given the required training and audio-visual material to carry out outreach activities.

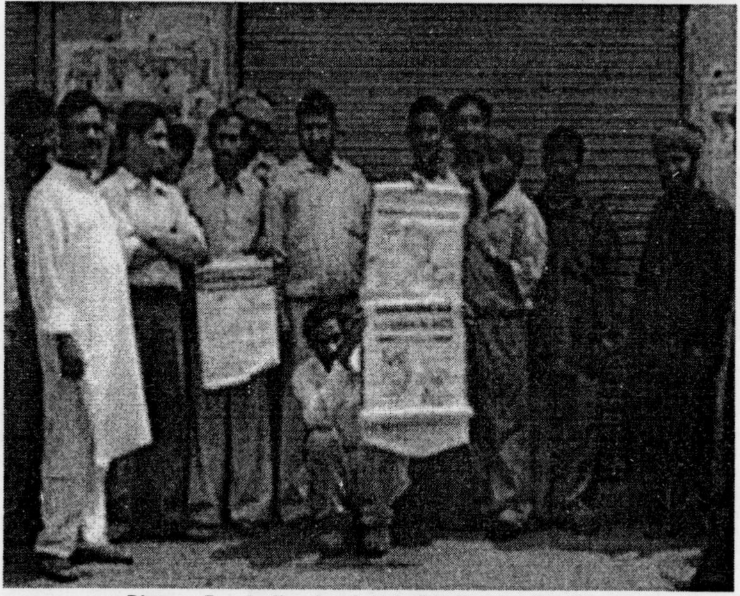

Picture 7 – Audio-visual Aids Display by Truckers.

Initially peer education activities were carried out under the supervision of the researcher but once the peer educators were confident they carried out the task all on their own. The outreach activities included:

1. Focus group discussions to promote safe behaviour.
2. Making the most of the audio-visual aids for creating HIV/AIDS awareness.
3. Acting as role models in street plays emphasizing different issues related to HIV/AIDS.

A total of nine individuals (i.e., three from each sample community) were trained as peer educators to further the cause of awareness generation among their friends and relatives. Regular and meaningful interactions were maintained with these peer educators throughout the course of intervention for getting the immediate feedback.

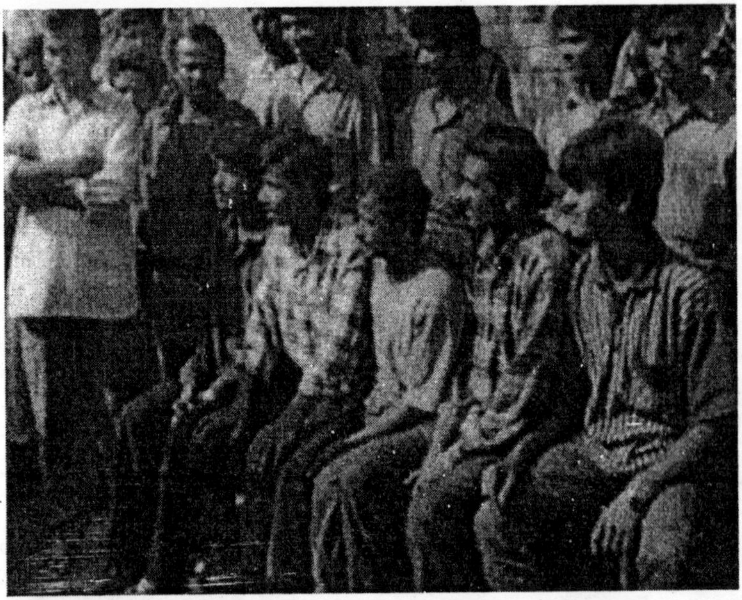

Picture 8 – Peer Education : Intense Listening of AIDS Awareness Message by a Group of Rickshaw Pullers.

It was premised that the peer educators could prove to be a valuable human resource, a vital link in the knowledge chain.

III. Communities participate by responding favourably to the intervention. The response of the three different communities under study was noted. The changes that were reflected through a post-intervention survey assessing KABP of the sample were documented.

Programme Evaluation

Despite the presence of a large number of HIV prevention programmes, the prevalence of HIV is escalating worldwide every year. The upsurging trend of the HIV infection has necessitated an urgency to develop evaluation methods that can effectively and reliably measure the impact of HIV prevention efforts. Westover et al. (1996) have emphasized on using research designs that enable effective evaluation of community level HIV prevention programme.

Evaluation techniques such as monitoring of knowledge and behavioural patterns by means of surveys, interviews and questionnaires administered before and after the campaigns have been widely used in various studies (Londero, et al., 1996; Chan, et al., 1996; Kagimu, et al., 1996). Pre- and post-awareness tests have been administered to determine changes in beliefs regarding sexual practices, frequencies of unprotected sex, and exposure to HIV/AIDS prevention (Ortiz, et al., 1996).

Similarly, various indicators have been used to quantify the impact of community level HIV prevention programmes. Indicators such as changes in behavioural practices, assertiveness regarding negotiation skills and incidence of STD have been used to evaluate the effectiveness of HIV prevention programmes (Chan, et al., 1996). The WHO has developed a set 10 prevention indicators (PI) with the objective of evaluating National AIDS Control Programmes (NACPs). These indicators were designed to evaluate achievements in respect of knowledge about preventive practices, availability, accessibility and actual use of condoms, quality of STD care and reduction in incidence of STD. The evaluation called Prevention Indicator (PI) Survey has been successfully conducted in 5 states viz. Maharashtra, Tamil Nadu, West Bengal, Delhi and Haryana (NACO, 1996).

In the present study the intervention impact was evaluated by using prevention indicators as used by the WHO (reported in NACO, 1996). These prevention indicators were used as parameters for assessing pre- to post-intervention changes. The prevention indicators were:

1. Knowledge about HIV/AIDS prevention practices.
2. Condom usage patterns.
3. Incidence of STD.

Other indicators that measured the programme impact included –

1. Negotiating skills related to condom usage such as frequency of condom use negotiations and success in these negotiations.
2. Behavioural change as measured by the percentage of respondents refusing sex without condoms (Chan, et al., 1996).

Besides these, other parameters as assessed by the KABP scale developed for the study were also used to measure the impact of the intervention. Significantly, these parameters included most of the core indicators used for behavioural surveillance survey 2001, by the Operations Research Group – Center for Social Research (as reported in NACO, 2001).

Phase III – The post-intervention Period

A. Evaluation Process

After the process of imparting AIDS awareness among the sample communities was completed, KABP were again assessed using the same methods that were employed to assess them at the pre intervention level. This marked the post-intervention period of the study. Further, the post-intervention assessment was conducted six months after imparting complete awareness regarding HIV/AIDS. The gap of six months for collecting post intervention data was justified by the fact that the sample needed sufficient time to switch over from one behaviour to another and to come of the inertia. Behaviours that individuals had been practicing for years were not so easy to change. Therefore, a shorter duration would not have been sufficient to show accurate levels of behavioural change. Pre-intervention and post-intervention data were compared to evaluate the impact of the programme.

Field-testing of the Audio-visual Aids

The three audio-visual aids developed during the course of the study were field tested with a group of 15 individuals (i.e., five individuals from each community viz. the CSWs, truck drivers and rickshaw pullers). These participants were not a part of the study sample.

The overall assessment of KABP was done by using the knowledge, attitude, behaviour and practices assessment scale, (concise form-Appendix VIII, XII and XIII respectively) prior and post-field-testing of the audio-visual aids.

The participants were interviewed separately for pre- and post-presentation assessment to overcome the problem of peer influences. The pre- and post-presentation assessment was conducted on the same day within each community to validate the impact of the audio-visual aids without any bias. The results are discussed in the proceeding chapter.

Data Analysis

The data was subjected to qualitative and quantitative analysis. The qualitative analysis was done through descriptive narrations and simple characterizations of day-to-day lives of the sample. Direct quotes of significant comments interspersed in the analysis represent the real world of the sample population.

The contents of each interview schedule were coded according to a coding plan developed for the purpose. The compiled data were entered into coding sheets and subsequently analyzed using SPSS (9.0) package at the Center for Study of Developing Societies (CSDS, Delhi). Percentages, averages and frequencies were computed for making simple classifications and comparisons. Simple descriptive statistical techniques were used to analyze high-risk behaviour patterns in relation to age, sex, occupation and other factors. In addition, data was graphically analyzed to establish meaningful relationships between variables and to determine differences between the three groups, which have been appropriately explained.

Further, triangulation technique (i.e., combining two methods for data verification (APAC – VHS, 2000)) was used to cross check the validity of data reported by the sample, wherever possible. For instance, the validation for consistent condom usage as reported by the sample was reasonably cross-checked by matching the number of sexual transactions of an individual with the number of condoms purchased by him. The technique was quite useful in consolidating the validity of self-reported data at a few crucial places.

't-test' was applied to measure the level of significance of the intervention. All data were treated at .05 level of significance. The gain in knowledge as well as changes in attitudes, behaviour and practices of the sample were reflected in the post-intervention scores of the sample. Results were analyzed primarily by comparing the pre-intervention and post-intervention data and by describing relationships among variables.

Problems Encountered During Data Collection

1. As the study delved into behavioural aspects especially those related with personal, private and intimate aspects of human body, it was a challenge. People had the tendency to avoid any query pertaining to their private lives.
2. The illegality of sex trade posed a major hurdle in gathering data from the CSWs. The lone researcher was seen as an object of suspect with some ulterior motive. The scenario gradually changed for the better.

3. The operating authorities like the agency owners for the truckers, rickshaw owners for the rickshaw pullers and brothel owners for the sex workers were the major bottlenecks, making data collection and the interventions indeed difficult.
4. There was an atmosphere of hostility to be seen, lest the trade secrets would be out.
5. Dirty and disease spreading environmental conditions also proved to be a working hazard for the researcher. The squalor and the sub-humane living conditions in the research locales too was a challenge beyond measure. All forms of infections (some even contagious) were prevalent in the study locations, but that was the reality to be highlighted.

These situations and the ground reality did not deter the determination and the commitment of the researcher but added greater vigour to the ongoing pursuit.

3

Results and Discussion

The present study was carried out as a small-scale intervention to create HIV/AIDS awareness among the selected communities. Community participation was an important component of the study. A set of audio-visual aids was developed keeping in mind the needs of the communities under study. The aim was to create awareness about HIV/AIDS amongst them in a simple and effective manner. The ultimate goal was to achieve HIV/AIDS prevention by generating awareness. The results and discussion are covered under the following heads keeping in line with the objectives of the study:

(i) Socio-demographic Profile of the Sample.
(ii) Living and Work Environment of the Communities.
(iii) Assessment of the Sample on Knowledge, Attitude, Behaviour and Practices (KABP) scale in relation to HIV/AIDS.
(iv) Development and Field-testing of the Audio-visual Aids.
(v) Case Studies –Focusing on HIV Vulnerability Factors.

The study portrays the socio-demographic profile of the commercial sex workers, truck drivers and rickshaw pullers who constituted the sample. An insight into their living and work environment with special reference to the socio-cultural ethos and health care has been covered and well documented. Emphasis was laid on studying all important aspects such as their myths, misconceptions, knowledge, attitudes, behaviour and practices in relation to their vulnerability to HIV/AIDS. The need to delve into the socio-demographic factors of the sample was necessitated by the fact that these characteristics have been known to strongly influence the epidemiological spread of the HIV (Fernandez, et al., 1996; Rosas, et al., 1996; Herkommer, et al., 1996).

Fig. 3.1 details out the range of information pertaining to each of these aspects that was gathered for the present study. This helped to delineate factors instrumental in increasing the sample's vulnerability to HIV/AIDS:

1. Socio-demographic Profile i.e.

Age, marital status, family composition, literacy & occupational status, monthly income, religious and regional trends of the sample groups.

2. Living and Work Environment viz.

Living conditions, work environment, occupational vulnerability of the sample to HIV/AIDS, familial & occupational problems, assessment of physical/substance abuse patterns, media exposure with regards to HIV/AIDS information and treatment seeking behaviour with reference to STD.

3. Assessment of the Sample on Knowledge, Attitude, Behaviour and Practices (KABP) Scale in relation to HIV/AIDS

This included "pre to post intervention" assessment of knowledge (including myths and misconceptions) and attitudes of the sample in relation to STD, HIV/AIDS, condom usage among the respondents practicing high-risk behaviour and the practice of sharing personal-use items such as blades, razors, needles and syringes. The intervention, which marked a transition phase, has also been discussed under this head.

4. Development and Field-testing of the Audio-visual Aids

This section covers the need to develop audio-visual aids, evaluation of a few existing audio-visual aids developed by various NGOs, specific characteristics of the designed audio-visual aids and field-testing of the same. It also includes evaluation of the ongoing HIV/AIDS prevention programme at the G.B. road.

5. Case Studies

Profiling a Commercial Sex Worker, a Truck Driver and a Rickshaw Puller with special focus on factors enhancing HIV vulnerability.

Fig. 3.1 : Information Pertaining to Study Sample.

HIV prevention campaigns must be appropriate to suit the socio-demographic needs of each group (Fernandez et al., 1996). This is extremely important especially while assessing the sexual risk-behaviour of people in a community-based programme. In fact, the social characteristics that influence the preventive measures, which the female sex workers take to reduce the risk of HIV infection and other sexually transmitted diseases (STD) have been identified (Rosas, et al., 1996).

As HIV has been truly recognized to be a behavioural epidemic largely fuelled by socio-cultural and demographic determinants, these become significant in relation to HIV vulnerability. In the present study, the socio-demographic profile of the sample helps in understanding the trends as well as the reasons for their indulgence in high-risk behaviour.

The following sub-sections highlight the respondents' profiles covering their age; family composition; marital, literacy, occupational and socio-economic status along with their religion as well as regional patterns.

Age Group

The age distribution of the sample is given in Table 3.1.

Table 3.1 : Age of the Respondents (in years)

Age Group	*CSWs*	*Truck drivers*	*Rickshaw pullers*
15 – 20	0	2	4
21 – 26	14	10	10
27 – 32	6	14	6
33 – 38	4	4	8
39 – 44	6	-	-
45 – 49	-	-	2
Total No.	30	30	30
Mean Age	**30.60**	**27.47**	**28.07**

Base: All respondents (N=90).

Overall, across the three different sample groups, the median age of the respondents ranged between 27 to 28 years. The mean age of the commercial sex workers was 31 years, of the truck drivers 27 years and for the rickshaw pullers 28 years. The entire sample belonged in the age group of 15 to 49 years. This age group has been recognized as the most productive and reproductive age group (NACO, 1996) and hence, its prevention from the dreadful HIV/AIDS epidemic becomes rather imperative.

Marital Status

Fig. 3.2 shows the marital status of the sample.

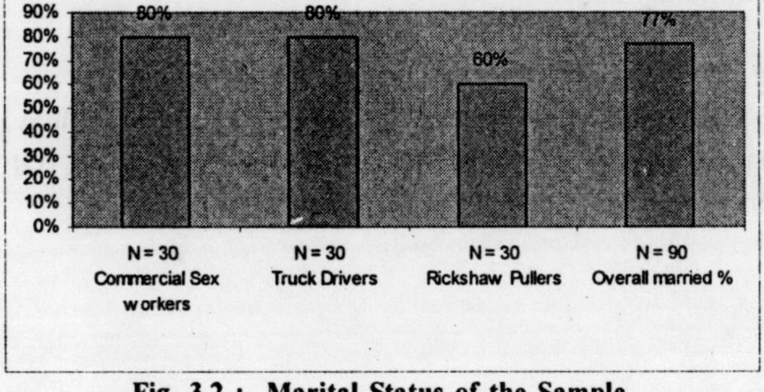

Fig. 3.2 : Marital Status of the Sample.

Majority of the sample (77 per cent) consisted of married respondents, accounting 80 per cent amongst the commercial sex workers (CSWs), 80 per cent amongst the truck drivers and 60 per cent amongst the rickshaw pullers. The study revealed that 67 per cent of the married CSWs had been either deserted or separated from their husbands prior to their entry into the sex trade. In fact, 58 per cent of these women cited desertion by their husbands as a major reason for entering into the sex trade.

Family Composition

The family composition of the sample was unique in the sense that the study participants from all the three groups comprising of CSWs, truck drivers and rickshaw pullers were living away from their families for most of the time.

Majority of the truck drivers and rickshaw pullers (86 per cent) were found to be having closely knit joint family with their parents, wives and children living together in their native villages. In the case of CSWs, 13 per cent of them had no contact at all with their families. The reason for severing of ties between these sex workers and their families (as reported) was the disowning of these sex workers by their respective families. The reasons being elopement of these women with their lovers and familial poverty. The rest 87 per cent of the sex workers had a moderate to minimal contact with their parents and/or children. These sex workers usually visited their families in a time period, ranging from once in every six months to two years.

The entire sample was found to be in either or both child bearing and child rearing stages. Sixty per cent of them had young children who were still dependent on the sample. The age of their children ranged between 6 months to 15 years. Most importantly, it was found that nearly 25 per cent of the sample represented individuals as the sole earning members for their respective families. The livelihood of the entire family was dependent upon the earnings of these members. Thus, their biological as well as productive existence was essential to maintain the socio-economic fabric of the community intact.

Literacy Status

The proportion of literate respondents among the sample was found to be very low (36 per cent). Fig. 3.3 presents the educational status of the three sample groups.

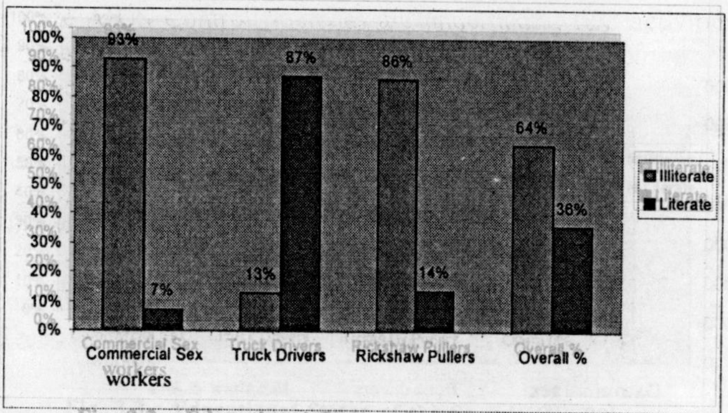

Fig. 3.3 : Educational Status of the Sample (N =90).

The level of illiteracy among the CSWs was as high as 93 per cent, and similar was the case for the rickshaw pullers (86 per cent). The largest proportion of literates was found among the truck drivers (87 per cent). More males were literate (50 per cent) than their female counterparts (7 per cent). This gender related difference in educational level was found to be 43 per cent.

Occupational Status

The entire sample was engaged in their respective occupations on a full time basis. Though, as reported by them, their earnings were not enough to make both ends meet; they seemed to have no other option. Thirty-seven per cent of the sample had previously worked in other occupational categories like working in a hotel as dishwasher (14 per cent), as unskilled labour in toy and bidi factories (13 per cent) and as domestic help (10 per cent).

The families of most of the individuals (78 per cent) were primarily engaged in agriculture in their native villages. Some families (22 per cent) were also working as unskilled labourers in the rural setting. Augmenting family income was very important for survival as majority of them were living in poor conditions.

Monthly Income

The monthly income of the respondents varied within as well as across the three different sample groups. Fig. 3.4 summarizes the average monthly income of the three sample groups.

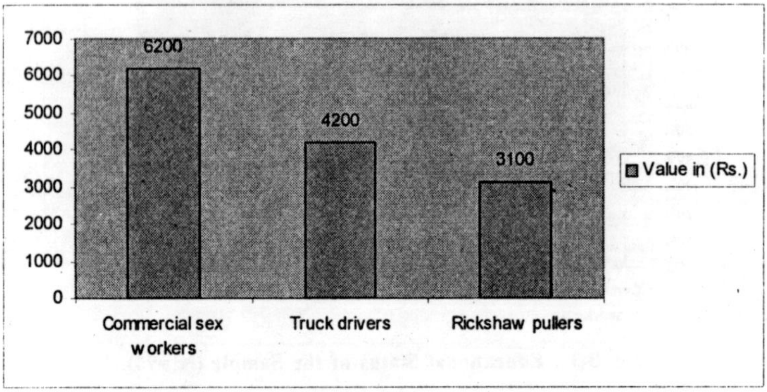

Fig. 3.4 : Average Monthly Income (N =90).

The mean income of the CSWs was Rs. 6200 per month, for the truck drivers Rs. 4200 per month and Rs. 3100 per month for the rickshaw pullers. It is further important to note that the earning status was not regular but on a daily basis. The daily income of the CSWs and the rickshaw pullers was dependent upon the number of customers they had per day. For the truck drivers, it was dependent upon the length of the route they travelled and the frequency of their travel. Whereas the CSWs reported that there was a sharp decline in the sex trade due to recent police raids, the truck drivers and the rickshaw pullers were worst hit during strikes and "*bandhs*" (i.e., call for a total close down on any kind of commercial work). During such lean periods, the sample has no choice but to borrow money from their friends/relatives to tide over the monetary difficulty.

Religious Conservatism

Various studies have shown that religious conservatism tends to make people more prone to high-risk behaviour. (Kemmegne, et al., 1996; DuBois, 1996; Bertinato, et al., 1996). While studying the role of theology and scriptures in context of HIV/AIDS, it has been observed that religious issues continue to be one of the significant obstacles to prevention and control of HIV/AIDS and also to any support to people living with HIV/AIDS (Frew, 1996).

Religion seemed like a major variable in the study because during the process of research, it was found to have a deep impact on the attitude of the sample with regards to their choice of adopting a contraceptive method. The method of contraception adopted by the sample needed to be delved into, to determine their condom usage behaviour, which was used as an

HIV prevention indicator in the later part of the research. The breakdown of the sample according to their religion is shown in Fig. 3.5.

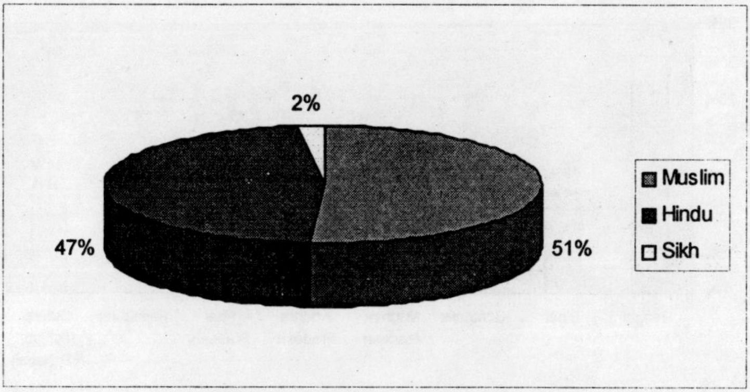

Fig. 3.5: Religion of the Sample (N = 90).

Fifty-one percent of the respondents were Muslim, 47 per cent was Hindu and a small proportion was represented by Sikhs (2 per cent). As far as religious variance was concerned it was found that individuals adhering to Muslim religion were less likely to opt for a permanent method of contraception due to their religious beliefs. For instance, 26 per cent of the Muslim sample had 3 or more children and 67 per cent of these admitted that although they wanted to adopt a permanent method of contraception but were unable to do so because of their religious belief. To quote, few of the rickshaw pullers had remarked, "Hamare mazhab mein aisae bacche rokna thik nahin maante" meaning, "In our religion stopping the birth of children like this is not acceptable". However, no such religious belief was cited by their Hindu and Sikh counterparts. They only cited lack of awareness regarding the procedure or irreversibility of the method as major reasons for not undergoing sterilization.

The data reflects the importance of religious beliefs in the lives of the sample communities. The findings suggest that since religious institutions, beliefs and spirituality were an integral part of many communities, these could be extensively used as an effective means for disseminating HIV/AIDS information in a positive and beneficial manner.

Regional Trends

The demographic profile of the sample is shown in Fig. 3.6.

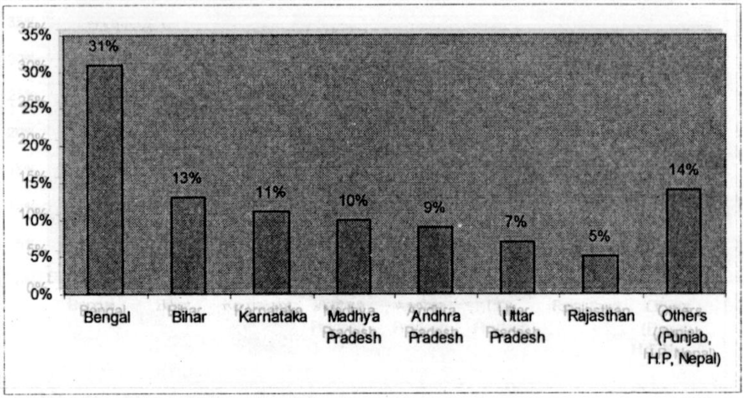

Fig. 3.6 : Demographic Profile (N = 90).

Regional trends indicated that the maximum number of respondents were from the state of Bengal (31 per cent) followed by Bihar (13 per cent), Karnataka (11 per cent) and subsequently, Madhya Pradesh (10 per cent). Considerable migration/mobility was also reported from other states like Andhra Pradesh (9 per cent), Uttar Pradesh (7 per cent) and Rajasthan (5 per cent). The major reason cited by the respondents for migration to Delhi was the lack of employment in their native villages. *The migratory/mobility pattern sheds light on the need to bring about adequate growth and development of rural areas to stop the continuous influx of migrants to the urban areas.* Rapid mobility and migration are increasingly being recognized as major factors enhancing the prevalence of HIV/AIDS by increasing high-risk behaviour among the mobile/migrant populations (UNAIDS/WHO, Dec., 2000). For instance, mobile populations have been known to have HIV prevalence rates up to ten times greater than the national average and they serve as a bridge from high-risk groups to the general population (Gates, 2002).

The regional trends in the present study also indicated low levels of HIV/AIDS awareness among the sample belonging to these states. These data can be used to plan and prioritize HIV/AIDS prevention programmes in selected states.

Living and Work Environment of the Communities

The living and work environment of all the three groups under study was appalling. This condition further aggravated the problem of HIV/

AIDS. An in-depth analysis of their living and work environment was taken up in this research so that the core issues could be addressed. The living and work conditions of the three sample groups and their role in increasing the vulnerability of the same to HIV/AIDS have been discussed as follows:

Commercial Sex Workers in Delhi – An Overview

India is identified as one of the worlds' worst offenders in trafficking of women. A report by the US State Department recognizes India as a country of origin, transit and destination for trafficked persons for purposes of sexual exploitation, domestic servitude and bonded labour (*India Abroad*, June –July, 2002).

Prostitution in our country is not a new phenomena and has long been practiced as "Devdasi system" in certain communities. It is formally defined as the sexual exploitation or abuse of a person for commercial purposes (ITPPA, 1986). The evolution of the "red light areas" where prostitutes were housed only for commercial purposes dates back to the British rule in India. During the British regime in India, there were instances when commanding regiment officers asked the cantonment magistrates to ensure that adequate numbers of women were housed in the brothel areas of the Regimental Bazars. These brothel areas were called as "*Lal Bazars*", the Hindi term probably coined for the "red light areas". There were protests from various missionaries against housing prostitutes in the cantonment area but British officers maintained that prostitution was fulfilling a socially needed function. After Independence, there were vigorous drives to eliminate this profession, but as Pt. Jawahar Lal Nehru rightly observed that prostitution existed from dawn of history and its elimination is a mere myth (Pran, *Hindustan Times*, undated).

Garston Bastion Road commonly known as the G.B. Road (i.e., Shradhanand Marg) denotes Delhi's red light area. According to the latest estimates, the number of brothels here has grown from five in the 1960's to presently a hundred, housing nearly 4500 sex workers. Of these, 3000 women reside here and practice sex work as the sole means of earning their livelihood whereas about 1500 of them comprise the "floating population" of casual sex workers, i.e., practicing sex work as and when needed and not on regular basis (Chatterjee, 2001).

Most of these women are from states and families with high levels of poverty and illiteracy. Local contacts in their villages lure these young girls/their parents with promises of marriage or a job and sell them for a handsome price at one of these brothels. The selling cost depends on the woman's age and her physical attributes. The younger a girl, the bigger is the price. The sex workers' network is well organized and consists of procurers, pimps, brothel owners, managers and sex workers as shown in Fig. 3.7.

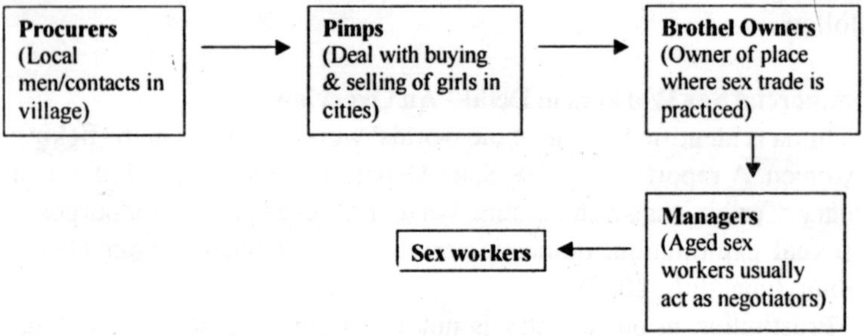

Fig. 3.7 : Sex workers' Network.

Every year, around 150 girls including many minors (i.e., girls aged less than 18 years) enter into this profession at the G.B. Road brothels (Chatterjee, 2001). According to a study conducted by the Center of Concern for Child Labour (1998), out of nearly 9 lac sex workers in India, about 30 per cent were below 14 years of age. Similarly, large-scale raids conducted in June-July 2001, at the G.B. Road brothels also confirmed that many minor girls were being forced into sex trade. During these raids some of the girls were found to be hidden in storerooms, cabins and even behind water tanks on the rooftops. It was also reported that some brothel owners were administering estrogen hormones to these minor girls for inducing maturity at an early age (TNN, 2001). This eventually helped the brothel owners to evade arrests as minor girls could be easily passed off as majors. Although, the long-term use of these hormones is known to have serious side effects like bone loss, cardiovascular damage and liver problems yet, their easy and cheap availability increased their misuse by commercial sex workers (*Times of India,* 2001).

The present study confirmed that as many as 13 per cent of the CSWs under study had entered into the sex trade as minors (under 18 years). Although, majority of these sex workers were extremely conscious about not reporting their correct age at the time of their entering into the sex trade. However, discrepancies could be detected by finding the difference between their present age and the number of years they had reportedly spent in this profession.

Fig. 3.8 shows the distribution of years in sex trade by CSWs.

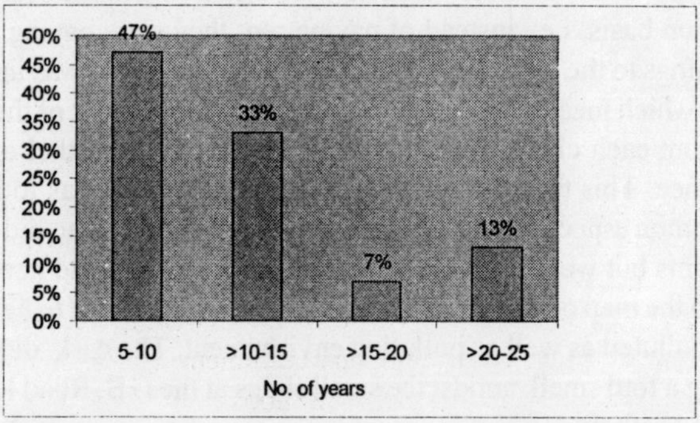

Fig. 3.8: Number of Years put into Sex Trade (N = 30).

Five to fifteen years appeared to be the case with 80 per cent of the CSWs. Poverty (47 per cent) and desertion by husband/lovers (40 per cent) appeared to be the cause for being driven into sex trade. Some of the sex workers (13 per cent) had run away from their homes with their lovers, who after abusing them thoroughly, had sold them for a decent price at these brothels.

Living Environment of the Commercial Sex Workers (CSWs)

Forty per cent of the sex workers under study were living in the brothels on a rental basis. They were paying around Rs. 200 as rent per month to their brothel owners. It was observed that there were usually 8-10 women in each brothel, who lived together as one family unit. The brothel owner was treated as the head to manage the affairs of the brothel including boarding, lodging and daily needs of the CSWs as well as offering suitable services to the customers as per their need and greed. The CSWs who stopped sex services due to their age, worked as brothel manager. They were called as "*mummy*" (meaning mother) by others in the brothel.

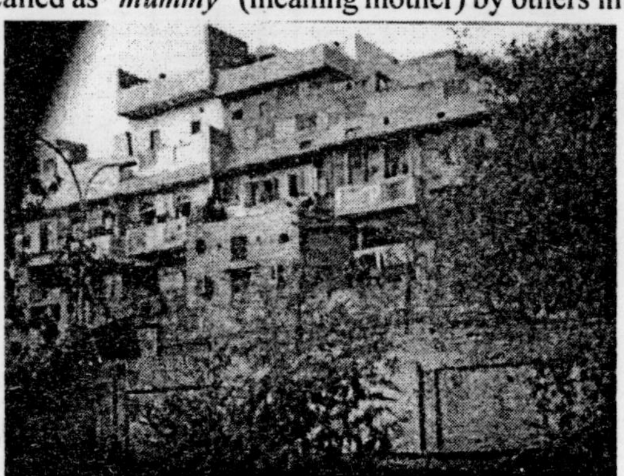

Picutre 9: A View of the Brothels at the G. B. Road.

Sixty per cent of the sex workers were also living in the brothels on a commission basis, i.e., instead of paying rent they were paying a part of their earnings to the brothel owners. The commission paid was in the ratio of 50:50, which meant that the sex workers kept 50 per cent of the amount earned from each client, and gave 50 per cent to the brothel owner for maintenance. This type of commission payment pattern was found to be more common especially among the elderly sex workers, who did not have many clients but were resourceful in the hunt for young and needy preys to fall into the map of sex deals. The sex workers were found to be living in a highly polluted as well as polluting environment. The dark, dingy stairs emanating a foul smell, amidst the small shops at the G.B. Road lead up to the actual brothels.

Most of the brothels were found to be operating at three floor-levels. Each floor usually housed 8-10 CSWs. The living area was very small as compared to the number of inhabitants. The rooms were generally 8 feet wide and 10 feet long and few were even smaller. Most of the sex workers were found to be sharing these rooms for their living needs and the spaces were partitioned for their work needs.

The lighting and ventilation were poor in these rooms. There was as such no strict demarcation between their living and work areas in terms of the infrastructure as shown below in Figure 3.9. Children could be seen roaming around freely. This is certainly not desirable for their normal growth and development.

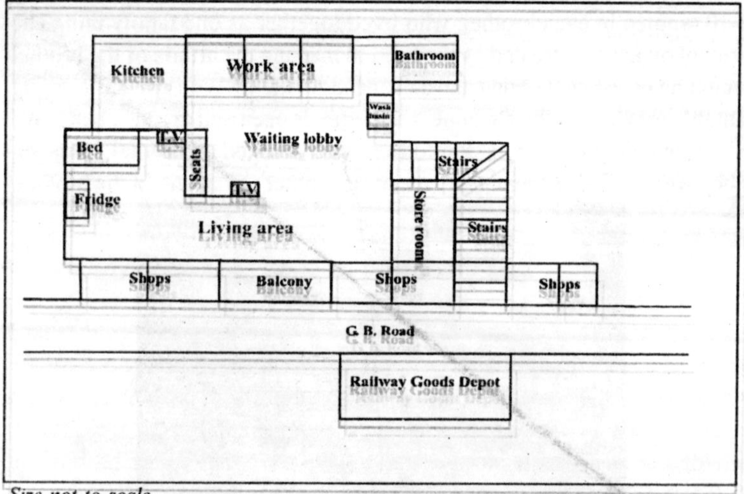

Fig. 3.9: Sketched Inner View of a Brothel (where the researcher worked for the present study) Showing Living and Work Areas.

The sanitary conditions in the brothels were equally appalling. Although, the sex workers were observed to be very beauty conscious and had many cosmetic provisions yet, the standard of personal hygiene was far from satisfactory. Seventy-three per cent of them were found to be practicing sex work even during their menstrual cycle although clinical studies have shown that sex during menstruation favours male to female transmission of HIV (NACO, 2000). Similarly, practicing sex work during periods can also be highly risky for the customers if the sex worker is HIV infected or is suffering from a STD. Some 20 per cent of the sex workers were in the advanced stages of pregnancy (5 months or more) yet, they too continued with the trade. It is critical to note here that a high frequency of unprotected sexual intercourse during menstruation and pregnancy is associated with an increased risk of mother to child HIV transmission (NACO, 2000).

Ironically, awareness about these crucial aspects was totally lacking among the sampled sex workers. The latest nationwide survey of female commercial sex workers conducted by the Operations Research Group (ORG) revealed that although most of the sex workers had heard of HIV/AIDS but many of them did not have adequate information on the prevention and risk of HIV transmission (NACO, 2001). Thus, all the CSWs who were part of the study were given the required information about HIV/AIDS and its manifestations. Focus group discussions were used as means to create awareness regarding safe practices during pregnancy. It was heartening to observe that most of the sex workers in childbearing age took keen interest and said that they would do anything in their capacity to ensure the health of their babies.

As a matter of routine, the day would start late for a typical sex worker. In the morning, they were found to be particularly shabby with unkempt hair, generously itching. The inmates of the brothels did brooming, mopping, cooking and cleaning of utensils as a routine. The duties were clearly divided among them, being overseen by the 'mummy'. At some brothels it was observed that the sex workers had kept a *"mundu"*, a servant for helping them with the household chores. The money was pooled to run the household day-to-day expenditure.

It was in the evening hours that the sex workers were seen gearing themselves up for their work. Usually around 5.00 p.m. in the evenings they would start getting dressing up and wearing the make-up. They would wear their sari, salwar-suit/jeans and a top in a provocative style to woo their customers. Prior to starting their work, most would do a "puja". They would burn incense sticks and do "aarti" in a traditional manner. Although, there were no strict working hours at the brothels, the number of customers during the daytime was fewer than at nights.

Occupational Environment of the CSWs

The number of clients for each CSW varied according to her age and physical appearance. Younger and good-looking sex workers were preferred to the ones who were not so. The distribution of average number of clients in a day is shown in the Fig. 3.10.

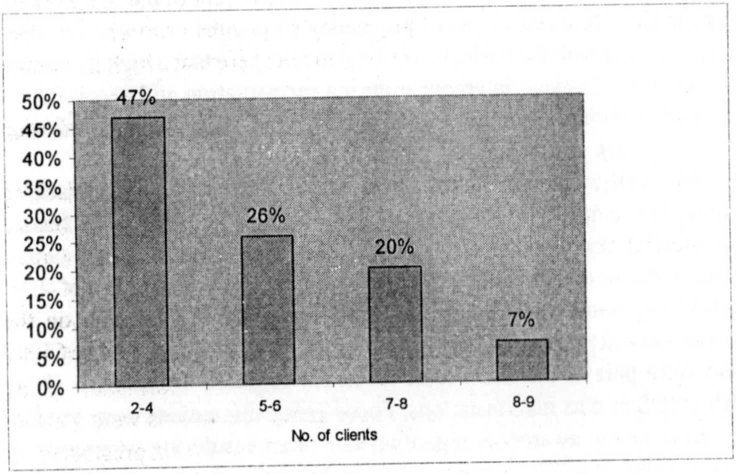

Fig. 3.10: Average Number of Clients/Day (N = 30).

Forty-seven percentage of the sex workers reported to have 2 to 4 clients per day, 26 per cent had 5 to 6 clients, 20 per cent had 7 to 8 clients and 7 per cent reported to have 8 to 9 clients each day. According to these workers the age of their clients ranged anywhere between 16 to 70 years. The mode of soliciting the clients was to sit on the stairs of the brothels and attract the customers by using body language and eye signals. Many a times, the sex workers were even seen approaching the passers by and proposing them directly. Further, many of their existing customers also helped the sex workers by bringing new clients to them. The sex workers reported that marital, occupational as well as socio-economic status were not the cutting factors in terms of their client class. Married and unmarried people from many occupations and diverse socio-economic status visited them. Among the prominent ones were truck drivers, auto drivers, rickshaw pullers and police and army personnel. Most of the sex workers said that barring a few; their clients treated them well.

The rate of services offered by the sex workers varied according to their age, type of sexual contact (i.e., vaginal/ anal/ oral) and the time spent with the client. The average rate per sexual transaction reportedly ranged from Rs. 50 to Rs. 500. The charges per transaction were higher for sexual contacts other than vaginal sex and also if the time spent with the client was more than the usual time of 10-15 minutes. Some sex workers also admitted that they were given tips by a few of their clients. The tip amount on an average ranged between Rs. 20-50 per client.

According to these sex workers winter was the peak time when they had maximum clientele whereas summer was the lean period. During the lean period when there were no earnings, the CSWs relied on their earlier savings. Some sex workers also said that they were dependent upon a nearby hotel owner who supplied them with food on credit basis during such times. Some of the sex workers were found to be saving money by operating chit system among them. Borrowing and lending money was a common practice during times of crisis.

Occupational Vulnerability of the CSWs

HIV/AIDS can be definitely addressed as an occupational hazard for CSWs. Without arguing on the issue of righteousness of the sex trade, it can be evidently concluded that CSWs are at a greater risk of acquiring HIV than people practicing other occupations by virtue of the nature of their work.

In the present study, 27 per cent of the sex workers said that their clients never asked for or initiated condom use with them prior to sexual transactions. Fifty three percent of the sex workers said that a few of their clients, i.e., roughly two out of every 10 (20 per cent) brought a condom with them to be used during sex. The reason cited by the clients for bringing their own condom was that the condoms supplied by the sex workers were not of good quality.

All the sex workers reported that they insisted upon condom use with each and every client. They also stated that while most of their customers agreed to do so, the ones who disagreed were sent back without offering any services to them. Although consistent condom usage (i.e., using a condom for each and every sexual transaction) was reported by 80 per cent of the sex workers yet, the presence of sexually transmitted diseases among them indicated that all of them were not using a condom for every sexual transaction.

All the sex workers said that almost 90 per cent of their clients had sexual transactions with them in an inebriated state. The sex workers also reported that many of their clients had alcohol at the brothel itself before having sex with them. Some of the workers (20 per cent) also said that few of their customers consumed some powdery preparation before having sex with them. This pointed to the probable intake of drugs like cannabis (*ganja*) by their customers.

It is important here to stress the fact that customers taking alcohol/drugs prior to sexual contact were found to be more violent and aggressive as compared to the sober clients during their sexual transactions by the sex workers. Studies have shown that excessive intake of alcohol loosens the sense of safety during sex (Alam, et al., 1996). Moreover, violent sex is more likely to transmit HIV because of the greater probability of genital injury as well as no condom use in such situations (UNAIDS, 1999).

Child Rearing Practices Among the CSWs

Sex workers in general were found to be very attached to their children. Seventy-five per cent of the mother sex workers had their children living with them. Most of these children were minor, with their age ranging from 10 months to 15 years. Majority of the sex workers (75 per cent) had their children born from their clients. Most of these sex workers were found to be treating one of their regular clients as their husband from whom they willingly had children. The need to have children was acutely experienced as the sex workers felt that in their old age they would have somebody to look up to. Contrary to this, it was ironic to see that some of the grown up children of these sex workers ill-treated and abused their mothers for getting money out of them or at being scolded for disciplinary reasons.

Twenty-five per cent of the mother sex workers were found to be sending their children to a nearby daycare center/school solely run by a NGO. These sex workers complained that their children were not treated well in public and government schools due to their familial background. Thus, 25 per cent of the mother sex workers had sent their children to their native villages for getting them educated over there. The remaining 50 per cent of the sex workers did not send their children to school as their children were either too young to go to a school (37 per cent) or they were found to be trying to earn their livelihood (13 per cent) by doing some petty jobs in the same area. Further, 27 per cent of the sex workers stated that they had not revealed about their profession to their families including their children. Besides, they also found it necessary to conceal the nature of their work from other villagers to avoid any sort of discrimination towards their children. It is noteworthy to find that 6 per cent of the sex workers were even able to send their children to a boarding school. Many of the sex workers had high aspirations of educating their children.

Most of the sex workers (87 per cent) said that they wished to continue with their present occupation of sex trade. The reasons to continue with the same work ranged from lack of education, skills, and job opportunities to lack of hope regarding their own selves. Many of them thought that they were not worthwhile any more. *"Ab jab kharab ho hi gayi toh aur kya karna hai*?" meaning "Now that I have been spoiled what else can I do?" was a common remark made by many of them. Commercial sex workers have been found to be resistant to change their sexual behaviour because of lack of sense of their utility to the society (Castro & Fleras, 1996; Silva, et al., 1996; Lewis, et al., 1996).

Truckers – An Overview

Trucks are a major means of goods transportation in India. As on March 1991, about 14,11,363 trucks were registered all over the country (Bansal, 1995) with Delhi alone estimated to have as many as 35,000 truckers (*Indian Express*, Dec.9, 2003). In trucks that are long distance bound, usually there are two drivers and a cleaner who is invariably an adolescent boy. Most of these truckers and cleaners stay away from their families and homes for long duration of time. Studies show that during these trips, drivers and cleaners visit sex workers as well as abuse substances (Bansal, 1995). Thus, it is not surprising that the HIV seropositivity rates have been found to be very high ranging from 7.27 per cent (Jayadekar, et al., 1997) to 8.33 per cent (Roy, et al., 1997) placing truck drivers as highly vulnerable to HIV, probably next to the commercial sex workers (CSWs) and injecting drug users (IDU) (Roy, et al., 1997).

Further, homosexual experiences were observed to be common among truckers (Ahmed, 1997; Jayadekar, et al., 1997). A study in Assam showed that 15 per cent of the truck drivers have had homosexual relations (Ahmed, 1997). In another study, describing sexual behaviour and substance use patterns amongst truck drivers, Bansal (1995) concluded that truck drivers' vulnerability to HIV/AIDS was on the rise due to substance abuse among them. Moreover, substance abuse has also been shown to encourage other risks like unplanned and unprotected sexual relations (Radford, et al. cited in Bansal, 1995).

Thus, practicing high-risk behaviour has resulted in a high incidence of STD as well as high levels of HIV seropositivity among the truck drivers. Different studies examining STD incidence rates show that as many as 36 per cent (Ahmed, 1997) to 50 per cent (Bansal, 1995) of the truck drivers may be infected at any given time in a sample group. The proceeding section brings to the fore some of the factors accelerating the truck drivers vulnerability to HIV.

Living and Work Environment of the Truck Drivers

The study revealed that the majority of truck drivers (60 per cent) were long haul drivers transporting goods to distant states. Fig. 3.11 shows the number of years put into the driving occupation by the relative percentage of truck drivers.

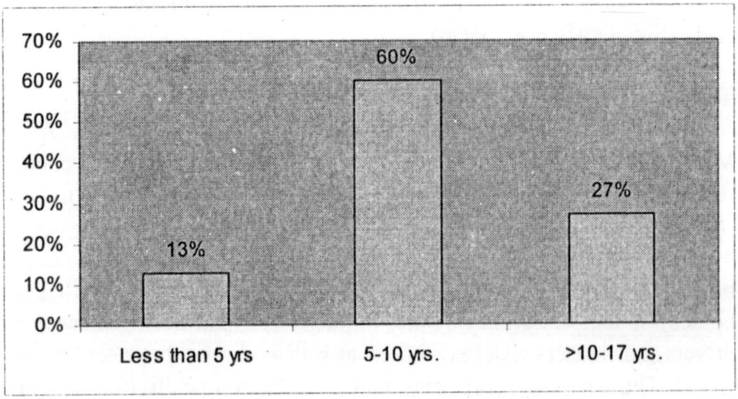

Fig. 3.11 : Number of Years put into Driving (N = 30).

A majority of the truckers (60 per cent) had been driving for the last 5 to 10 years. All the truck drivers excluding one said that truck driving was their occupation by choice. Only one driver mentioned that he took to driving because he was not able to get any other suitable job. Eighty-seven per cent of the truck drivers were working on a salary basis in different transport agencies that owned the trucks, while 13 per cent of the drivers had their own trucks and were working on a commission basis with these transport agencies. To clarify, each driver who owned a truck was found to be paying 5 per cent of his earnings per trip to the transport agency as commission, in lieu of getting contracts from them for transporting goods. Most of the drivers were transporting goods on long routes from Delhi.

The major routes taken by these truckers from Delhi are shown in Fig. 3.12.

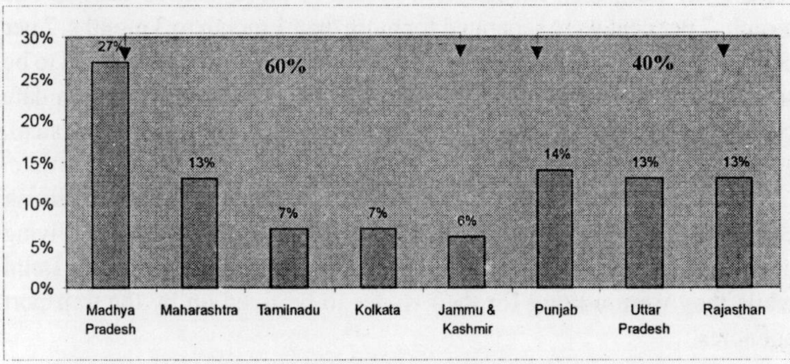

Fig. 3.12 : Major Routes taken by the Truckers from Delhi (N = 30).

It is quite evident that 60 per cent of the truck drivers were traveling long distances to distant states like Madhya Pradesh (27 per cent), Maharashtra (13 per cent), Tamil Nadu (7 per cent), Kolkatta (7 per cent) and Jammu & Kashmir (6 per cent). This necessitated a long separation time from their families and homes, which has been recognized as an important reason for their visits to commercial sex workers (Bansal, 1995; Shubhandha, et al., 1997). The rest 40 per cent of the truck drivers were transporting goods to comparatively near by states from Delhi like Punjab (14 per cent), Uttar Pradesh (13 per cent), and Rajasthan (13 per cent).

Fig. 3.13 shows the average separation time of the truck drivers from their families.

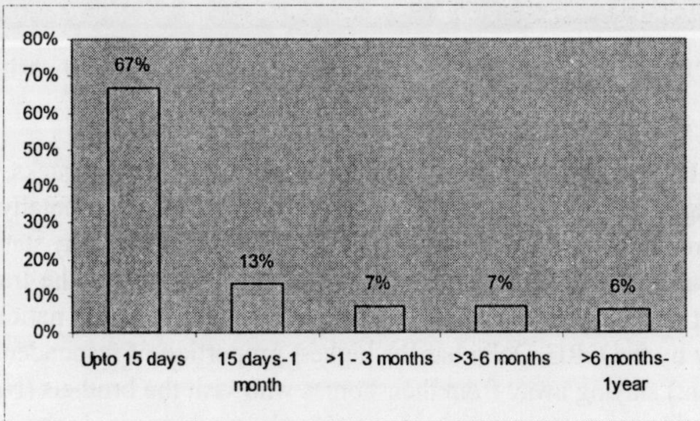

Fig. 3.13 : Average Separation time of the Truck Drivers at a Stretch (N = 30).

At a stretch, 67 per cent of the truckers were on an average staying away from their homes for a period of upto 15 days, 13 per cent of them were away from their homes for a period of more than 15 days to one month, 7 per cent were separated for more than 1 month to 3 months, 7 per cent for more than 3 months to up till 6 months and 6 per cent stated to be separated from their families even up till one year. This separation data clearly suggests that these drivers were profoundly lacking physical, emotional and psychological support of their families for most of the time.

All the truck drivers said that they missed their families. The living conditions of the truck drivers further pointed out that they were living under constant stress. There was no fixed place for them to stay in Delhi while they were waiting for their routes to be fixed up by the transport agencies.

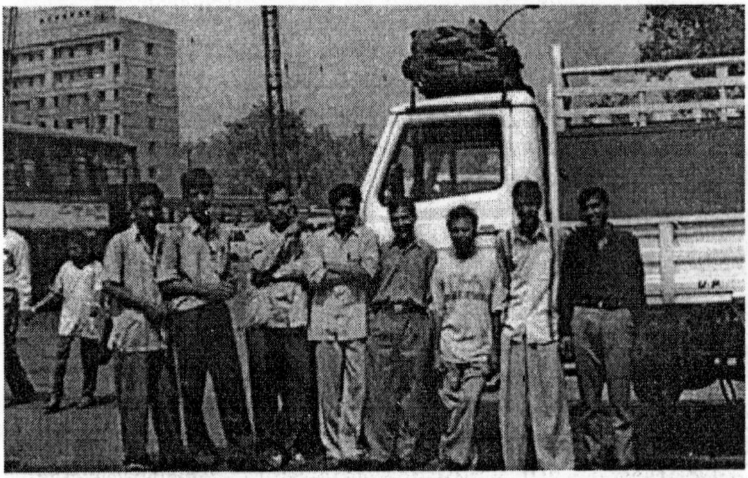

Picture 10 : Patient wait by Truckers Prior to Leaving for their Destination.

All the truck drivers were found to be putting up in their trucks, while parking in the parking lot of New Delhi railway station. Incidentally, G.B. Road red light area is in close vicinity to the New Delhi railway station. It was during these waiting periods that about one-third of the truckers visited the brothels at the G.B. Road. According to a recent nationwide survey by the ORG, Delhi has the highest proportion of respondents (43 per cent) staying away from their homes who visit the brothels (NACO, 2001). The most common reason cited by the truck drivers in the present study for visiting sex workers was separation from their families. These truck drivers commonly remarked, "Parivar se door aur vanchit rehne se dimag mein bahut tension hota hai" meaning "Staying away and separated from the family causes a lot of tension". Factors suggestive of underlying psychological stress have been found to be strongly associated with high-risk behaviour (Strathdee Steffanie, et al., 1996).

Long driving hours coupled with excess of exposure to noise and air pollution during nights further added to their stress. Traffic rules permit truck drivers to operate for the purpose of transporting goods only during late evening and night hours. Thus, they had to keep awake and drive on their routes through the entire nights. This called for great alertness.

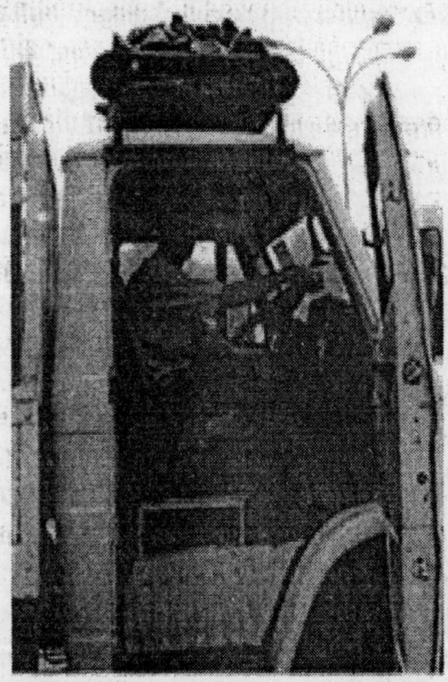

Picture 11 : What is to be a Truck Driver!

During transit, the truck drivers would stop by at specific "*dhabas*" (the roadside eateries). The commonly cited reasons by them for stopping at specific eateries were – enjoying a good rapport/closeness with the eatery owner, receiving help from the eatery owner in situations like minor accidents, truck breakdowns etc. and being provided with good food at these places. Twenty per cent of the truck drivers also agreed that they had an access to sexual partners at these eateries, which was an additional advantage.

Rickshaw Pullers in Delhi – An Overview

It is estimated that in Delhi nearly 5 lac cycle rickshaws ply on the roads (*Hindustan Times*, Sept.11, 2001). These cycle rickshaws are manually pulled and the men doing this strenuous job are called "rickshaw pullers". The rickshaw pullers are usually migrants from poor states such as West Bengal, Bihar and Uttar Pradesh. Poverty coupled with large family sizes, low educational levels and lack of employment opportunities force many of these young people to migrate from rural areas to urban industrialized cities in search of work. Once in a big city like Delhi where living cost is exponentially high and employment prospects stiff, these migrants are left with no choice but to settle for jobs that do not require any educational or skillful prerequisites. Thus, pulling rickshaw becomes a viable option.

Further, low earnings of these pullers diminish the prospect of bringing their families and living with them in cities. Majority of the rickshaw pullers live on pavements in Delhi. They were subjected to various other adversaries due to illiteracy and poverty. Till recently, law required all rickshaws plying in Delhi to be licensed by Municipal Corporation of Delhi (MCD). Yet, it was found that out of 5 lac rickshaws only 73,000 were having licenses (*Hindustan Times*, Sept.11, 2001). The pullers plying non-licensed rickshaws were being subjected to undue harassment by law enforcing authorities. Such rickshaws were seized by the MCD and destroyed, which were later sold as scrap. The MCD has already sold around 60,000 rickshaws as scrap in the past three years (*Hindustan Times*, Sept.11, 2001).

With the situation taking a deteriorating turn, resulting in an intervention from the Prime Minister's Office, the MCD has passed a resolution, which now does not require licensing of the cycle rickshaws. The rickshaws are only to be registered in a person's name and under the existing scheme, there is no ceiling on the number of rickshaws that can be registered in an individual's name. Thus, the move reportedly brings relief to some politicians too, who are earning several thousands of rupees per month by renting out their cycle rickshaws (*Hindustan Times*, Sept.11, 2001).

Despite such resolutions and moves, the situation of the rickshaw pullers remains unchanged. Many of them are exploited, mostly financially, by the cycle rickshaw owners, customers and the police as well. High rent charges of cycle rickshaws charged by rickshaw owners, low plying charges paid by customers and some amount of money reportedly taken by police personnel on various accounts leaves the pullers with little earnings. The present study focused on an in-depth situational assessment of the living and work environment of the rickshaw pullers in relation to their HIV vulnerability.

Living and Work Environment of the Rickshaw Pullers

Majority of the rickshaw pullers constituting the study sample had been staying in Delhi for many years. Fig. 3.14 indicates the number of years spent by the rickshaw pullers in Delhi.

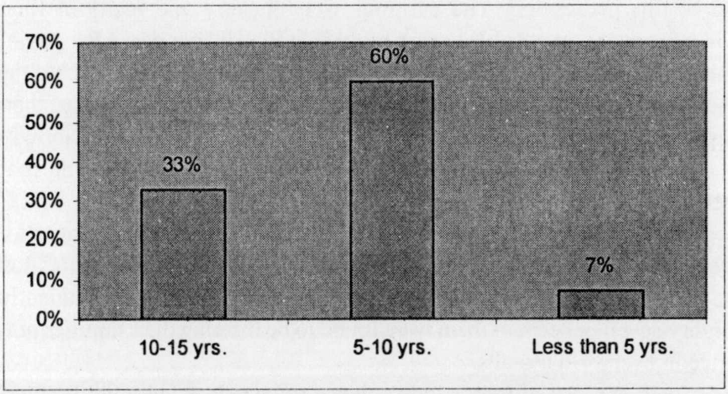

Fig. 3.14 : Number of Years Spent in Delhi (N = 30).

Thirty-three per cent of the rickshaw pullers had been living in Delhi for the last 10-15 years, 60 per cent had been here since the last 5 to 10 years and the rest 7 per cent had been living in the capital for a period of less than 5 years. All of them stated that they had come to Delhi in search of employment, as there was no work for them in their native villages. Since all these pullers were extremely poor, they were living on the road pavement of the Chitra Gupta Road.

The average number of years each puller put into rickshaw pulling is shown in Fig. 3.15.

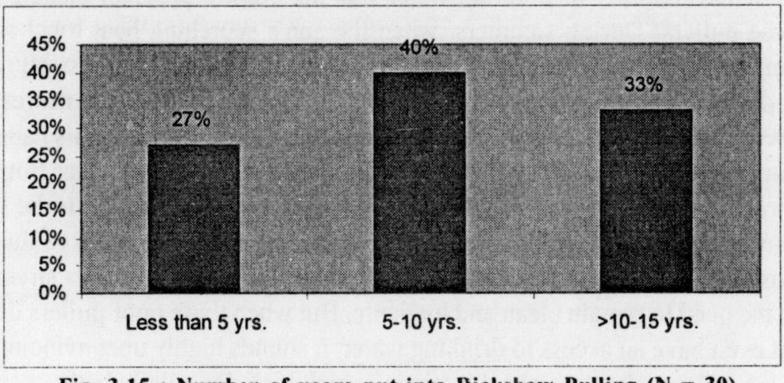

Fig. 3.15 : Number of years put into Rickshaw Pulling (N = 30).

Twenty seven per cent of the rickshaw pullers had been into this occupation for less than 5 years, 40 per cent of them had been working as pullers for the last 5 to 10 years, and the rest 33 per cent of them had been pulling rickshaws for more than 10 to 15 years. All the rickshaw pullers were pulling rented rickshaws and the rent per day was Rs. 22 for each rickshaw. Rickshaw pulling was not an occupation by choice for these pullers. All of them said that since they had nothing else to do they took up to this profession. The earnings were meagre and many of them (34 per cent) were not able to earn more than Rs. 100 per day. After paying the rent for rickshaw and spending on food and other basic necessities they were not able to save more than Rs. 30 to Rs. 40 per day. All of them reported that they could not afford to keep their families in the city with such kind of low income as they themselves were living on the road pavement. *"Gharwali aur parivar ko road peh kaise rakh sakte hain?"* meaning "How can I keep my wife and family on the road?" was a question frequently encountered by the researcher. It was also revealed that most of the rickshaw pullers were not able to visit their families frequently. Eighty-seven per cent of them were found to be meeting their families only once in every 4-6 months.

Even the lack of public convenience toilet was acutely felt by these pullers. All of them had to travel a distance of about 1-1/2 kilometers to reach to the nearest public toilet. Most of them were found to be using the Sulabh Shauchalya complex (i.e., public convenience services on nominal payment basis) in the Motia Khan area to relieve themselves. But this was also an expensive task since each puller had to pay Rs. 3 every day for relieving himself as the service fee for using the Sulabh Complex. These service charges were applicable on every entry made by a puller. Thus, all of them were found to be using the Sulabh Complex only once in the morning.

Unavailability of drinking water was the biggest problem faced by these pullers. During summers, when the sun's scorching heat touched temperatures up to 108 degree Fahrenheit, these pullers had no accessibility to drinking water. All of them had to rely on a hand pump, the nearest being ½ kilometer from their place of dwelling. Unfortunately, this hand pump too was not working for most of the time. Drinking cold water from a trawler meant parting 50 paisa for each glass, which seemed to be a heavy price to these pullers to pay. Here, it is important to observe that most of the sexually transmitted diseases prevention programmes stress on the need to remain clean and hygienic. But when these poor pullers do not even have an access to drinking water, it sounds highly unconvincing to teach them about personal hygiene, which includes a daily bath.

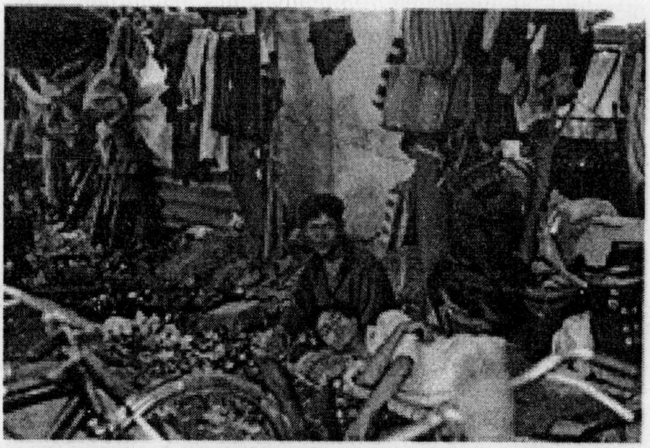

Picture 12: Rickshaw Pullers Living by the Roadside.

Shelter was another major hurdle. Their rickshaws were the only shelter to protect them from heat, wind, rain and cold. All of them complained that they were not able to sleep properly on their rickshaw seats, which were just 1.5 feet long and 1 foot wide. These seats were temporarily placed on their rickshaw handles by the pullers as shown in picture 13 to make some extra space for sleeping. The constant fear of falling down prevented the poor pullers from turning sides.

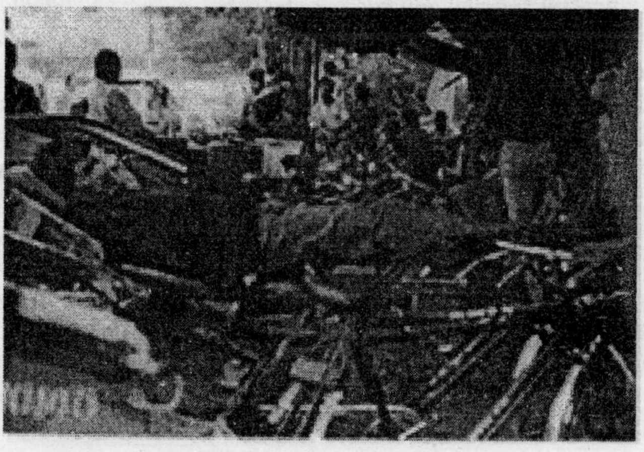

Picture 13 : Seat as a Humble Bed.

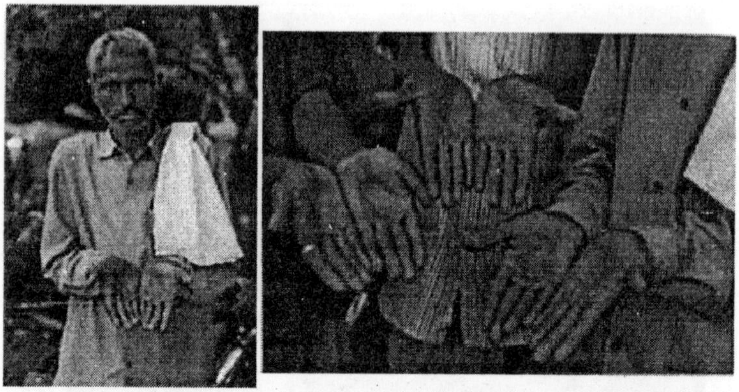

Picture 14: Corns Ridden Hands of Rickshaw Pullers.

All the rickshaw pullers baring one wished to change their occupation. Fifty-three per cent of them said that rickshaw pulling was a very tiring and strenuous job with little money coming from it. The plight of the poor pullers can be realized from the fact that 40 per cent of them had corn formation (hardening of skin) as shown in picture 14 in their hands while 13 per cent of them were reportedly suffering from neuro-muscular problem of legs. These conditions were a result of the excessive pressure exerted on the hands and legs of the rickshaw pullers.

All the rickshaw pullers said that they missed being with their families but since they had no other alternative to earn, they had now become used to such kind of distant living. Most of them had remarked, "*Yaad toh ghar ki, bachon ki bahut aati hai, par kya karen. Kamayenge nahin toh khayenge kya.*" meaning "I remember my family and children a lot but what to do? If I don't earn, how will they eat and live?"

Twenty-seven per cent of them were found to be visiting commercial sex workers. Overcoming loneliness and stress were cited as the basic reasons for their visits to the brothels. The findings are in line with the social behaviour hypothesis given by Bronfman & Rubin–Kurtzman (1996) which states that "migrants are likely to engage in high-risk sexual practices which increase their risk of HIV infection because they seek companionship to compensate for the alienating aspects of the migration experience, there are fewer constraints or social controls on their behaviour, they are exposed to sexual behaviours and practices unknown or unacceptable to them and precarious economic circumstances compel some migrants to exchange sexual services for food, lodging or money (survival sex)".

Familial Problems

Since the contact of all the three sample groups was limited with their families, 60 per cent of them reported that their families had problems because of such kind of a distant living. Most of the truck drivers and rickshaw pullers reported that they had young children; some had ailing parents/wives who needed their regular attention. Yet, they were not able to stay back and look after them because of the nature of their work. Similarly, few of the sex workers (25 per cent) who had kept their children in native villages with their own parents said that they had no idea how their children were doing.

The sample was found to be staying away from their families for long periods of time and the frequency of communication between the sample and their families was also found to be quite low. Most of them (54 per cent) were calling their families only once in every two months. This was primarily because of the lack of telephone facilities in their villages and secondly, because of relatively high costs of interstate-calling services Thus, 42 per cent of them were found to be communicating only through letters whereas 4 per cent of the entire sample (comprising of CSWs) had no contact at all with their families.

Ninety-three per cent of the sample individuals were found to be sending money and goods such as clothes, oil, soap, biscuits and "namkeen"(traditional Indian salted snacks) to their families either through their friends or taking these things themselves during personal visits. Seventy-three per cent of the sample said that their families objected to/ did not like this kind of living but because of the lack of other options they had no other way out.

Occupational Problems

Different occupational problems were reported by different individuals but the most prominently reported problem was that of the police harassment, reported by 78 per cent of the sample.

Forty per cent of the sex workers said the very same police that used their services and exploited them also harassed them to the point of stopping their profession. It was also reported that some customers did not honour the promised payment leading to avoidable problems. Forty-seven percent of the sex workers said that a few of their customers had on certain occasions made false complaints to the police even after availing their services. As a result, the sex workers had to pay "harzaana", i.e., monetary fine either to the police personnel or to that customer. Here it is interesting to note that contrary to this, some of the truck drivers and rickshaw pullers also complained that sex workers stooped to overcharging and were never satisfied as such.

The truck drivers as well as the rickshaw pullers also reported harassment by the police as a common problem faced by them. An overwhelming majority of truckers (93 per cent) and 40 per cent of the rickshaw pullers said that police personnel fined them for various reasons like not having valid documents of the vehicle or non-possession of the driving license or driving into no entry zones etc. Many of them complained that most of the time the reasons for fining them were not valid and were only meant to make some extra money.

Thus, the socio-demographic profile of the sample along with their living and work environment gives a clear and reasonable understanding of the issues that affect high-risk behaviour in these communities. Issues such as poverty, illiteracy, migration, and separation from families need to be assessed before developing an effective HIV/AIDS intervention. Knowledge of factors that make people more prone to HIV/AIDS can help a long way in combating the same.

Assessment of Physical and Substance Abuse Patterns Amongst the Sample

HIV/AIDS prevention programmes must address the critical role played by physical and substance abuse in increasing the community's vulnerability to HIV/AIDS. People subjected to physical or substance abuse are more likely to contribute to risky behaviour by virtue of their association with substance use and depression (Morrill & Ickovics, 1996).

In context of the present study, sexual and substance abuse were found to be significantly prevalent amongst the three sample groups. For instance, 16 per cent of the sample reported to have been sexually abused either during their childhood or in their youth. It was shocking to know that 71 per cent of the abusers were somehow related or known to the families of their victims. On being asked as to why was the abuse not reported to their parents, 57 per cent of the abused sample said that they were afraid to do so since the abuser was well known to their family.

It is also ironic to note that 58 per cent of the married commercial sex workers stated that they had been physically and/sexually exploited by none other than their own husband. Thirty-three per cent of such sex workers revealed that they had themselves run away from their husbands due to intolerable exploitation and abuse. Majority of these women felt that social, cultural, economical and legal barriers prevented them from taking their own decisions. All of them experienced that they had been brought up in a manner, which accepted male domination/oppression over women in all respects as an accepted socio-cultural norm.

Ironically, various studies have shown that women who have been exploited lent themselves to unprotected sex. For instance, Pinel (1996) while studying the patterns of intra-personal dynamics of women that influenced their decision to practice unprotected sex with their partners, observed that emotionally oppressed women manifested their anger in aggression towards themselves and/their sexual partners by practicing unsafe sex with them.

Thus, it becomes imperative to review and redefine the status accorded to women, the concept of masculinity and the process of socialization with special emphasis on curbing gender-based inequality in order to prevent the further spread of HIV. AIDS prevention strategies need to understand, question and re-elaborate the values that limit women's capacity to choose and make decisions about their sexuality and about their access to handling of information (Bascunan & Ana, 1996).

Sexual and physical abuse were found to be traumatic by some individuals in the present study. Fifty-seven per cent of the abused individuals said they had developed a feeling of insecurity, 29 per cent of them felt being oppressed with a loss of self-esteem and 14 per cent of these said they had been emotionally hardened. It is also important to observe that there existed an association between sexual abuse and the tendency to indulge in high-risk behaviour among the sample. Sexually abused individuals were more likely (71 per cent v/s 50 per cent) as compared to non- abused individuals to describe that having homosexual/ premarital/extramarital sex was something normal and that there was nothing wrong in it.

Substance use/abuse patterns were also assessed among the sample in order to reduce the HIV risks related to their intake. Heavy alcohol and drug use have been known to be strongly associated with risky sexual behaviour (Woody, et al., 1996). Likewise, clinical studies have shown that heavy drug use suppresses the body's immune system and decreases its ability to cope up with the AIDS virus (Bagasra, et al. cited in Bansal, 1995). Thus, it was necessary to study these determinants amongst the sample in order to assess the intake patterns and reduce their heavy use if detected, in order to decrease the sample's vulnerability to HIV. Overall, 76 per cent of the sample was found to be addicted to various substances such as tobacco, cigarette, *bidi* (tobacco rolled in a betel leaf), alcohol and drugs like cannabis (*ganja*) and opium (*afim*).

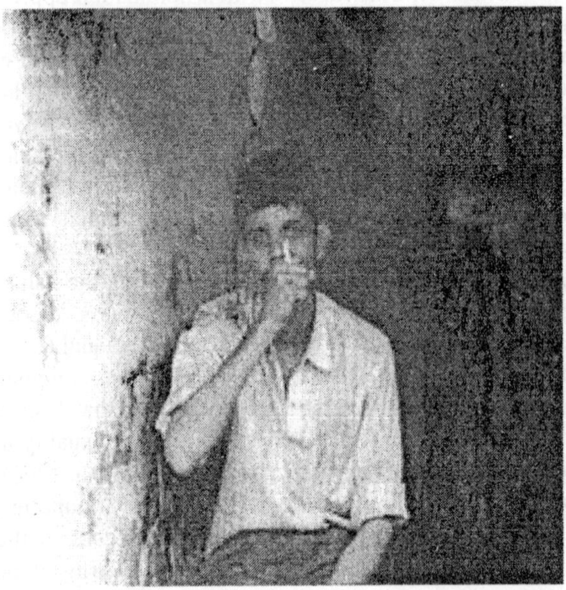

Picture 15 : One of the Common Addictions.

Majority (74 per cent) had been addicted for about 8 to 10 years and admitted that it was difficult for them to give up the use of these substances. Although the daily intake of these substances was reported to be moderate, yet 21 per cent of the addicted individuals agreed that sometimes (on an average 2 to 3 instances reported per month) the use was heavy, depending upon their earnings or their mood.

The substance use pattern among the three sample groups is shown in Fig. 3.16.

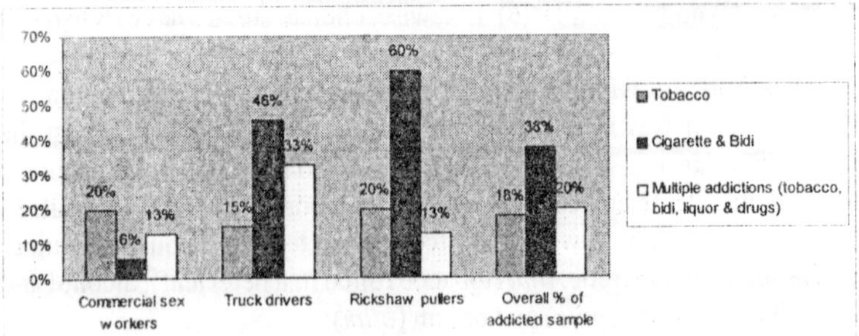

Fig. 3.16 : Substance use Pattern among the Three Groups (N = 90).

About 40 per cent of the commercial sex workers were in the habit of chewing tobacco, pan and smoking bidi. The reasons as given by them were to get some momentary pleasure, to relieve themselves of stress and some even said that tobacco helped them digest their food. The truck drivers were found to be the most heavily addicted amongst the three groups. Consequently they were wasting a lot of money. Sixty per cent and a little over truck drivers had addiction for tobacco, cigarette and bidi while 33 per cent of them had multiple addictions like tobacco, *bidi*, liquor and drugs. The major reasons cited for substance intake were to remain awake and alert at night while driving (64 per cent), to overcome feelings of stress and loneliness (29 per cent) and to relieve themselves of tiredness (7 per cent). One of them had remarked, "*Mood kharab ho toh pauaa le ke baith jata hoon*" meaning "When I am upset I take a quarter bottle of liquor and start drinking".

The rickshaw pullers were mostly (60 per cent) smoking bidi/cigrattes, chewing tobacco and a small per cent indulged in multiple addictions. All of them said that they felt active/energetic (93 per cent) and good (7 per cent) after taking these substances.

The average monthly spending pattern of the sample on their addictions is shown in Fig. 3.17.

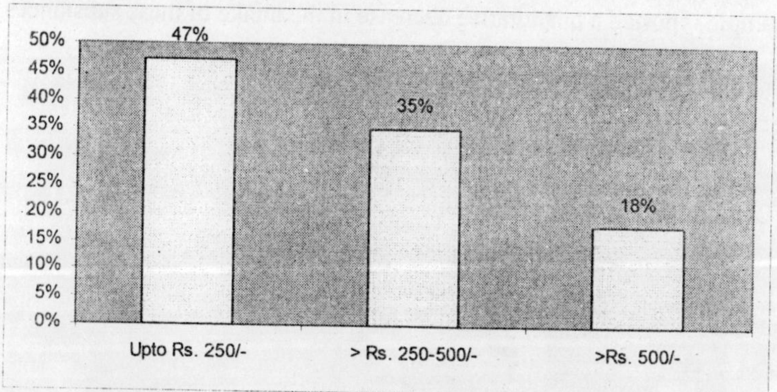

Base : Sample addicted to various substances (N = 68)

Fig. 3.17 : Average Monthly Spending Pattern.

Overall, 47 per cent of the individuals addicted to various substances were spending up to Rs. 250 per month on their substance use, 35 per cent were spending up to Rs. 500 and 18 per cent were found to be spending more than Rs. 500 per month. Further, the average expenditure on substance use for a CSW worked out to be Rs.100, for a truck driver Rs.500 and Rs. 200 for a rickshaw puller per month.

It is critical to observe that 67 per cent of the individuals taking alcohol and drugs reported that the use of these substances was mostly followed by sexual transactions. More significantly, men taking alcohol and/drugs were more likely (100 per cent v/s 63 per cent) to indulge in pre-marital and/ extra-marital sex as compared to those not taking these substances. This was apparently due to the effect of substance abuse, which is known to lead to poor decision-making. Similar findings documenting an association between substance use and tendency to indulge in high-risk behaviour have been reported by Dawson et al. (1996).

Most of the ongoing HIV/AIDS prevention programmes have somehow overlooked the impact of substance abuse on an individual's behaviour. Since substance use impairs judgment capacity and decreases enforcement of safer sex option (NACO, 2000), this information needs to be integrated into HIV/AIDS awareness programmes. The present study focused on the role of substance use in relation to high-risk practices and the respondents were educated accordingly. Efforts were made to motivate them to bring down levels of their addiction, if giving up of the same was not possible. It is significant to note that in the post-intervention period 10 per cent of the respondents especially the drug users were willing to totally give up their substance abuse, while 23 per cent of the addicted sample reported a quantitative decrease in the intake of these substances.

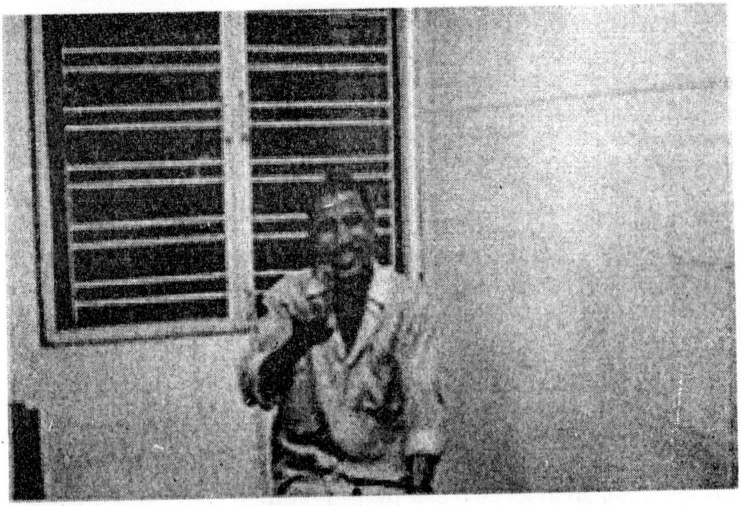

Picture 16 : Semeruddin Stating the Impact of Intervention – "From Three to One" (Cannabis Intake).

Media Exposure of the Sample with Regards to HIV/AIDS Information

This section deals with the frequency and the extent to which the respondents were exposed to mass media with regards to HIV/AIDS information. Although NACO is trying to generate HIV/AIDS awareness by the extensive use of different mass media channels such as television, radio and print material, yet, majority of the sample was found to be untouched by such strategies. The reasons for this lack of media exposure among the respondents need to be carefully examined. This information can in turn help in modifying the present mass media strategies wherever required and thus increase their effectiveness.

Fig. 3.18 shows the relative percentage of sample in relation to their accessibility to electronic mass media.

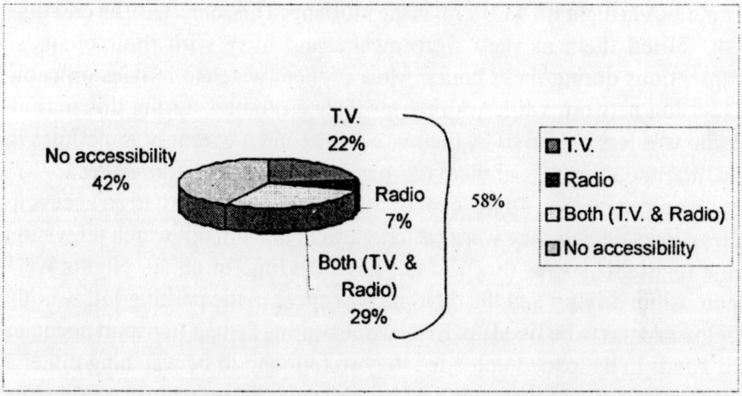

Fig. 3.18 : Accessibility of the Sample to Electronic Mass Media (N = 90).

Twenty-two per cent of the sample was found to have an access only to television, 7 per cent had an access only to radio and 29 per cent were having an access to both television and radio either in their homes or in their work environment. Here, it is very important to observe that 42 per cent of the sample did not have access to any mass media. Further, the actual viewership/listenership rates varied among the three sample groups. Fig. 3.19 summarizes the percentage of sample along with media viewership/listenership patterns.

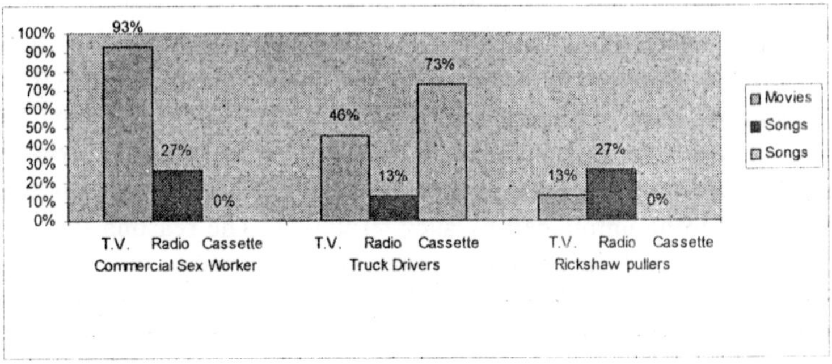

Fig. 3.19 : Viewership/Listenership Patterns (N = 90).

Maximum television viewership rates (93 per cent) were noted among the commercial sex workers who said that they watched television between 12 o'clock at night till 4.00 a.m. in the morning. This, otherwise an odd time slot, suited them as they were awake and busy with their business transactions during these hours. Most of them watched movies on cable television network while waiting for their customers during this period. Radio was less preferred by the sex workers and it was only sometimes in the afternoon that few of them (27 per cent) listened to film songs.

Contrary to this, 46 per cent of the truck drivers who had an access to television said that they were casual viewers and did not watch television on a regular basis, as they did not have the time to do so. Nights were spent while driving and the daytime was spent in the parking lot, waiting for their routes to be fixed up. Even while waiting at their transport agencies for goods to be loaded/unloaded they were found to be watching either a Hindi movie or a cricket match. Similarly, radio listenership was quite low (13 per cent) as these truck drivers were traveling most of the time and since different states have radio programmes in different languages these drivers were not able to understand the contents of the messages being aired. Thus, most of the truck drivers (73 per cent) were found to be listening to audiocassettes while driving. The truck drivers also reported that when they visited their families after a long touring period they preferred to spend time with their families instead of watching television.

As far as the rickshaw pullers were concerned 73 per cent of them were found to be having neither a television nor a radio in their homes. The study also revealed that 54 per cent of these pullers were living in villages where there was no supply of electricity. Thus, as pointed out by these pullers possessing a T.V. or a radio was not of any use due to the unavailability of electricity. Only 13 per cent of the rickshaw pullers were found to have a battery operated T.V while 27 per cent of the pullers had a radio in their homes. Further, all of the rickshaw pullers who owned a T.V. said that they usually watched Hindi movies while the ones who owned radio said that they were fond of listening to new movie songs.

It was also observed that while living in Delhi unlike the commercial sex workers and the truck drivers, none of the rickshaw pullers had a direct access to a television or a radio since all of them were staying on the road pavement. There was only an indirect access to a radio which was owned and usually tuned in by a nearby roadside tea stall owner. Further, subject to the accessibility of a radio, 53 per cent of the rickshaw pullers said that they were only interested in listening to new film songs while 47 per cent of them said that they were interested in listening to news as well as new movie songs. All the rickshaw pullers reported that there were no fixed hours for listening to radio programmes. It was only while they were resting during the afternoon time that they could listen to radio programmes, subject to the condition that the tea stall owner had switched it on.

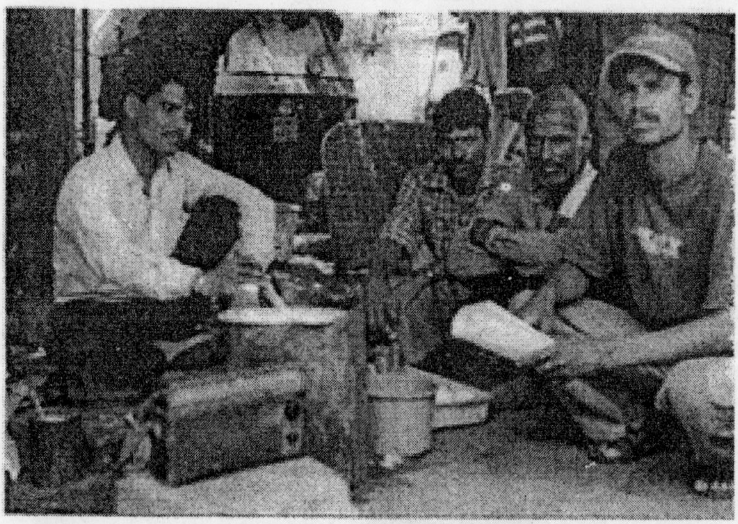

Picture 17: Few of the Rickshaw Pullers Listening to Manglu's Radio.

According to NACO, from effectiveness point of view it is assumed that individuals who listen to radio at least once a week (or more frequently) have a more realistic chance of being exposed to some mass communication message on sexually transmitted diseases and HIV/AIDS than those who listen less frequently (NACO, 2001). However, the present data makes it amply clear that many of the respondents did not have an access to electronic mass media channels and even those who had an access were not interested in any other programme except Hindi movies, film songs and news. Thus, the probability of the sample being exposed to HIV/AIDS prevention messages became all the more remote.

Fig. 3.20 shows the relative percentage of the sample in respect to their exposure to HIV/AIDS prevention information through various mass media channels.

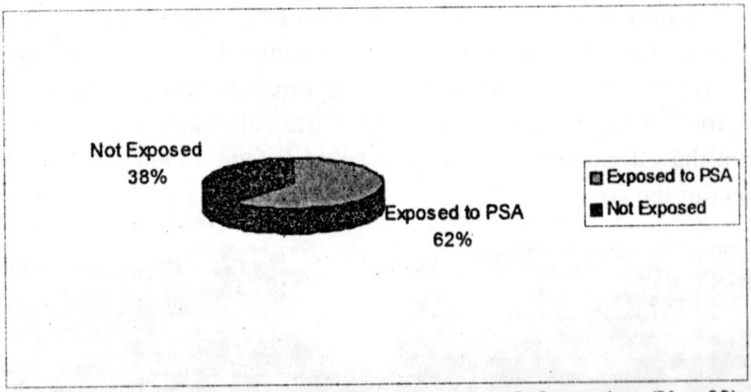

Fig. 3.20 : Exposure to HIV/AIDS Prevention Information (N = 90).

Overall, only 62 per cent of the entire sample reported to have seen/ heard any public service information/announcement (PSA) regarding HIV/AIDS while the rest 38 per cent denied having been exposed to any such source of information. Further, the break up of the sample in accordance to the type of mass media channels to which they had been exposed pertaining to HIV/AIDS information is shown in Fig. 3.21.

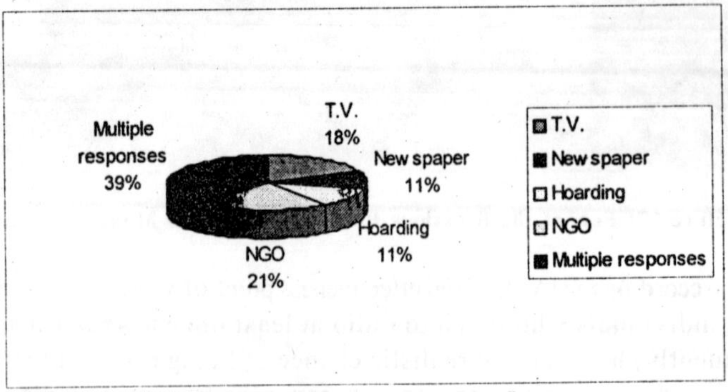

Base : Sample exposed to HIV/AIDS information (N=56)

Fig. 3.21 : Exposure to Different Types of Mass Media Channels.

Eighteen per cent of the sample that had been exposed to HIV/AIDS information, reported to have seen a HIV/AIDS information shot on T.V. whereas none of the respondents remembered having listened to any HIV/AIDS prevention message on radio. As far as newspapers, magazines or any other print material readership was concerned, it is important to note that since 64 per cent of the sample was illiterate; they could not read any of these. Thus giving HIV/AIDS information through print media is of no use for such population. Among the three sample groups newspaper readership was registered only among 18 per cent of the sample (comprising only of the truck drivers) and that too occasionally. Thus, as was evident, out of the entire sample that had been exposed to any public service AIDS information message, only 11 per cent reported to have read some information about the disease in the newspaper. As per Indian Readership Survey (IRS) 2001 data, the three media in terms of their exposure to the masses have been ranked as television, followed by print media and radio (NACO, 2001). Thus, the IRS 2001 findings corroborate the findings of the present research.

As regards to other sources of HIV/AIDS information, 11 per cent of the sample that had been exposed to AIDS information said that hoardings and posters put by roadsides or on bus stops were their source of information, while 21 per cent of such sample reported that one of the non-governmental organizations was their primary source of HIV/AIDS information. Multiple responses regarding source of information like newspaper, television and a NGO were registered by 39 per cent of the respondents.

It was also observed that apart from these conventional mass media channels, friends and peers were also found to be a source of acquiring HIV/AIDS information. For instance, out of 38 per cent of the sample that had never been exposed to a public service AIDS information message through any mass media channel, 18 per cent of these reported that their primary source of AIDS information was one of their friends. This information highlights the fact that since friends and peers can also play an important role in spreading HIV/AIDS information, their potential in doing so needs to be extensively and effectively tapped.

Further, it was observed that all the respondents who had been exposed to some kind of mass media HIV/AIDS prevention messages, were not fully aware about the disease and all of its preventive aspects. For instance, barring a single truck driver none of the respondents that had been exposed to HIV/AIDS prevention message/s were aware about all the four modes of HIV transmission as well as the symptoms of AIDS. Most of these individuals (78 per cent) only knew that AIDS was a disease primarily caused by sex. This sounds reasonable in light of the fact that comprehending sexual transmission of HIV was much easier for them given their poor educational background as compared to other modes of HIV transmission, which required some comprehension ability on part of the respondents. Thirty-two per cent of such respondents were able to relate AIDS disease with the picture of a nude man and a woman in a compromising position (e.g., picture 18).

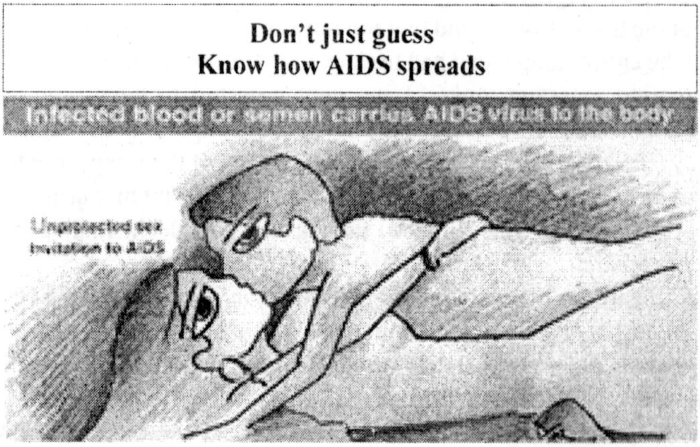

Picture 18 : Picture Commonly Used in HIV/AIDS Information Messages.

Such pictures were highly explicit of the reason for contracting HIV/AIDS. Other modes of HIV transmission required some comprehending ability on the part of the respondents. This highlights the urgent need for mass media programmes to develop strategies that would create awareness regarding other modes of HIV transmission too apart from sex as well as the symptoms of HIV/AIDS.

It was also observed that apart from the sex workers (for whom a few NGOs are working at the G. B. Road and a single truck driver no other study participant (64 per cent) had ever received any form of inter-personal communication on HIV/AIDS. Ninety-seven per cent of the truck drivers and rickshaw pullers agreed that they all could be better informed on HIV/AIDS through interactive and interpersonal communication approach. Majority of them felt that other mass media approaches like television, radio and print material were not totally effective, as they could not clear their doubts through such media.

Therefore, the analysis of media exposure of the sample concludes with the result that majority of the sample was not exposed to mass media channels as frequently as needed and more so to the desired HIV/AIDS prevention programmes. Moreover, since majority of the sample were illiterate, text material messages were not of much help. Thus, inter-personal communication channels in the form of community educators, peer educators and audio-visual aids need to be harnessed by the policy-makers for such vulnerable communities. Keeping all these crucial factors in mind, the study effectively developed and used audio-visual aids for creating AIDS awareness amongst the sample.

Awareness of the Sample Regarding Sexually Transmitted Diseases (STD)

As clinical studies continue to confirm that the presence of sexually transmitted diseases (STD) enhance the risk of acquiring HIV infection (WHO, 1997), it was vital to assess the samples' awareness regarding STD and their prevalence amongst them. This section uncovers the awareness level regarding STD, self-reported prevalence of STD and the treatment seeking behaviour of the sample. Self-reported STD prevalence implies to the proportion of respondents who reported genital discharge or ulcer/ sore or both within the reference period (NACO, 2001), which was 6 months prior to the data collection for the present study.

Fig. 3.22 shows the awareness level regarding transmission modes and symptoms of STD as well as their self-reported prevalence among the three different groups.

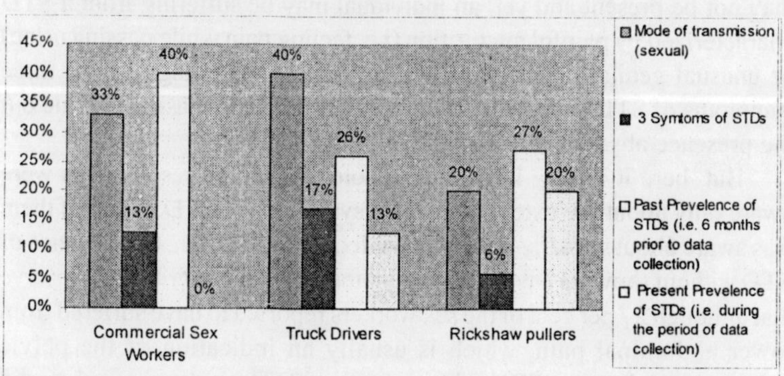

Fig. 3.22 : Awareness of the Sample Regarding STD (N = 90).

Contrary to the general assumption that majority of the sex workers must be having sufficient or rather high levels of STD awareness due to their exposure to various programmes run by different NGOs working in their area, the study revealed that only 33 per cent of the sex workers were aware about a single mode (sexual) of STD transmission. The rest 67 per cent of them were found to be harbouring various misconceptions regarding the causes of STD. For example, 50 per cent of these said that STD were caused as a result of excessive heat generation in the body, 40 per cent said that STD was prevalent only among people who remained dirty whereas 10 per cent cited blood or salivary infections as causative factors for STD. Low awareness regarding STD among the sex workers at the G.B.Road has also been confirmed by Ahmad (1996), who reported that only 8 per cent of the commercial sex workers in his study sample knew about STD.

In the present study too, significantly low level of awareness was recorded regarding symptoms of STD amongst the sex workers. For instance, only 13 per cent of them were able to report at least three correct symptoms of STD. Majority of the sex workers (67 per cent) were only aware about itching while few (20 per cent) also said that genital sores could be an indication of STD.

The knowledge regarding not one or two, but at least three correct symptoms of STD was assessed in order to have an in-depth understanding of the sample's awareness level regarding the same. This was necessary because many a times the two most commonly known/observed symptoms of STD to the masses viz. itching and/presence of sores in the genital area may not be present and yet, an individual may be suffering from a STD characterized by painful micturition (i.e. feeling pain while passing urine) or unusual genital discharge. Thus, awareness regarding at least three symptoms of STD was crucial amongst the sample to reasonably rule out the presence/absence of the same.

But, here it is very important to note that all the respondents were aware only about the externally visible symptoms of STD. None of them was aware about sexually transmitted infections (STI), i.e., the presence of STD without showing any external symptoms. Thus, it is critical to observe that although 27 per cent of the sex workers reported to have suffered from lower abdominal pain, which is usually an indication of the pelvic inflammatory disease (PID) and a symptom of STD yet, the sex workers did not take it as a STD because of the lack of externally visible symptoms. Further, it was observed that the sex workers due to their professional norms were less likely as compared to the truck drivers and rickshaw pullers to admit the occurrence of STD among them. All of them were rather cautious not to reveal the prevalence of STD amongst them and said that they were neither suffering (i.e., during the data collection period) nor had previously suffered from a STD in the last 6 months prior to data collection. Their concern to convince about their good health status was obvious since they did not want to lose their customers by disclosing their illness.

Another important revelation was that most of the sex workers referred to STD as *"gandgi ki bimari"* meaning dirty disease. Since the business of selling sex required sex workers to be good looking and healthy, no sex worker was ready to accept that she could have a "dirty disease". In-depth probing regarding symptoms of the illnesses from which the sex workers usually suffered from, revealed that approximately 40 per cent of the sex workers under the study had suffered from a STD. The high prevalence of STD among the sex workers at the G.B. Road was also confirmed by the paramedical staff of the NGO "Shakti Vahini" which was primarily involved with the distribution of medicines and condoms among these sex workers. It was also reported by these paramedics that they were mainly providing medicines only for common ailments whereas the sex workers suffering from STD were referred to a nearby government hospital for treatment purposes. Similarly, although various other researchers have also documented STD prevalence rates as high as 37 per cent (Khan & Sharma, 1997) among the sex workers in the G.B. Road area yet, the same have been contradicted by these workers mainly due to occupational reasons.

However, the present data on the prevalence of STD represents only the symptomatic cases of STD as reported by the sample whereas the presumed asymptomatic ones have been excluded to avoid any over reporting of the prevalence.

As far as the truck drivers were concerned, awareness regarding STD and their preventive aspects was found to be high among them (refer to Fig. 3.22). Forty per cent of the truck drivers were aware about the sexual mode of STD transmission. 17 per cent of them knew about at least three symptoms of STD. Twenty-six per cent of the truck drivers had reportedly suffered from a STD in the past 6 months prior to data collection, while 13 per cent were found to be suffering from a STD at the time of pre-intervention data collection. The study also revealed that 60 per cent of the truck drivers were not aware about STD and thus even if they had or were suffering from one at any time, they were totally ignorant about it. This was verified in case of 18 per cent of the truck drivers who were as such ignorant about STD. However, on being asked if they had ever suffered from genital sores, burning pain during urination or a discharge problem, (which are all symptoms of STD) they replied positive.

Similarly, among the rickshaw pullers (refer to Fig. 3.22) only 20 per cent of them were aware about a single (sexual) mode of STD transmission through an infected partner and as few as 6 per cent of them could state at least three symptoms of STD. Majority of the rickshaw pullers (80 per cent) were totally ignorant about STD and many of them said that STD were caused only by having sex with sex workers (67 per cent), and because of excessive body heat (13 per cent). Twenty-seven per cent of the rickshaw pullers had in the last 6 months prior to the data collection suffered from a STD whereas 20 per cent were found to be suffering from one, at the time of pre-intervention data collection.

Overall, 49 per cent of the entire sample believed that STD could be cured, 16 per cent said that STD were not curable while 35 per cent were not at all aware about the treatment aspect. None of the respondents knew that the presence of STD could facilitate HIV transmission. Further, it was found that STD prevalence was more likely to be reported by truck drivers and rickshaw pullers (57 per cent) who indulged in pre/extra-marital sexual contacts as compared to those (11 per cent) who did not indulge in them. The high prevalence rate of STD among the sample indulging in pre/extra-marital sex may be explained due to their indulgence in risk behaviour (i.e., unsafe sex) with commercial sex workers as well as casual sex partners. Similar findings associating the prevalence of STD with high-risk behaviour have also been reported by Ahmed (1997); Singh, et al., (1994) and Bansal (1995).

During the course of intervention the sample was thoroughly explained about the relationship between the presence of STD and their role in enhancing HIV vulnerability. The sample was counselled to seek immediate treatment on the occurrence of STD. This was of prime importance in order to reduce the HIV vulnerability amongst those practicing high-risk behaviour.

Treatment Seeking Behaviour

STD prevalence amongst the sample was supplemented by information on treatment seeking behaviour. The treatment seeking behaviour studied the type of treatment sought by the sample especially those who reported to have suffered from a sexually transmitted disease, the preferred source of treatment and adherence to the treatment undertaken. These aspects were important to realize, in order to bring down the prevalence of STD among the sample.

A common treatment-seeking pattern was observed among all the three sample groups. The study revealed that a large number of respondents had no access to proper diagnosis and treatment facilities for any of their ailments including STD. Three basic reasons were encountered for this lack of accessibility to appropriate health-care facilities which are as follows:

Firstly, majority of the sample did not seek treatment for any of their illnesses as long as it was manageable. For instance, 60 per cent of the sample suffering from a STD at the time of pre-intervention data collection did not take any treatment in the hope that the condition would soon get better. Secondly, many of them tried self-medication to cure their illnesses. For instance, 20 per cent of the truck drivers who ever suffered from a STD were found to be using dettol/soda water for cleaning their genitals with the aim of treating their STD. Similarly, 73 per cent of the commercial sex workers were found to be douching/cleaning themselves with dettol at night with the purpose of protecting themselves from STD. Lastly, the entire sample irrespective of the type of their ailments did not visit a government hospital or a dispensary for availing treatment. It is critical to observe that 68 per cent of the sample that ever reported to have undergone treatment for the presence/symptoms of STD was found to be seeking treatment only from private medical practitioners. Similar trends of preference of private hospitals over government hospitals by CSWs as well as their clients have also been observed by the ORG in their nation wide survey (NACO, 2001). Although the survey has not enlisted the reasons for their preference pattern, yet, the same need to be delved into in order to increase the accessibility of such facilities to the masses. The basic reason mentioned by the truck drivers and rickshaw pullers for not availing treatment from government hospitals was the lack of time. All of them complained that in government healthcare facilities a lot of time (an average reported time of 3-4 hours) was wasted while waiting in the queue. This meant a loss in their earning time, which they were unable to afford. Moreover, the treatment meted out by the hospital staff was reported to be inappropriate. Eighty per cent of the commercial sex workers in the present study complained to have been discriminated against/ treated badly by government hospitals' staff. Ironically, although countering discrimination of marginalized groups is known to prevent occurrence of new HIV infections by increasing their accessibility to HIV prevention services yet, only 36 per cent of the countries have legal measures in place to prohibit discrimination against such populations (UNAIDS, 2003). The majority of nations that are not able to provide a protective environment to their vulnerable populations need to enforce measures to reduce HIV/AIDS related stigma and discrimination which is so very essential in containing the further spread of the HIV.

Thus, as is evident from the above mentioned findings, the entire sample due to some or the other reason was found to be visiting only private medical practitioners for getting their treatment. It is critical to observe that many of these private practitioners were not even specialized for the type of ailments they were visited for. Ironically, few of the rickshaw pullers (6 per cent) were even found to be taking medicines on the prescription of a nearby chemist whom they thought to be a doctor since he sold medicines. Further, 58 per cent of the entire sample said that they visited only one particular doctor for all of their ailments. The reasons cited for sticking to one particular doctor were that either the sample in course of time knew that doctor or the doctor charged reasonable amount of money as his fee. It also came to light that since the doctor belonged to the same state and spoke the same language as that of the sample, it was easy for them to communicate with him.

Regarding follow up of the treatment, it was noticed that 69 per cent of the sample undergoing/having undergone treatment for a STD did not adhere to the full treatment schedule due to their ignorance as well as a lack of monetary resources. Many of them stopped their medication once the symptoms of their disease disappeared. Thus, relapse of their medical problem was frequent and called for. This in turn led to a vicious cycle of ailments accompanied with medical expenses at frequent intervals of time. The details of medical expenditure incurred on an average in a month on treatment of sexually transmitted diseases (STD) as and when they occurred, by the sample are shown in Fig. 3.23.

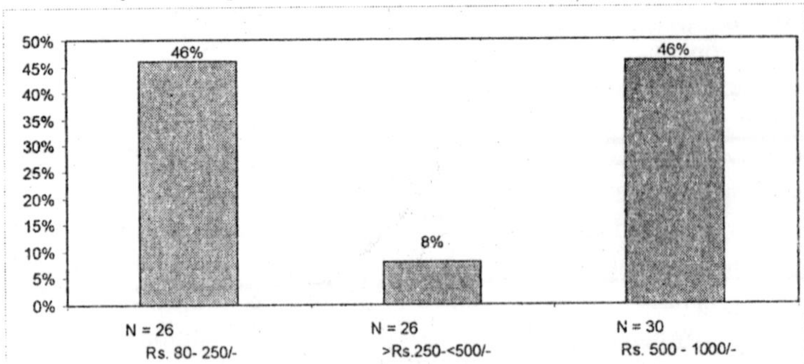

Base : Sample reported to have suffered from STD.

Fig. 3.23 : Average Monthly Expenditure on STD.

Forty-six per cent of the sample who agreed to ever have suffered from a STD reported to have spent anywhere between Rs. 80 to Rs. 250 in a month on seeking STD treatment while 8 per cent of such sample had spent more than Rs. 250 but less than Rs. 500 in a month. Although the CSWs did not categorically admit to be suffering from a STD at any time which was most probably due to the fear of loss of customers, yet, 46 per cent of them reported to be spending anywhere between Rs. 500 to 1000 in a month on getting treatment for various ailments. The symptoms cited by these workers for their illnesses included pain in the lower abdomen and itching in private parts of the body which pointed to the possible prevalence of STD. Further, the high expenditure incurred by the commercial sex workers on seeking treatment can be justified by the fact that of all the three groups they were most exposed to infections by virtue of their occupation.

It is also significant to observe that 63 per cent of the sample who ever suffered from a STD were found to be having sexual transactions as usual during their period of infection. Since STD are highly contagious, the sample was convinced to practice abstinence during such periods. The lack of awareness about these issues shows that such details have been overlooked by the ongoing HIV/AIDS prevention programmes. These need to be explained extensively to the most vulnerable sections of the society.

The audio-visual aids developed during the course of intervention tried to address some of these critical issues with the goal of creating awareness regarding them. For example, the modes and symptoms of STD, the myths and misconceptions related to STD, the need to resort to early treatment on occurrence of STD were all stressed in the photo-script.

Further, the study recommends on-site treatment facilities for minor ailments including STD for such communities, which are highly vulnerable to infections and yet have limited access to healthcare services due to various reasons. A team of mobile medical staff visiting these areas/communities even once a month could bring about a significant change in the overall health status of these individuals as well as help in bringing down STD rates and subsequently HIV/AIDS prevalence on a large-scale basis.

Assessment of the Sample on Knowledge, Attitude, Behaviour and Practices (KABP) Scale

The knowledge, myths & misconceptions, attitudes, behaviour and practices of the sample were assessed on a knowledge, attitude, behaviour and practices (KABP) scale to determine the pre to post intervention changes regarding HIV/AIDS. Significant findings and level of changes related to KABP were observed during the pre to post intervention period, which have been discussed separately for the purpose of maintaining a logical and sequential order.

The percentages calculated for certain aspects on the KABP scale may seem to vary for the pre- and post-intervention periods due to the difference in the total number of valid sample for a few aspects during these two phases of intervention. For instance, the percentage of sample which knew that condoms could provide protection against HIV/AIDS during the pre-intervention period was registered to be 45 per cent (i.e., 34 individuals out of a total of 76 individuals were considered, as only 76 individuals prior to the intervention were aware about the advantages of using a condom and thus could comment on this issue). Whereas, while comparing the pre- and post-intervention results the percentage of such sample that knew about condom's ability to protect from HIV/AIDS during the pre-intervention period has been calculated to be 38 per cent (i.e., 34 individuals have been considered out of a total of 90 individuals which was the entire sample size). The computation of percentages out of the entire sample size (N = 90) was necessary in order to compare the overall difference brought about as a result of the intervention. However, for clarity purposes, the base sample has been clearly mentioned at all such places where it's size was variable which means their familiarity/awareness on a given issue, however marginal that may be. Those who did not have any clue about the issue that was deliberated were not called a part of the base sample.

Similarly, the correct response for the concept of fatality of AIDS was calculated to be 42 per cent during the pre-intervention period (i.e., 30 individuals out of a total of 72 individuals have been considered as only 72 individuals prior to the intervention had heard about HIV/AIDS, while the rest 18 were unaware about the disease and thus could not comment the same). But during the post-intervention period, while comparing the pre- and post-intervention results the percentage of such sample that knew about fatality of AIDS has been calculated to be 33 per cent (i.e., 30 individuals have been considered out of a total of 90 individuals which was the entire sample size) in order to reflect the complete difference between the two phases of intervention.

Here, it is also worth mentioning that although the strategy for carrying out the intervention in terms of different methods deployed for creating HIV/AIDS awareness through community participation such as conducting of general and focus group discussions, development and presentation of the audio-visual aids, short stories and skits as well as the training and role of peer educators in bringing about the desired changes in context to HIV/AIDS have been elaborately discussed in the "*Methodology*" chapter, still a review of the same has been written entitled 'The intervention – a review' before discussing post intervention scores for knowledge, attitude, behaviour and practices scales. This was considered necessary in order to brush up the strategies mentioned earlier as well as to portray the types of strategies that helped in bringing about the specific changes. The findings during the pre- and post-intervention periods have been discussed as follows:

Knowledge Assessment Scale

The knowledge assessment scale measured the extent of correct knowledge regarding HIV/AIDS amongst the three different sample groups. Various aspects such as HIV/AIDS/STD, their etiology, transmission routes, serological testing facilities and methods of prevention were assessed by using this scale. It comprised of 11 questions and a maximum score of 20 marks (Appendix VIII). The findings along with the scores secured by the sample are discussed as follows:

Knowledge Assessment : Pre-intervention

The knowledge of the sample regarding HIV/AIDS was found to be considerably low. Fig. 3.24 shows the mean scores of the three sample groups on knowledge assessment scale.

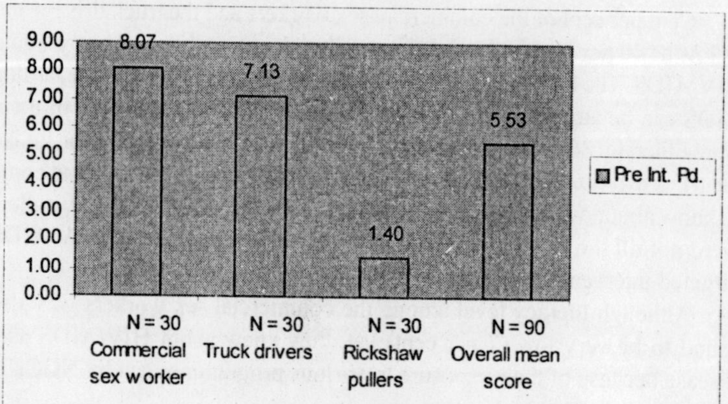

Fig. 3.24 Mean Scores on Knowledge Scale.

During the pre-intervention period the mean score was 8.07 for the commercial sex workers, 7.13 for the truck drivers and 1.40 for the rickshaw pullers out of a total of 20. The overall mean score for the entire sample was 5.53 out of a total of 20.

Overall, a very high proportion of the sample (80 per cent) had heard about HIV/AIDS. However, here it is important to note the inter-group differences amongst the three sample groups regarding their exposure to HIV/AIDS information due to wide variations in their educational status as well as accessibility to ongoing HIV/AIDS prevention programmes. Fig. 3.25 shows the relative percentage of individuals amongst the three different groups who reported to have heard about HIV/ AIDS.

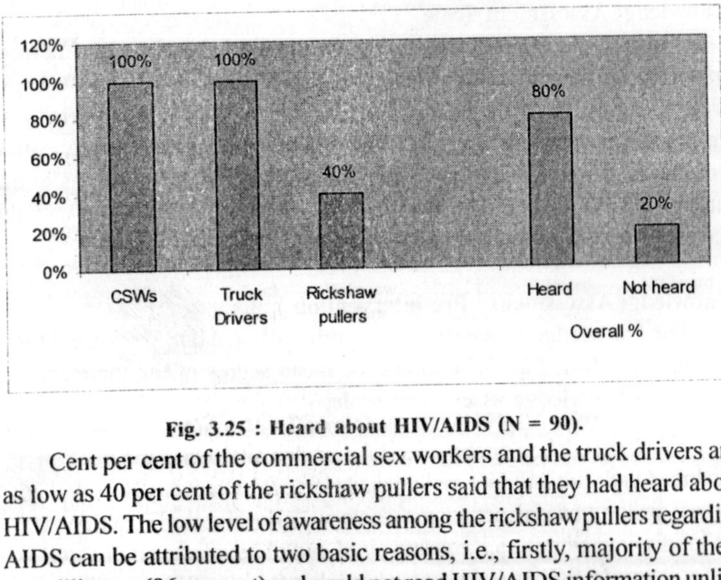

Fig. 3.25 : Heard about HIV/AIDS (N = 90).

Cent per cent of the commercial sex workers and the truck drivers and as low as 40 per cent of the rickshaw pullers said that they had heard about HIV/AIDS. The low level of awareness among the rickshaw pullers regarding AIDS can be attributed to two basic reasons, i.e., firstly, majority of them were illiterate (86 per cent) and could not read HIV/AIDS information unlike the truck drivers who were educated and thus 20 per cent of them had come to know about AIDS through newspapers. Secondly, these rickshaw pullers were not till the time of intervention covered by any ongoing HIV/AIDS targeted intervention/programme.

Although literacy level among the commercial sex workers was also found to be very low (7 per cent) yet, they knew about HIV/AIDS as a disease because of their exposure to various programmes run by NGOs in their area and also to television.

The entire sample that had heard about AIDS knew that it was a disease but not a single respondent knew what causes AIDS. None of them had heard about HIV and thus very often the cause of AIDS, i.e., HIV was mixed up with the mode of transmission by the respondents and many of them replied that AIDS is caused by having sex. Further, 71 per cent of the truck drivers and rickshaw pullers who had heard about AIDS were of the opinion that only having sex with commercial sex workers could cause AIDS. The reason given behind this was that commercial sex workers were dirty and indulged in wrong/immoral acts. They were thus, the primary source of acquiring HIV/AIDS. Majority of the truck drivers and rickshaw pullers had remarked, *"Galat aurton ke saath samband rakhne se AIDS ho jata hai"* meaning "AIDS is caused by having sexual contacts with commercial sex workers".

Similarly, except for a single truck driver none of the individuals was aware about any symptoms of HIV/AIDS. On the contrary, many individuals were found to be harbouring various misconceptions like AIDS manifests itself in the form of fatigue and weakness (35 per cent), itching (28 per cent), sores and pain in private body parts (15 per cent), inability to perform sex (11 per cent) and changes in facial looks of a person (9 per cent). Some of them also said that AIDS was just like any other fever accompanied with cough and cold (19 per cent). The responses add up to more than 100 per cent because of multiple responses given by a few individuals. Only one truck driver was aware that chronic diarrhoea/chronic fever were the symptoms of AIDS disease. This particular truck driver was aware about symptoms of AIDS, as few members of his near family had recently died of the disease.

Similarly, the level of awareness regarding all the four modes of HIV transmission was found to be very low amongst the sample. Fig. 3.26 shows the percentage of sample in relation to their awareness regarding different modes of HIV/AIDS transmission.

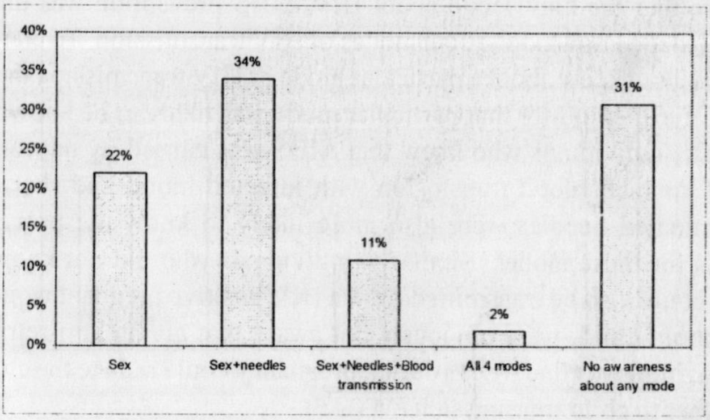

Fig. 3.26 : Awareness Regarding Modes of HIV Transmission (N = 90).

Twenty-two per cent of the entire sample was aware only about the sexual mode of HIV transmission, 34 per cent of them were aware about sexual mode as well as needle sharing risks, 11 per cent knew about blood transfusion related risk in addition to sexual and needle sharing mode and only 2 per cent of the sample knew about all the four HIV transmission modes viz. sexual, needle sharing, blood transfusion by contaminated blood and the vertical mode, i.e., transmission from a HIV positive mother to her unborn child before or during child-birth. Awareness regarding HIV transmission through breast-feeding was lacking among all the respondents. Overall, 31 per cent of the entire sample was found to be completely unaware about any mode of HIV transmission. Thus, the data clearly portrays an alarming lack of awareness regarding all the four modes of HIV transmission amongst the sample. Similar findings showing a lack of awareness regarding HIV transmission modes have also been widely confirmed by various reports (Chhabra, 2003; *Times of India*, Jan.4, 2002; Gates, Nov., 2002). Further, 62 per cent of the sample was not aware about the testing procedure for HIV/AIDS. As few as 38 per cent of the entire sample knew that a blood test by a doctor could reveal the HIV status of an individual. Although increased access to treatment (including diagnostic facilities) has been recognized as one of the most powerful incentives for individuals to learn about their HIV status (UNAIDS/WHO, Dec., 2003) yet, the present study showed that 51 per cent of the sample was totally unaware about the availability of HIV/AIDS testing facilities in various hospitals whereas only 49 per cent of them knew that the presence of disease could be tested in a few hospitals.

Regarding methods of preventing HIV/AIDS, it is important to observe that the knowledge about HIV/AIDS prevention was directly related to the knowledge about modes of HIV transmission. To clarify, if an individual knew about a particular mode of HIV transmission then the preventive method for that particular mode was likely to be known. For example, individuals who knew that AIDS was caused by unprotected sexual contact, blood transfusion with infected blood and sharing of contaminated needles were also more likely to know the preventive aspects for these modes. Similarly, individuals who did not know that AIDS could also be transmitted from a HIV positive pregnant woman to her unborn child, were obviously not aware that giving anti-retroviral drug (azidothymidine -AZT) during pregnancy could reduce the chances of mother to child transmission (MTCT).

The awareness level of the sample regarding different HIV/AIDS preventive methods is shown in Fig. 3.27.

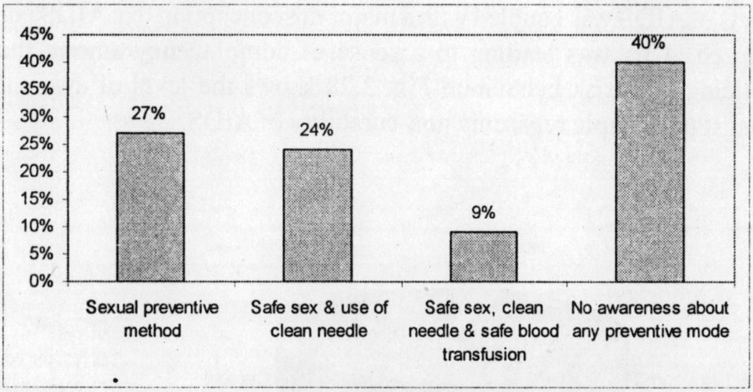

Fig. 3.27 : Awareness Regarding HIV/AIDS Preventive Methods (N = 90).

Overall, 27 per cent of the sample was aware only about the sexual preventive mode, i.e., either having sex with one uninfected partner (usually the spouse) or using a condom in case of multi partner sex. Many truck drivers and rickshaw pullers (23 per cent) said that not having sex with commercial sex workers was the most important method of HIV prevention because according to them only commercial sex workers were the transmitting source of HIV. Here it is important to stress that casual sex partners (i.e., sexual partners other than CSWs) were not seen as a potential source of HIV infection by these truck drivers and rickshaw pullers. Moreover, consistent condom usage was not known to these individuals as a preventive method to avert sexual HIV transmission during the pre-intervention period of the study.

In contrast, (93 per cent) of the CSWs cited condom usage as a HIV prevention method. The high percentage of sex workers giving this response can be apparently explained because of the condom promotion and distribution activities undertaken by various NGOs in the red light area.

Twenty-four per cent of the sample was aware about two prevention modes pertaining to safe sex as well as the use of clean injecting needles and syringes, and only 9 per cent of the individuals were aware about three preventive modes pertaining to safe sex, use of clean needles and syringes and safe blood transfusion if required. Preventive aspect related to mother to child transmission was not known to any respondent during the pre-intervention phase of the study, although most of them were in the childbearing stage besides being vulnerable to HIV/AIDS due to their indulgence in risky behaviour. Overall, 40 per cent of the sample was not aware about any of HIV/AIDS preventive mode.

The low awareness level of the sample population regarding different aspects of AIDS was coupled with a major misconception that AIDS could be cured. This was leading to a sense of complacency among those practicing high-risk behaviour. Fig. 3.28 shows the level of awareness amongst the sample regarding non-curability of AIDS.

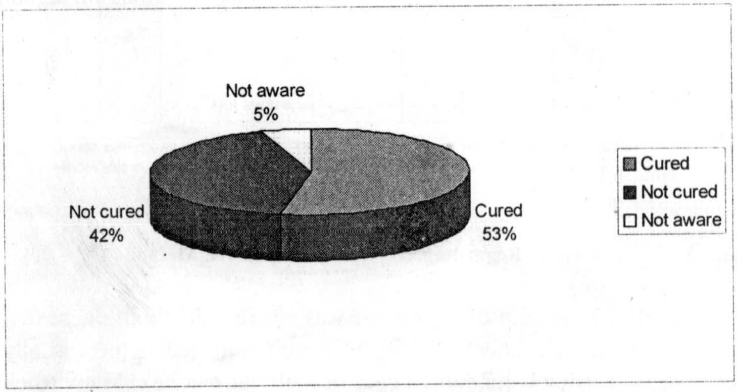

Base: Sample that had heard about HIV/AIDS (N = 72)

Fig. 3.28 : Awareness Regarding Non-curability of AIDS.

Fifty-three per cent of the sample that had heard about AIDS said that AIDS could be cured with treatment. Further, 35 per cent of these individuals said that a person with HIV/AIDS could live for long like any other normal person if treated properly. In fact, none of the respondents was aware about the correct survival time of an individual infected with HIV/AIDS. Only 42 per cent of the sample that had heard about AIDS knew that the disease could not be cured, while 5 per cent of such sample was unaware about the treatment aspect and thus could not comment on the same.

Another important aspect delved by the research was the perceived vulnerability of the sample to HIV/AIDS. Although majority of the study sample had been exposed to high-risk behaviour in various forms such as indulgence in pre/extra marital sex (80 per cent) and being injected for medical reasons with used needles (24 per cent) yet, 47 per cent of them said that they did not perceive themselves to be at risk of HIV/AIDS. Their answer was justified due to their lack of awareness regarding HIV/AIDS. It is obvious that an individual in the absence of knowledge regarding all the four modes of HIV transmission cannot correctly judge his/her vulnerability to HIV/AIDS despite being exposed to those modes of transmission.

The perception of the commercial sex workers was further blurred by misconceptions such as taking shots (mostly penicillin) could protect them from HIV/AIDS. Thirteen per cent of the sex workers said that they had got themselves injected against AIDS. Manju (name changed) a 26-year-old sex worker determinedly stated, "*Mujhe AIDS nahin ho sakta. Mein AIDS ka sui lagwa ke aai, paanch sau rupaye mein*" meaning "I can't get AIDS as I paid Rs. 500 and got myself injected against AIDS". Apart from complacency of the sample, this also shows beyond doubt that many local medical practitioners whom the sex workers visited were giving them a false sense of security against AIDS by giving them some shots just for the sake of making some quick money. Such issues need to be stringently dealt with a sense of utmost urgency to combat AIDS.

Similarly, undergoing HIV testing was wrongly perceived as a preventive method to protect oneself from AIDS. Six per cent of the truck drivers said that they had already undergone HIV testing a couple of months ago and since their HIV status was negative at that time, they presently too thought themselves to be protected of the disease irrespective of their continued indulgence in risky behaviour.

Overall, the data regarding HIV/AIDS knowledge, gives a clear impression that misconceptions about the disease still exist among a large proportion of the vulnerable communities. Similarly, a recent report by the Operation Research Group showed that only 23.5 per cent of the people questioned in a study in Delhi, knew correctly how HIV was transmitted (*Indian Express*, April 4, 2002). The present findings highlight the need to implement HIV/AIDS interventions aggressively with a special emphasis on eliminating myths and misconceptions of the masses.

The Intervention – *A review*

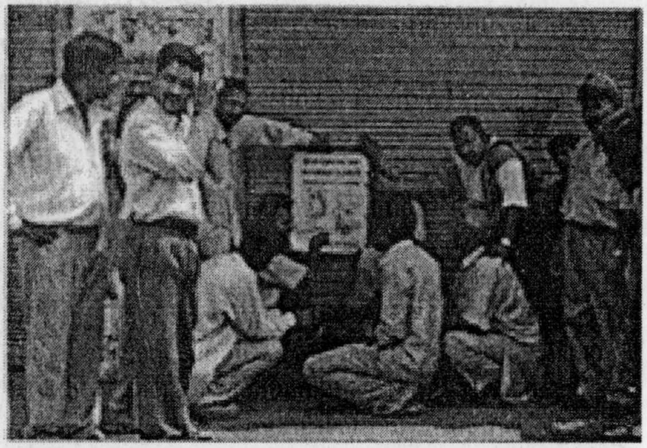

(a)

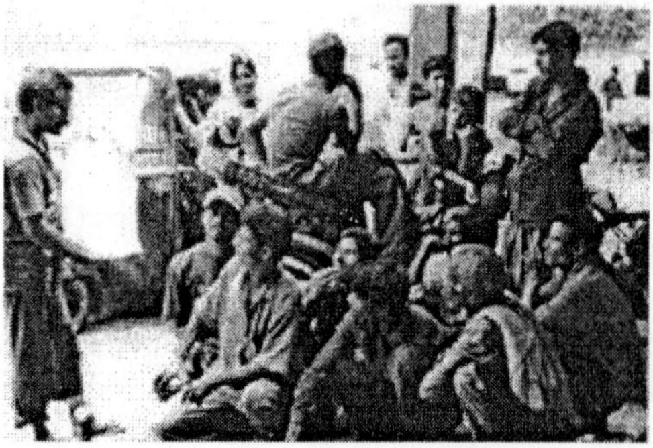

(b)

Picture 19 : Peer Educators Disseminating AIDS Awareness among Truck Drivers.

Based on the pre-intervention knowledge assessment, an awareness campaign was created for the benefit of the sample. Knowledge with regards to HIV/AIDS was imparted by using various audio-visual aids designed by a few HIV/AIDS prevention organizations (listed in Appendix XI) as well as through the use of audio-visual aids specially designed during the period of study, keeping in mind the needs of the sample communities. Simple pictures and charts highlighting the modes of HIV transmission, symptoms of HIV infection and prevention from HIV/AIDS (incorporated in the photo-script) were crafted and extensively used in accordance with the needs of the sample.

Similarly, short stories and skits related to different aspects of HIV/AIDS were staged before the sample in order to present the otherwise raw and complex information in an easy to understand as well as humourous manner. The sample took keen interest in viewing these presentations as they could easily identify themselves with the story characters. For instance, during the presentation of the photo-script many truck drivers and rickshaw pullers identified themselves to be in same circumstances as the hero of the story and admitted that they now perceived themselves to be at risk of acquiring the disease due to their continued indulgence in unprotected behaviour with non-regular partners just like the script-hero. Such presentations apart from filling some excitement and humour in the lives of the sample also helped the sample to retain the information conveyed through such modes.

Similarly, the poster developed during the study period depicting a few happy-looking truck drivers was effectively used with the sample in order to motivate them to be happy in a similar way after acquiring knowledge regarding HIV/AIDS. Overall, the impact of the intervention on the sample was significant in terms of the increase in their knowledge level as described in the proceeding sections.

Knowledge Assessment : Post-intervention

The results show that the sample exhibited a significant increase in knowledge regarding various aspects of HIV/AIDS from the pre- to post- intervention period. The changes in knowledge level as reflected by the difference in mean scores scored by the three sample groups during the pre- and post-intervention periods are shown in Fig. 3.29.

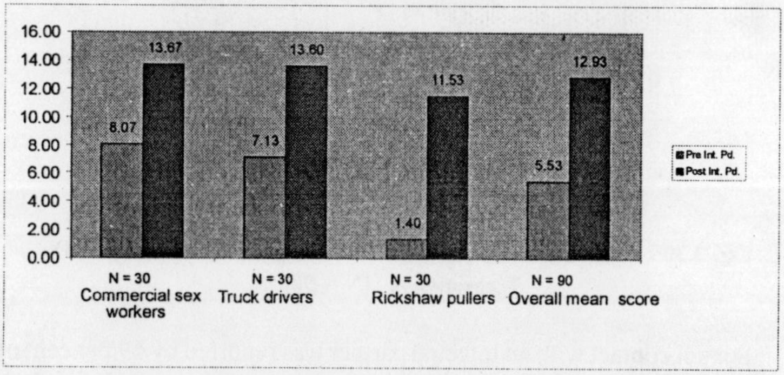

Fig. 3.29 : Mean Scores during Pre- and Post-intervention Period.

The post-intervention evaluations showed that the intervention had a positive impact on the sample's knowledge level regarding HIV/AIDS and the mean score rose to 13.67, 13.60 and 11.53 for the commercial sex workers, truck drivers and rickshaw pullers respectively. The overall mean score for the entire sample rose from 5.53 to 12.93 out of a total of 20. Considerable improvement was recorded in the overall score for each participant. Some of the major changes recorded on the knowledge scale have been described as follows:

Twenty per cent of the sample, which was totally unaware about AIDS prior to the intervention, was now aware of it. The awareness level of AIDS as a disease rose from 80 per cent in the pre-intervention period to a total of 100 per cent in the post-intervention period.

The knowledge regarding modes of HIV transmission also showed a significant increase in terms of the number of modes known to the sample.

As compared to the pre-intervention data in which only 47 per cent of the sample knew about other modes of HIV transmission apart from sex, in the post-intervention data, 100 per cent of the sample reported other HIV transmission modes too, apart from sex. This was very vital as it helped in increasing the sample's perceived vulnerability to HIV/AIDS through other modes of HIV transmission. Fig. 3.30 portrays the marked difference in the sample's awareness level regarding different modes of HIV transmission during the pre- and post-intervention stages.

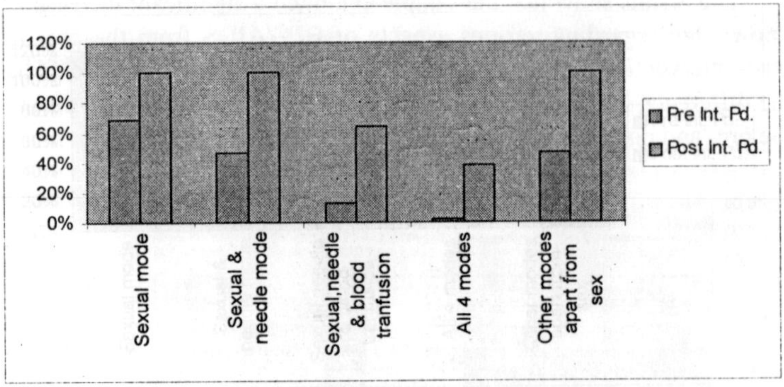

Fig. 3.30 : Changes in Awareness Level Regarding Modes of HIV Transmission (N = 90).

Sexual contact with an infected partner was reported by 69 per cent of the sample as a HIV transmission mode during the pre-intervention period, whereas 100 per cent of the sample reported it as a transmitting factor in the post-intervention period. Similarly, two modes which are sex with an infected partner and use of a contaminated needle for injecting purposes were reported by 47 per cent of the sample as HIV transmitting agents in the pre-intervention period, and by 100 per cent individuals in the post-intervention period. The level of awareness regarding three modes of HIV transmission viz. sexual contact, use of contaminated needle and by transfusion with infected blood rose from 13 per cent to 64 per cent during the course of intervention. It is important to notice that prior to the intervention only 2 per cent of the respondents were aware about all the four HIV transmission modes whereas after the intervention 38 per cent of the respondents showed awareness about all the four HIV transmission modes.

Maximum changes were observed in the knowledge levels related to the symptoms of HIV/AIDS. As compared to a single truck driver (2 per cent) having knowledge about the symptoms of the disease prior to the intervention, 62 per cent of the sample could recall at least one symptom during the post-intervention period whereas 18 per cent were able to mention two or more symptoms. This crucial change was brought about as a result of role-play presentations given before the sample. For example, three individuals enacting the symptoms of prolonged fever, diarrhoea and weight loss were presented before the sample indicating the onset of AIDS disease. Such presentations made it easier for the study participants to remember symptoms of AIDS, which otherwise appeared so difficult to them to memorize. This knowledge was of prime importance in helping the sample for initial self-assessment purposes related to the onset of the disease if and when it occurred. Only 20 per cent of the sample comprising mostly of the CSWs and rickshaw pullers was not able to recall any symptom of the disease. The reason for this could be best explained in view of extremely high levels of illiteracy amongst these two groups (90 per cent) coupled with low memorizing capacity.

The awareness regarding HIV testing procedure as well as the availability of these services in various hospitals rose from 38 per cent to 95 per cent and from 49 per cent to 100 per cent respectively. This helped the sample in putting aside their fears that HIV testing was a difficult and expensive procedure. Further, the concept of fatality of AIDS was registered among 82 per cent of the entire sample as compared to only 33 per cent during the pre-intervention period. The complacency of the sample that AIDS could be cured needed to be put to rest in order to bring down their risk behaviour. Although no fear-based messages were used to address the fatality of the disease yet, it was emphasized that AIDS was incurable and would surely lead to death. Hence, prevention as a prime necessity was stressed upon.

HIV preventive methods were most emphasized during the entire period of intervention as the study was all about HIV/AIDS prevention. The rise in knowledge regarding various HIV transmission modes was accompanied by a similar rise in awareness regarding HIV prevention from those modes.

In contrast to the pre-intervention notion, held by 23 per cent of the truck drivers and rickshaw pullers that avoiding sex with commercial sex workers was an effective way of HIV prevention, the post-intervention results showed that 72 per cent of the truck drivers and rickshaw pullers had started perceiving casual sex partners too as a source of HIV. Thus, all of these agreed that safe sex was to be practiced as a preventive measure with all the sexual partners outside marriage. Similarly, the level of awareness regarding other HIV prevention methods increased considerably as is shown in Fig. 3.31.

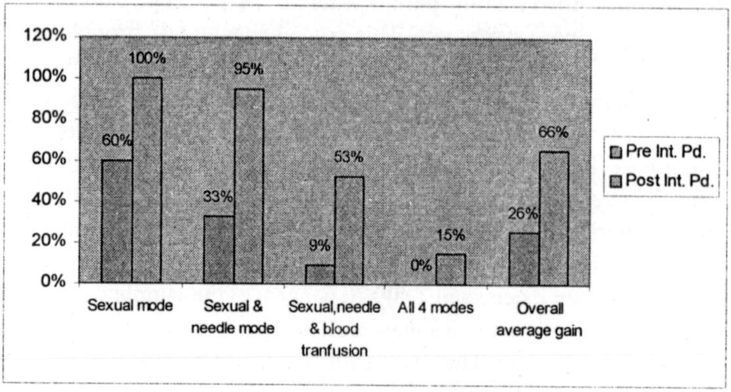

Fig. 3.31 : Changes in Awareness Level Regarding Methods of HIV Prevention (N = 90).

During the post-intervention period 100 per cent of the sample was aware that practicing safe sex could prevent HIV transmission in contrast to 60 per cent of the sample during the pre-intervention period. Similarly, 95 per cent of the sample was aware about two HIV preventive modes (i.e., safe sex and use of clean needles) as compared to 33 per cent in the pre intervention study and 53 per cent was aware about three prevention modes (i.e., safe sex, use of clean needles and safe blood transfusion if required) in contrast to 9 per cent prior to the intervention. It is significant to observe that the awareness level regarding all the four preventive modes including prevention of mother to child transmission rose from a base of zero to 15 per cent. An overall average gain of 40 per cent i.e., from 26 per cent to 66 per cent was recorded from the pre- to post-intervention period in the sample's awareness regarding various HIV prevention methods.

The sample's perception of acquiring HIV/AIDS showed a major shift. Along with HIV/AIDS awareness came the realization amongst the sample that they were not immune to the disease, irrespective of any shots or the HIV testing they had gone through. This aspect was powerfully staged before the sample with a view of putting an end to their complacency regarding the acquiring of disease. Two peer educators (i.e., one acting as a doctor and the other as a person practicing high-risk behaviour) were prepared to present a short skit. A scene showing the doctor emphasizing the fact to a person practicing high-risk behaviour that inspite of his being tested HIV negative previously he still was at risk of acquiring the disease by virtue of his continued indulgence in unsafe behaviour with non-regular partners was very effective in communicating the futility of HIV testing procedures as it's preventive method amongst the sample groups. Fig. 3.32 shows the difference in the level of perception related to HIV/AIDS vulnerability during the pre- and post-intervention periods amongst the sample exposed to various forms of high-risk practices.

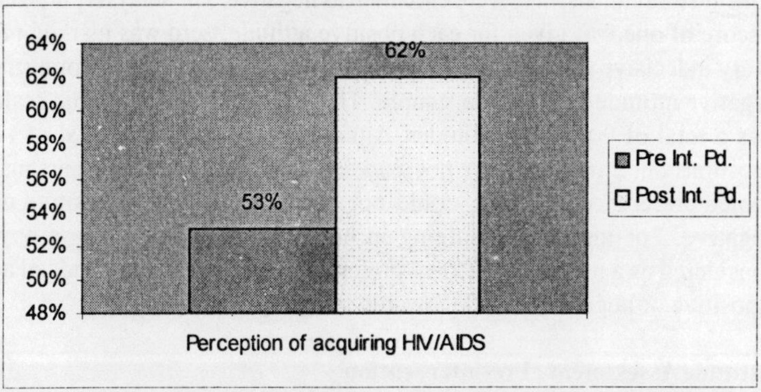

Base : Sample exposed to various high-risk practices (N = 76)

Fig. 3.32 : Changes in Level of Perception Regarding HIV/AIDS Vulnerability.

Overall, the perception of acquiring HIV/AIDS amongst the sample exposed to various forms of high-risk practices was only 53 per cent prior to the intervention. However, in the post intervention period, 62 per cent of such sample indicated that they now perceived themselves to be at risk of HIV/AIDS due to their indulgence in various risky practices.

Although there were major and significant overall changes in the pre- and post-intervention data yet, it was observed that majority of the respondents (98 per cent) were unable to recall the name of the virus, i.e., HIV as AIDS causing factor. The reason behind this was the English pronunciation of the word, which seemed complex to the sample to comprehend because of their illiteracy. Hence, no undue stress was placed on them to memorize the name of the virus. However, 2 per cent of the sample was able to mention "virus" as the source of HIV infection in the post-intervention period.

Attitude Assessment Scale

The attitude of the sample regarding sex and sexuality, gender based differences and towards people living with or affected with HIV/AIDS (PWHA) was assessed on the attitude assessment scale (Appendix IX). The attitudes were classified as positive if they favoured HIV risk reduction and prevented stigma towards PWHA. Contrary to this, if they were found to be increasing HIV vulnerability or social discrimination of infected or affected individuals, they were classified as negative. For analysis purpose, a score of one was given for each positive attitude, zero was marked for every indecisive response while a score of minus one was given for every negative attitude held by the sample. The maximum score on this scale was a total of 9 positive attitudes. Although the scale had a total of 11 questions but 2 of these were not marked as they were a matter-personal choice/preference and thus, could not be judged as being positive or negative. For instance, indulging in homosexual relationship is now considered as a matter of personal preference and thus can't be judged as a positive or negative attitude towards sexuality.

Attitude Assessment : Pre-intervention

The attitudes of the three different groups regarding various aspects of HIV/AIDS were varied and complex.

Fig. 3.33 shows the mean scores of positive attitudes held by the three sample groups.

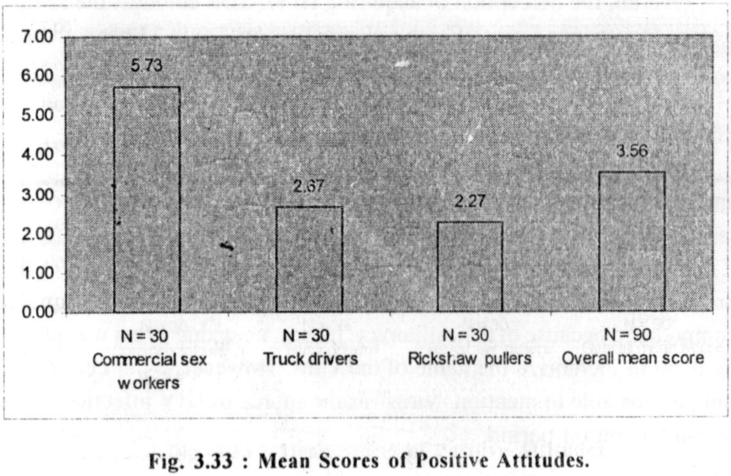

Fig. 3.33 : Mean Scores of Positive Attitudes.

The mean score for the commercial sex workers was 5.73, for truck drivers 2.67 and for rickshaw pullers it was a mere 2.27 out of a total of 9. The overall mean score for the entire sample was 3.56 out of a total of 9. Commercial sex workers scored a fairly high score in having positive attitudes primarily because of gender-related differences. These women had positive attitude for most of the queried aspects because harbouring any negative attitude would have affected them adversely. The women were at the receiving end for most of the negatively held attitudes. This concept becomes clearer in the proceeding findings.

It was heartening to see that (76 per cent) of the sample was of the opinion that education regarding sex, HIV/AIDS and STD should be given to the masses including appropriately aged children in schools. The sample also felt that there was a lack of services, which could deliver such information.

Almost the entire sample (96 per cent) said that they came from rural settings where talking about sex and sexuality still remained a big taboo. Bharat (cited in Mathai, et al., 1997), in her related study has minutely observed the same - "Young girls often observe older women and follow the same trend". Thus, this model of knowledge transmission continues being followed from generation to generation. The "culture of silence" thus prevails (Mathai, et al., 1997). In order to contain the spread of HIV, it is vital to break this culture of silence and talk freely about all the information that is needed to protect precious lives from HIV/AIDS. Contrary to the general assumption that talking about sex and sexuality exposes young children to adult behaviour at an early stage, it has been found that such programmes may successfully change attitude towards sex and the promiscuous behaviour (Baldo, et al., 1993; Brooks-Gunn & Paikoff, 1992; Kirby, 1992 cited in Mathai, et al., 1997).

However, 24 per cent of the sample in the present study comprising mostly of the truck drivers and rickshaw pullers said that women and children should not be given sexual, HIV/AIDS and STD education. The reason cited for this attitude being that children are too small to understand such issues whereas women are barred by socio-cultural factors to discuss sexual matters. Some of the rickshaw pullers had conclusively remarked - "*Aurtein hamare samaaj mein aisee baat nahin kartin*" meaning "Women in our society do not talk about all this". Although, various such inequities are known to contribute to the vulnerability of women yet, nearly 1/3rd of countries lack policies ensuring women's equal access to critical prevention and care services (UNAIDS, 2003). Some 65 million girls worldwide are kept out of school, increasing their risks of suffering from extreme poverty, dying during childbirth or from AIDS and further passing these dangers to future generations (UNICEF cited in *Times of India*, Dec.12, 2003). Contrarily, an effective response to contain the spread of HIV/AIDS requires enforcement of policies, which while addressing gender dimensions also ensure an equal access of basic prevention services to women too.

Regarding attitude towards having homosexual, premarital and extramarital relationships, it was surprising to see that several respondents had liberal views, given their conservative rural and socio-cultural background. Fifty-three per cent of the sample felt that there was nothing wrong in having such relationships provided they were done by mutual consent. The present data shows that individuals, who ever had or were still during the pre-intervention period indulging in homosexual/premarital/extramarital sex, were more likely (75 per cent v/s 29 per cent) to endorse these relationships as a matter of personal choice rather than considering them as wrongful deeds in comparison to the sample who had not indulged in such acts. Here it is important to add that in the case of CSWs their indulgence in pre/extramarital sex with regards to their condoning of such behaviour was considered prior to their entry into the sex trade, as practicing sex work by them now which too accounted for pre/extramarital sex, was considered to be an economic necessity rather than a matter of personal choice.

The responsibility of using a contraceptive during sexual relationship was an aspect, which showed vast gender-based differentiation. Fig. 3.34 depicts the difference in attitude of men and women regarding responsibility to use a contraceptive.

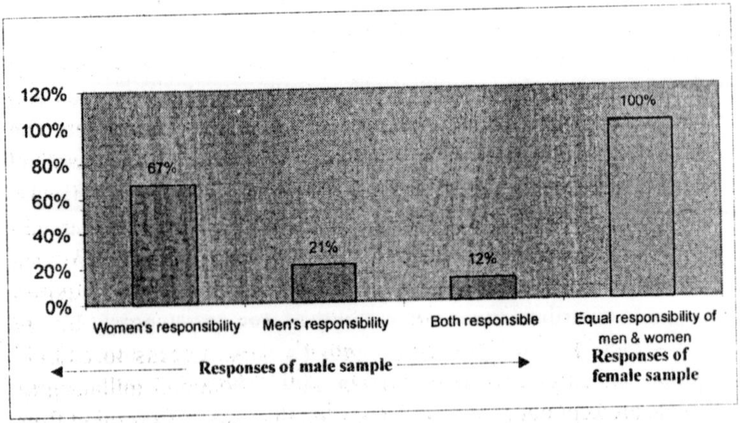

Fig. 3.34: Difference in Attitude Regarding Responsibility to Use a Contraceptive (N = 90).

Sixty-seven per cent of the men said that it was only women's responsibility to use a contraceptive, 21 per cent said that only men were responsible for the same, whereas only 12 per cent of them agreed that either of the partners could use a contraceptive on the basis of mutual consent. On the other hand, the entire female sample comprising of all the sex workers said that using a contraceptive should not only be a women's liability all the time and that men should also be equally responsible for the same.

The unreasonable and unlimited male dominance is evident from the fact that when asked as to who should take a decision regarding when and which contraceptive was to be used, 78 per cent of the men said that it was a man's prerogative to decide when and which contraceptive was to be used. This in essence means that men wanted women to use a method of contraception which men liked and also at the time when they liked. So deeply ingrained is the problem of gender inequality in our society that according to a recent Human Development Report cited in *Times of India* (Dec.12, 2003), it may not be tackled before the year 2050.

As far as the vulnerability to HIV/AIDS and STD was concerned it was observed that there were again vast gender-based variations. Men and women held each other responsible for their vulnerability to such diseases. Fig. 3.35 depicts the attitude of men and women with regards to vulnerability to HIV/AIDS and STD.

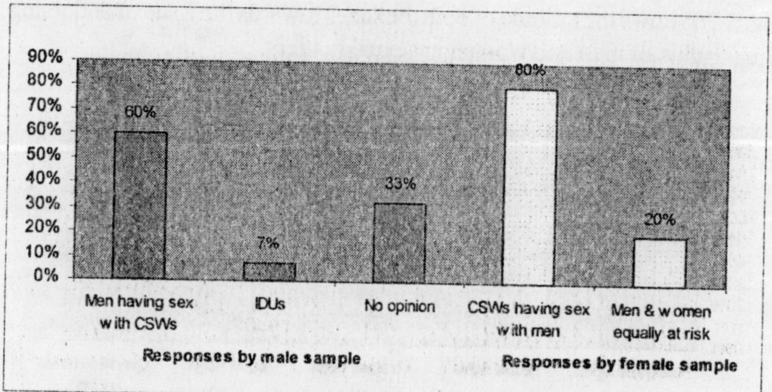

Fig. 3.35: Attitude with Regards to Vulnerability to HIV/AIDS and STD (N = 90).

Sixty per cent of the male sample said that men having sex with commercial sex workers were only prone to HIV/AIDS and STD since commercial sex workers mostly had such diseases. Seven per cent of the men said that injecting drug users (IDUs) could also be vulnerable to HIV/AIDS because of needle sharing practices. Except these two categories no other category was reported by men to be vulnerable to HIV/AIDS and STD. Further 33 per cent of the male sample could not opine regarding the vulnerability aspect related to HIV/AIDS and STD due to their lack of awareness regarding these diseases. Here it is important to note that contrary to the male sample, majority of the commercial sex workers (80 per cent) were of the firm opinion that it was not men who were at the risk of contracting HIV/AIDS and STD by virtue of their having sex with commercial sex workers, rather it was the sex workers who were at risk of acquiring various infections as these men had various diseases. However, 20 per cent of the CSWs (representing only 7 per cent of the entire sample) said that men and women were equally at risk of acquiring HIV/AIDS due to various factors.

Thus, the data clearly shows that the attitude towards HIV/AIDS vulnerability was divided on the basis of service provider and service user status. The service providers, i.e., the sex workers felt that they were exposed to HIV/AIDS risk because of their clients whereas the clients (i.e., the service users) felt that they were at the risk of contracting HIV/AIDS because of the sex workers.

Another major gender based difference was realized in the attitude regarding rights of men and women in matters related to sex and sexuality. Fig. 3.36 shows the attitude of both the sexes towards the issue of endorsing equal rights of men and women in sexual matters.

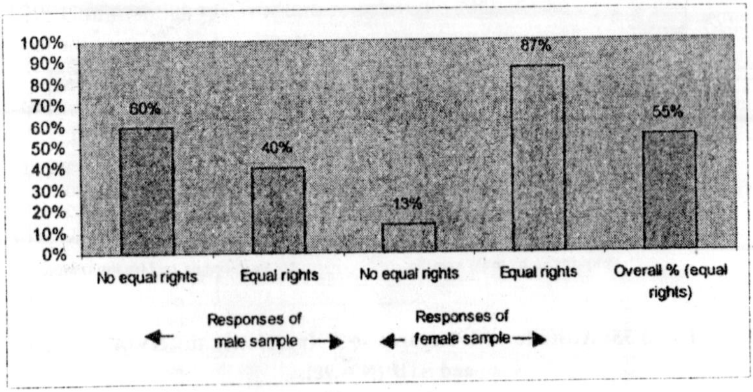

Fig. 3.36: Attitude Endorsing Equal Rights of Men and Women (N = 90).

On being asked if women should have equal rights as men to take decisions and assert themselves in sexual matters, 60 per cent of the men replied in the negative. Various reasons pertaining to socio-cultural ethos were cited for maintaining this inequality, which primarily included social and cultural factors. Fifty-six per cent of these men said that their culture did not approve of women talking about sex or sexual rights. As a matter of fact, they reiterated their stand by observing that no such knowledge, information or experiences endorsing women's equality in sexual matters were passed on to them traditionally. All of them agreed that they belonged to conservative families where women were not expected to address issues like sex and sexuality, methods of contraception, STD, condom use etc. Their culture demanded especially women to be religious minded, morally upright and barred them from expressing their sexuality. Taboos on sexuality and religious influences are stronger in poor women (Bianco, et al., 1996). Thus, talking about and asserting their sexual rights still remains a distant possibility for such women. Similar findings have also been reported by Maine & Maitra (cited in Mathai & Hira, 1997) who have identified the cultural stereotypes about gender appropriate sexual behaviour as a constraint to HIV/AIDS prevention.

Thirty-three per cent of the men condoning inequality of women's sexual rights also said that apart from their culture, the society in which they live did not endorse the idea of women having equal sexual rights as men. According to them, women have always been subordinate to men and at best they can make good homemakers. All vital decisions have been taken by men, they said so. Thus, sexuality for them was also a man's domain. Eleven per cent of such sample said that since men were more experienced in different aspects of life as compared to women thus, they needed to have more rights as they could exercise them in a rightful manner. This was applicable to all aspects including sexual matters.

The overall view that emerges from these findings is that men have been socially and culturally conditioned in a manner, which upholds their dominance over women in all aspects of life including sex and sexuality. It therefore appeared that the spread of HIV/AIDS could not be contained without bringing about a radical change in the anti-women attitude, still persisting among the male society. Only 40 per cent of the male sample was in favour of granting equal sexual rights to women as men.

Contrary to the men's attitude, 87 per cent of the sex workers said that women should have equal rights as men regarding matters related to sex and sexuality while 13 per cent of the sex workers maintained that women could not be at par with men in context of such rights. Overall, only 55 per cent of the entire sample endorsed equality of sexual rights among men and women.

Rights of people living with HIV/AIDS (PWHA) was a critical issue taken up during the course of study. Ironically, according to a recent ILO research some 70 per cent of people living with HIV/AIDS in India reported to have faced discrimination, most commonly within families and in health care settings. Discrimination and stigma remain one of the greatest barriers to preventing further infections, providing adequate care, support and treatment, and alleviating the epidemic's impact (UNAIDS/WHO, Dec., 2003). Hence, it becomes vital to eliminate all forms of discrimination against, and ensure equal rights to PWHA. With a view of mobilizing community support towards PWHA, the equality of rights of PWHA was touched upon in the present study. A significant trend pointing towards discrimination of people living with HIV/AIDS was observed among the sample based on their myths and misconceptions regarding the disease. Fig. 3. 37 shows the attitude of the sample towards rights of people living with HIV/AIDS.

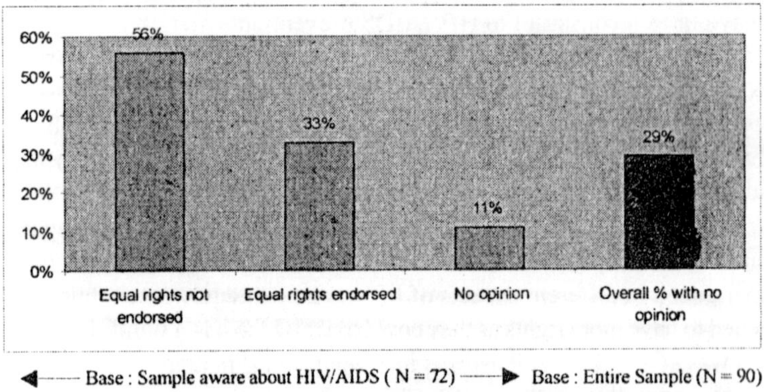

Fig. 3.37 : Attitude towards PWHA.

Fifty-six per cent of the sample who was aware about HIV/AIDS was of the firm opinion that people living with or affected by HIV/AIDS should be segregated in the better interest of the larger society and that they should not have equal rights as compared to an uninfected individual. Many reasons were given for advocating inequality of rights along with segregation of infected people. Most of the reasons were based on myths and misconceptions of the sample regarding HIV/AIDS.

For instance, 55 per cent of such sample said that since HIV/AIDS spreads through air thus, an HIV infected person needs to be isolated from others. Similarly, misconceptions like HIV could spread by sitting with an infected person (45 per cent) and by sharing utensils, clothes, soap, food, water, and cigarettes (40 per cent) were commonly cited as reasons supporting isolation of HIV positive individuals. The responses add up to more than 100 per cent because of multiple responses registered in case of some individuals.

Only 33 per cent of the sample that was aware about AIDS opined that HIV infected people should have similar rights as any uninfected individual while 11 per cent of them were unable to give any opinion due to their lack of awareness regarding this aspect of HIV/AIDS. Here it is important to note that overall 29 per cent of the entire sample was not able to opine about the equality of rights of HIV/AIDS infected people due to their lack of knowledge regarding the disease.

Similarly, it is very important to observe that 50 per cent of the sample who had heard about HIV/AIDS felt that if one of the spouse tested HIV positive then, he or she should be abandoned by the other partner. The decision of leaving one's positive partner stemmed from the fear of getting infected. This was again based on myths/misconceptions like HIV/AIDS could spread by a mere touch or by living with an infected person. Similarly, 25 per cent of the sample that had heard about AIDS said that they were not sure as to what would they do if their spouse tested HIV positive. Ironically, 67 per cent of the sample that knew about AIDS as a disease believed that AIDS was a God's way of punishing people for their infidelity and thus people abandoned on the basis of their HIV status rightfully deserved their fate. As far as the rights of children living with HIV/AIDS were concerned, 55 per cent of the sample that had heard about AIDS said that HIV positive children should not to be allowed to study with HIV negative children because of the risk of HIV transmission through casual contact.

Thus, it is evident that an attitude of discrimination stemming from various myths and misconceptions was prevalent amongst the sample against people living with HIV/AIDS. Discrimination based on myths and misconceptions in similar communities have also been reported by Sehgal (1997); Bhave, et al. (1995) and Singh, et al. (1994). Kashyap (2002) while highlighting the issue of discrimination against people living with HIV/AIDS reported that misconceptions about the disease had only added up to the problems of those living with or affected by HIV/AIDS. A recent report revealing the denial of admission by various schools to HIV positive children (*Times of India*, July 18, 2003) shows the intensity of discrimination being practiced presumably on the basis of misconceptions even by educationists as well as educational institutes. Some of these children are still forced to take school lessons and write their exams at home, despite appeals from several high-ranking officials. A lack of knowledge about the virus (often flanked by denigrating attitudes towards PWHA) remains an important factor in fuelling discrimination (UNAIDS/WHO, Dec., 2003).

Consequently, more efforts are needed to dispel myths and misconceptions of such communities to decrease levels of discrimination towards PWHA. Further, IEC programmes also need to effectively address the fears and the baseless apprehensions of the people. This is as important as the knowledge regarding HIV transmission.

On being asked as to whose responsibility was it to protect the family from HIV/AIDS, it is interesting to note that 43 per cent of the truck drivers and rickshaw pullers who had heard about AIDS promptly replied that both husband and wife were equally responsible for safeguarding their family from HIV/AIDS. Although, the attitude was positive as it gave equal opportunity and power to each husband and wife to protect their family from HIV/AIDS, in reality the women did not enjoy the right or the freedom to practice safe sex. Fig. 3.38 depicts the onus (attitude) of the sample towards protection of their family from HIV/AIDS.

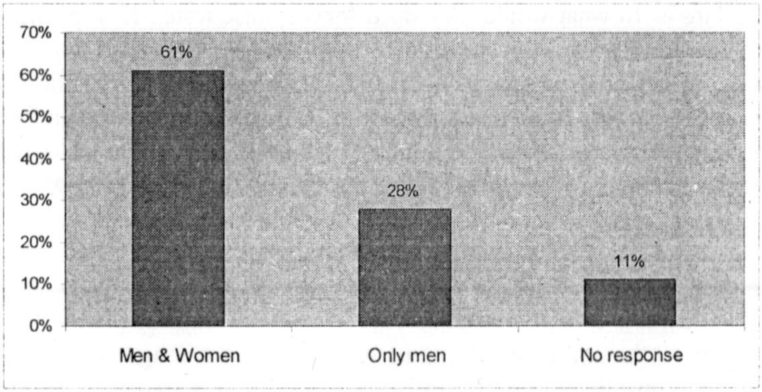

Base : Sample that had heard about HIV/AIDS (N=72).

Fig. 3.38: Onus of Protecting One's Family from HIV/AIDS.

Overall, the responses regarding the responsibility of protecting one's family from HIV/AIDS amongst the sample who had heard about the disease were recorded in the order as responsibility of both men and women 61 per cent and only men's responsibility 28 per cent. No response could be registered for 11 per cent of the sample during the pre-intervention period, as they were unable to comment on this issue.

The intention to get oneself HIV tested was recorded to be quite low among the sample due to their ignorance regarding modes as well as the chances of acquiring HIV. Only 31 per cent of the entire sample during the pre-intervention period indicated that they wanted to be tested for HIV. Further, the intention to get oneself HIV tested was found to be directly linked to the perceived vulnerability of the sample to HIV/AIDS. Individuals who did not perceive themselves to be at risk of HIV/AIDS were less likely (13 per cent v/s 71 per cent) to opt for voluntary HIV testing as compared to those who perceived vulnerability to the disease. Observation depicting a similar relationship between perceived vulnerability to HIV/AIDS and the intention to get HIV tested has also been reported by Kurth, et al. (1996). Thus, the findings suggest that increasing sample's perception to HIV vulnerability can help a lot in raising their intention to get HIV tested.

Similarly, value formation among the sample has been recognized as a crucial factor leading to behavioural change. According to Josefina & Tayag (1996) values form the basis of an individual's behaviour and provide norms and guidelines for his/her choices in life. In her study on sex workers, the value system upheld by the sex workers was found to determine their choices of work as well as adoption of high-risk practices in regard to HIV/AIDS and STD. Similarly, low self-esteem resulting from low self-worth has been identified as a major determinant to HIV prevention in various studies (Halloran, et al., 1996; Koo, et al., 1996). Thus, keeping in mind the importance of value framework and it's impact on high-risk behaviour the present study tried to delve into some of the relevant values held by the sample with special reference to their families.

Seventy-three per cent of the sample was found to have a positive attitude towards their lives and valued goals such as rearing their children into good human beings and making their families comfortable and at ease. They all said that they wanted their families to lead a good life and were working hard to achieve this goal. This concept of giving a good life to their family members was later used as a collectivist theme focusing on wife, children and other family members for creating HIV/AIDS prevention awareness among them. Unfortunately, 27 per cent of the sample was found to possess a negative attitude in terms of feelings of helplessness and frustration perceived in their lives. Efforts were directed to incorporate amongst them a positive value formation component, which stressed on the need to lead a meaningful and responsible life. The basic idea was to gear up HIV/AIDS prevention by increasing a sense of self-esteem, worthiness and responsibility amongst them.

The intervention – ***a review***

Focus group discussions and group talks were effectively used to address issues like sex and sexuality, gender-based differentiation in various aspects, cultural stereotypes and sexual orientation, with the aim of bringing about desired changes in the attitudes of the sample regarding the same in context to HIV/AIDS. Similarly, hypothetical questions were raised while presenting short stories/skits (i.e., provocative theatre) to the sample in order to challenge their deeply held attitudes that were found to be promoting gender-based discrimination with reference to HIV/AIDS. For example, a recent report of a woman being stoned to death due to her HIV positive status (*Hindustan Times,* July 10, 2003) was taken up as an issue with the sample. It was hypothetically asked if men also deserved the same fate as women on the basis of their seropositivity. To this, when most of the men replied negative, then the appropriateness of discrimination against HIV positive women was duly questioned. Such thought-provoking efforts helped the sample realize the futility of irrational attitudes. Similarly, attitudes towards various issues like rights of children and people living with HIV/AIDS, equality of both genders in matters pertaining to sex, sexuality and reviewing of cultural stereotypes were elaborately discussed to bring about the desired changes in the same.

Attitude Assessment : Post-intervention

Post-intervention results showed major changes in attitudes of the sample regarding various issues related to HIV/AIDS. Fig. 3.39 shows the level of change in attitudes among the three sample groups from the pre- to post-intervention period.

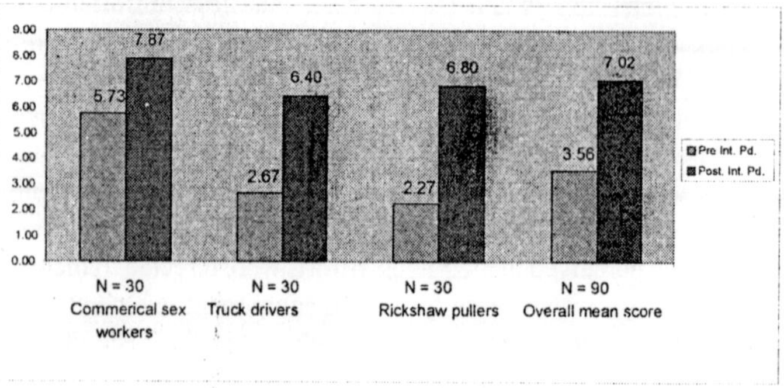

Fig. 3.39 : Level of Change in Attitudes among the Three Sample Groups as shown by the Mean Scores.

The mean score on the attitude assessment scale was recorded to be 7.87 for the CSWs, 6.40 for the truck drivers and for the rickshaw pullers it was 6.80 out of a total of 9. The overall mean score for the entire sample rose from 3.56 in the pre-intervention period to 7.02 during the post-intervention period out of a total of 9. The major changes observed in attitudes of the sample are described as follows:

Out of 24 per cent of the sample who were against giving HIV/AIDS education to women and children during the pre-intervention period, 20 per cent got convinced during the post intervention period and agreed that such information should be given to women and children as well to ensure their protection from the virus. Yet, it was observed that 4 per cent of such sample still maintained that giving HIV/AIDS, STD and sex education to women and children could do more harm than any good. The data shows that elderly people (i.e., aged 35 years and above as compared to the younger sample in the present study) were more likely (33 per cent v/s 20 per cent) to believe that sex education need not be given to women and children, as they feared this would expose them to immoral behaviour. Similar findings documenting rigidness and conservative opinion related to sexual matters among the elderly people have also been reported by Krizansky, et al. (1996). Policy-makers need to realize that HIV prevention requires a deep attitudinal change and this process must start early in life. The older a person gets, the more difficult becomes the process to change his/her attitude.

The attitude regarding having homosexual/pre/extra-marital sexual relations also showed a considerable change as shown in Fig. 3.40.

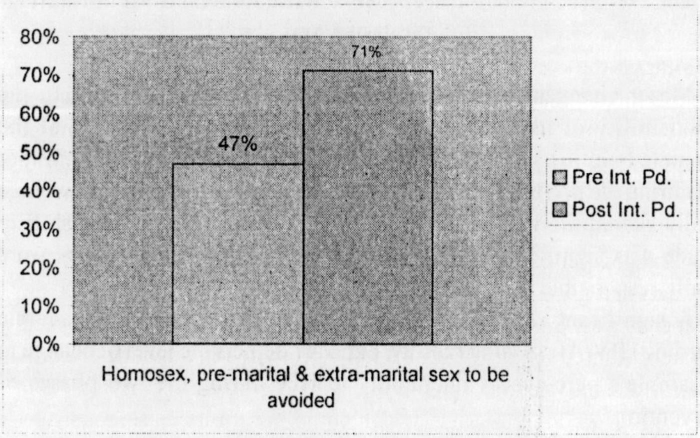

Fig. 3.40: Attitude regarding having Homosexual, Pre/extra marital Sexual Relations (N = 90).

The percentage of sample that believed that homosexual, pre-marital and extra-marital sexual relations should be avoided rose from 47 per cent during the pre-intervention period to 71 per cent in the post-intervention period. This change reflected an increase in awareness level of the sample that indulgence in such behaviours could enhance HIV transmission risk.

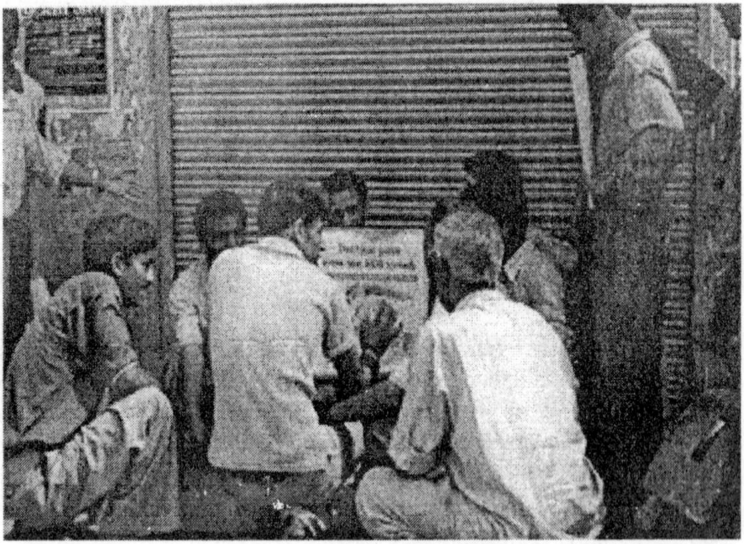

Picture 20: Focus Group Discussions to Raise Awareness against having Unprotected Sex.

Major changes were also observed in the attitude related to the responsibility of using a contraceptive. Seventy-five per cent of the respondents in the post-intervention period as compared to only 42 per cent during the pre-intervention period now believed that men and women equally shared the responsibility of using a contraceptive. This shift in attitude was significant in terms of recognition by men that they were equally responsible in matters pertaining to contraceptive usage.

A significant change was noticed in the perception of the sample regarding HIV/AIDS vulnerability. Fig. 3.41 depicts the level of change in the sample's perceived vulnerability to HIV during the two phases of intervention.

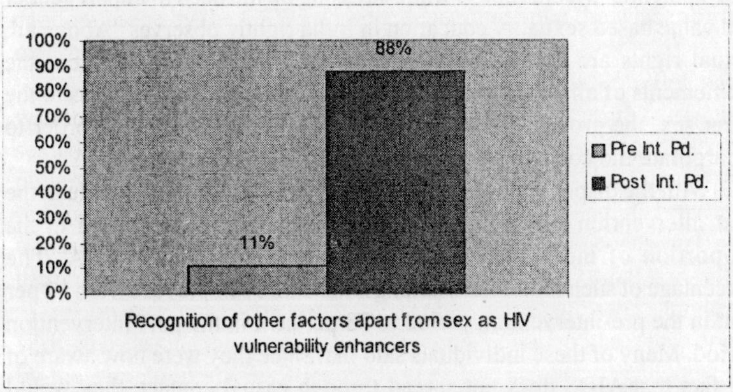

Fig. 3.41 : Change in Perceived Vulnerability to HIV/AIDS (N = 90).

During the post-intervention period 88 per cent of the sample as against only 11 per cent during the pre-intervention period had realized that only individuals having sex with CSWs were not at risk of STD, HIV/AIDS and that sex was not the only factor enhancing HIV vulnerability. The other modes of HIV transmission like contaminated needle and syringe sharing, transfusion by infected blood and mother to child transmission were equally seen as HIV vulnerability enhancers. This change in perception would help a long way in warding off the stigma attached to HIV/AIDS as a disease caused by sex with sex workers.

Regarding equality of rights in matters related to sex and sexuality, 84 per cent of the sample in the post-intervention period as against 55 per cent during the pre-intervention agreed that women should have similar rights as men in sexual matters. Another important finding related to this aspect was that men indulging in pre/extramarital sexual acts were more likely (33 per cent v/s 11 per cent) to condone gender-based inequality as compared to those who did not indulge in such acts. This was expected of them, as advocating equal sexual rights would have meant giving women too the similar right to indulge in pre/extramarital sex which by no means was acceptable to them.

Contrary to this, still in many societies across the globe, fulfilling sexual needs outside marriage is generally accepted for men whereas women are ostracized for the same behaviour (Bharat, 1996). The issue highlights the need to put an end to gender-based inequality especially in matters pertaining to sexuality, in order to contain the further spread of the

HIV epidemic. Mehra (2003) while stressing on the need to impart gender and value based sexuality education in India rightly observes "Above all, sexual rights are human rights and not privileges or favours, but the entitlements of all young women and men." Thus, to yield fairness to the fairer sex, the process of socialization needs to be modified in order to incorporate the concept of equality of both genders in all respects.

With the dispelling of myths and misconceptions of the sample in the post intervention period, a considerable increase was recorded in the proportion of individuals advocating equal rights for PWHA. The percentage of such individuals amongst the entire sample rose from 27 per cent in the pre-intervention period to 73 per cent in the post-intervention period. Many of these individuals said that since they were now aware of the fact that AIDS does not spread through casual contact, they would not discriminate against any person living with HIV/AIDS. Similarly, the idea of separating from or deserting a HIV+ spouse showed a major decline. Seventy-six per cent of the sample during the post-intervention period as compared against mere 25 per cent prior to the intervention, said that a HIV+ spouse need not be abandoned but rather looked after by the other partner. This change was a result of the fact that casual contact was no longer considered as a threat of HIV/AIDS.

It was further observed that the protection of one's family from HIV/AIDS was no more considered to be only a man's domain. Eighty-nine per cent of the entire sample in the post-intervention period as compared to only 49 per cent prior to the intervention agreed that men and women should be equally responsible to protect their families from HIV/AIDS. This awareness is expected to help men in realizing that women have a right to ask them for safe sex in the interest of the family. Similarly, it is also expected that women will seriously think about their duty to protect their families from HIV/AIDS and thus take necessary action including assertion of their right for safe sex with their sexual partner/s.

The intention of the sample to opt for voluntary HIV testing showed a significant increase during the post intervention period. Fig. 3.42 shows the level of change among the sample in terms of their option for voluntary HIV testing as well as perceived self-vulnerability to HIV/AIDS.

Sixty-nine per cent of the sample in the post-intervention period opted for HIV testing as against 31 per cent during the pre-intervention period. This increase substantiates the fact that the sample's perception of self-vulnerability to HIV/AIDS increased as a result of the present intervention. The level of perceived self-vulnerability to HIV/AIDS amongst the entire sample rose from 31 per cent to 64 per cent during the course of intervention.

These results suggest that the sample had now started showing abilities to introspect their behaviour in context of acquiring the HIV infection.

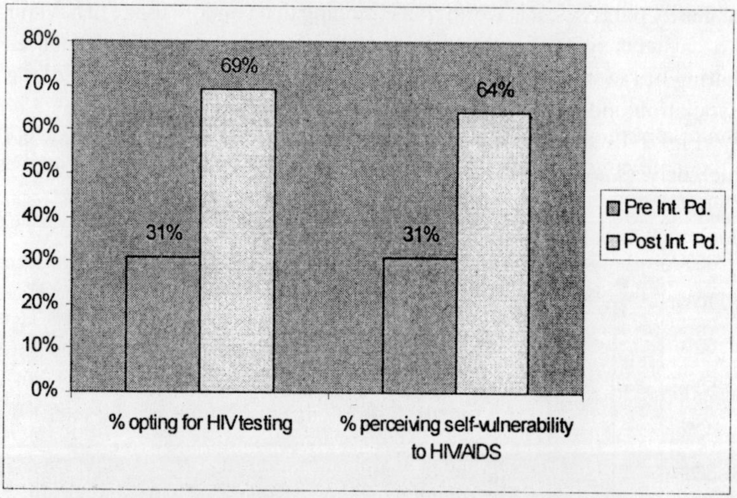

Fig. 3.42: Changes in Option for Voluntary HIV Testing and Perceived Self-vulnerability to HIV/AIDS (N = 90).

Condom Usage Behaviour Assessment – Pre-intervention

Consistent condom usage that is using a condom at all times during sex with casual partner/s has been recognized as the best preventive measure against HIV infection. But various studies have revealed that people especially those practicing high-risk behaviour are not using condoms due to various reasons (Wolf and Dejong, 1996; Maticka-Tyndale, et al., 1996). Chabbra, R. (2003) while arguing on the "condomisation of society" observes, "Despite years of effort and hundreds of crores already spent on condom promotion and subsidies, condom usage has not gone up in terms of real numbers-covering only 3 per cent of those using contraception." Therefore, the barriers to condom use need to be studied and overcome in order to increase the condom usage among communities, as a part of effective interventions.

In the present study, condom usage behaviour and practices assessment scale (Appendix X) was used to assess the knowledge regarding advantages of using a condom as well as the actual use of condoms by the three sample groups. Further, the difference in level of condom usage during the pre- and post-intervention period was used as an indicator to measure the impact of the study. Variations by gender, age, type of community and other factors with regards to condom usage were investigated and have been described in the proceeding sections. Here for clarity purposes, it is worth re-mentioning that condom usage behaviour (i.e., aspects related to condom usage) and general practices such as sharing of razors, blades, etc., were assessed on one scale because of the association and overlapping of behavioural and practices aspects.

Fig. 3.43 shows the condom use behaviour in marriage among the truck drivers and the rickshaw pullers who constituted the sample.

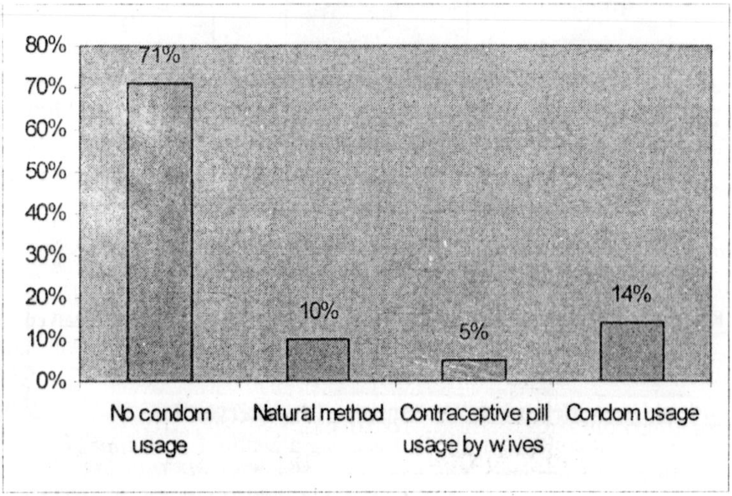

Base : Married male sample (N= 42).

Fig. 3.43 : Condom usage Behaviour in Married Men.

Overall, 71 per cent of the married men reported of not using condoms while having sex with their wife. It was given to understand that it was the birth right of a husband to have uninterrupted sex with his wife. Ten per cent of the men said that they were practicing the natural method of contraception (i.e., non-ejaculation in the vagina) whereas 5 per cent of them reported that their wives were taking oral contraceptive pills. As little as 14 per cent of the men reported condom usage with their wives as a contraceptive method. Various reasons were cited by the sample, for not using a condom with their wives. For instance, 56 per cent of such men said that a condom acted as a barrier and interfered in sexual pleasure, 11 per cent of them reported that condoms were subject to bursting during use while 33 per cent did not use a condom with their wife, as they were totally unaware about it.

Fig. 3.44 shows the awareness level of the sample regarding advantages of using a condom.

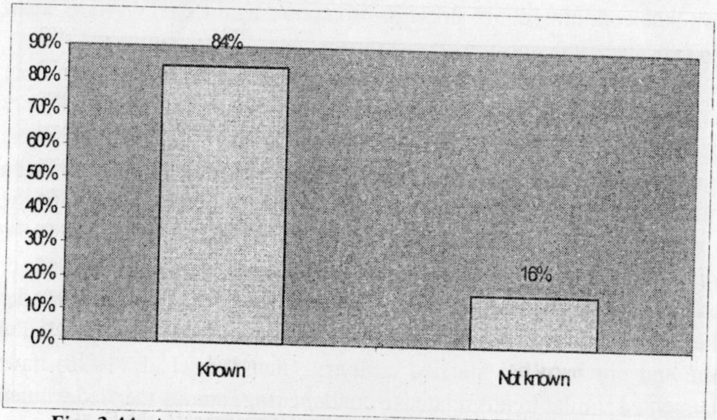

Fig. 3.44: Awareness Regarding Advantage/s of Using a Condom (N = 90).

The advantage/s of using a condom were known to 84 per cent of the entire study sample whereas 16 per cent of the sample was not aware about any of the advantages of using a condom. Further, the different types of advantages of using a condom as known by the sample are shown in Fig. 3.45.

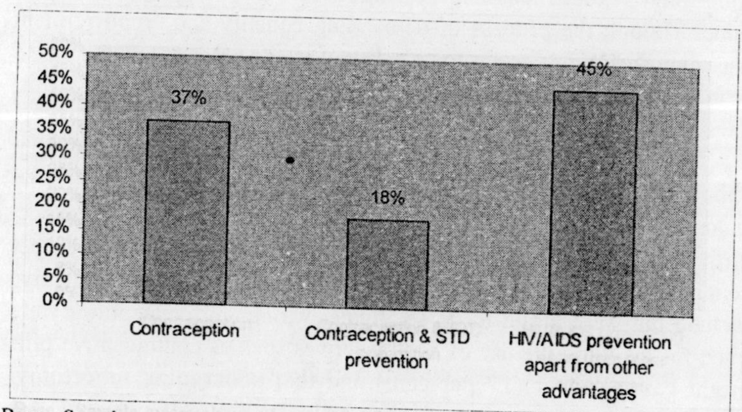

Base : Sample aware about advantage/s of using a condom (N=76).

Fig. 3.45: Different Advantages of Using a Condom.

Out of the entire sample who knew about any of the advantages of using a condom, 37 per cent of them cited condoms only to be a method of contraception, 18 per cent said that condoms apart from providing contraception could also protect from STD and only 45 per cent of them knew that condoms could provide protection against HIV/AIDS apart from other advantages.

Significant variation was observed regarding condom use behaviour with regards to the type of sexual partner. For instance, the entire 80 per cent of the married women sex workers on being asked about condom use behaviour with their spouse promptly replied that they had never used a condom with their husbands as it was against the social norm. One of the sex workers had defiantly reasoned out, "*Gharwale ke sang condom kabhi nahin istemaal kiya, woh toh ghar ka aadmi hai*" meaning "I have never used a condom with my husband, as he is my own man". This reaffirms the belief that condom usage was mainly seen in context of sex outside the home and not between married partners. Chandlok et al. (1996) have documented similar trends related to condom usage among married women in their study on comprehensive intervention programmes for women.

Although, 42 per cent of the married women in the present study reported that their husband had pre-marital/extra-marital sexual relations, yet they were unable to ask them for condom use due to socio-cultural inhibitions as well as their economic dependence on their husbands. Again, it is important here to stress the fact that women need to be educated about their sexual rights and be empowered to ensure equality of the same. Though the process of demanding equality and empowerment regarding such rights seems to be a distant reality yet, a beginning has to be made and in context of HIV/AIDS the sooner we are able to realize this, the better are the chances to contain the spread of this infection.

Apart from condom use behaviour, it is important to observe that although 33 per cent of the male sample had completed their child bearing stage and had three or more children yet, they were unable to exercise a birth control method due to their lack of awareness. Twenty-seven per cent of such sample said that their wives wanted to adopt a contraceptive method but were afraid to do so. Again, various misconceptions were cited for avoiding the use of contraceptives such as contraceptive pills might cause cancer (17 per cent) and that undergoing tubectomy/vasectomy may cause serious illnesses including death (10 per cent). It is ironic to note that some of the fears of the sample were not merely based on false notions but on real life experiences. For example, 4 per cent of the sample confirmed that few women in their villages who had undergone tubectomy had suffered from critical illness and three of them had reportedly died. This could be presumably because of septic conditions as related by the sample. One of the rickshaw pullers also reported that in spite of taking oral contraceptive pills, his wife had conceived and they were now expecting their fourth child irrespective of their desire as well as poverty.

The data strongly suggests that family planning measures including condom usage need to be practically promoted and operationally strengthened in the overall interest of such communities. Further, the quality of such services delivered especially in the rural areas, needs to be greatly improved in order to revive the trust of communities in such facilities.

As far as the commercial sex workers were concerned it was observed that most of them were aware of different methods of contraception due to their exposure to various NGOs. In the present study, 54 per cent of the sex workers said that they used condoms as a method of contraception, 33 per cent reportedly took oral contraceptive pills while 13 per cent of them had undergone sterilization for contraception purpose.

Condom Usage Behaviour Assessment among Sample having Pre/extra-marital Sex

The base for scoring condom usage behaviour consisted only of the sample that reported to have ever indulged in premarital and/extramarital sexual relationships. Although indulging in pre & / extra-marital sex have been categorized as having sex with non-regular partner (NACO, 2001) yet, in the present study pre- and extra-marital sex have been categorized and studied separately with a view of achieving an in-depth analysis regarding the extent as well as various aspects related to these two different kinds of relationships. The selection of base is justified in view of the fact that only individuals practicing sex with non-regular partners (i.e., sexual partner/s other than the spouse) were at risk of acquiring HIV through sexual contact and thus, needed to use a condom in all such transactions and be assessed for the same. However, individuals not having pre/extra-marital sexual relationships were not bound to use a condom with their presumably uninfected spouse for purposes related to HIV prevention. Hence, their inclusion as sample for condom usage behaviour assessment was not justified, as it may have led to a biased scoring in terms of their being under-scored for eventually not using a condom with their spouse even when it was not a criterion for the present research.

The condom usage assessment scale aptly applied to the commercial sex workers as well, since the sex work that they were practicing was either before or after their marriage had taken place resulting in being justified as premarital or extramarital sex for the purpose of HIV prevention.

In condom usage behaviour assessment scale, scoring proceeded and was thus marked in a logical sequence. For example, if an individual was not at all using a condom with a commercial sex worker in the first place then he was marked zero on the next aspect asking him how successful he was in condom use negotiations because, he lost the probability of success initially, by not negotiating condom use at all. The maximum score on the condom usage behaviour assessment scale was a total of 20.

Fig. 3.46 shows the mean score on condom usage behaviour scale for individuals of the three sample groups having pre/extramarital sexual relationships during the pre-intervention period.

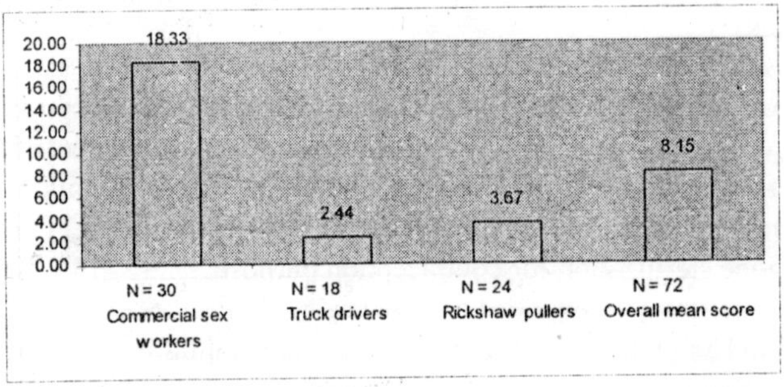

Base: Sample indulging in premarital/extramarital sex (N = 72).

Fig. 3.46: Mean Scores on Condom Usage Behaviour Scale.

The mean score for the commercial sex workers was 18.33, for the truck drivers 2.44, and for the rickshaw pullers it was 3.67 out of a total score of 20. The overall mean score for the entire base sample was 8.15 out of a total of 20. Commercial sex workers registered a higher score on condom usage behaviour scale as compared to the other two sample communities because of their exposure to various ongoing HIV/AIDS prevention programmes in the red light area, which promoted condom usage.

Fig. 3.47 shows the relative percentage of sample who had ever indulged in premarital sex (PMS) and/extramarital sex (EMS).

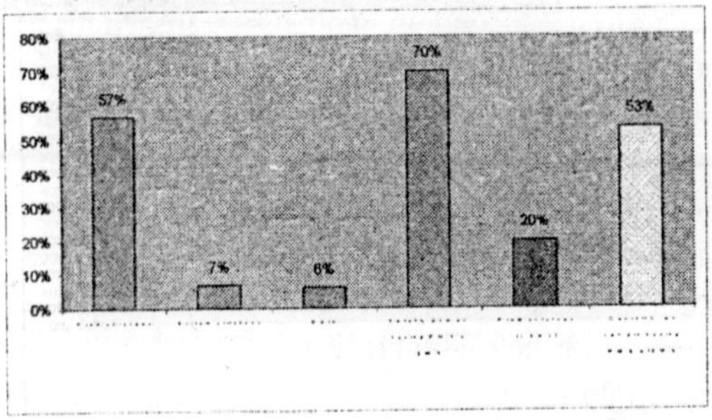

* Prior to practicing of sex trade

Fig. 3.47: Percentage of Sample Indulging in PMS/EMS (N=90).

The study revealed that 57 per cent of the male sample had indulged in pre-marital sex, 7 per cent of them had extra-marital sexual relationships and 6 per cent were found to have both pre-marital as well as extra-marital sexual relations thereby totaling up to 70 per cent of the entire male sample having indulged in pre-marital and/extra-marital sex. Such high percentage of the sample having indulged in sex outside marriage reveals that inspite of the traditionally transmitted socio-cultural norms, which stress on abstinence for the unmarried and fidelity for the married individuals, practices such as pre-marital and extra-marital sex were taking place on significantly high levels. Similarly, it was found that 20 per cent of the sex workers had pre-marital sexual relations before entering into the sex trade. Here, it is critical to observe that all of the sex workers who reported to have indulged in pre-marital sex said that they had been coerced into such sexual acts by their lovers (7 per cent), strangers (7 per cent) and employers (6 per cent). Further, the level of condom usage in such transactions was found to be extremely low among the sample. For instance, none of the women who had pre-marital sex prior to their entry into the sex trade reported condom use by their male partners. Similarly, condom usage was found to be significantly low among the truck drivers and rickshaw pullers indulging in sex with non-regular partners. Fig. 3.48 shows the condom usage among men having pre-marital and/extra-marital sexual relations.

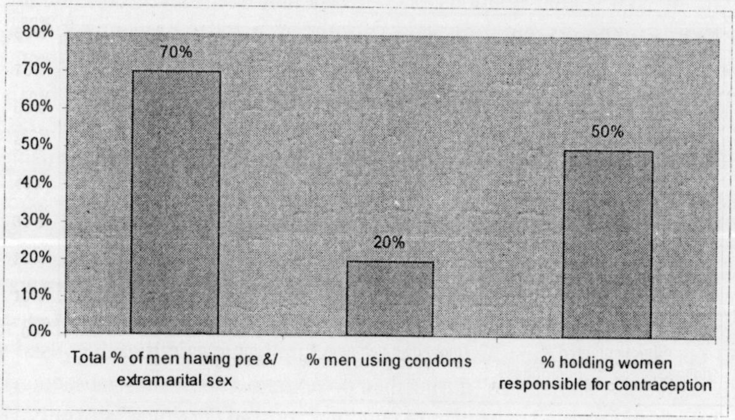

Base : Male Sample (N = 60).

Fig. 3.48: Condom Usage among Men having PMS/EMS.

Out of 70 per cent of the men having premarital and/extra marital sex, only 20 per cent were found to be using a condom with their sexual partners. The rest 50 per cent expected women to be responsible for contraception and thus expected them to act accordingly. Further, the reasons for using a condom with their sexual partners differed for different individuals and have been shown in Fig. 3.49.

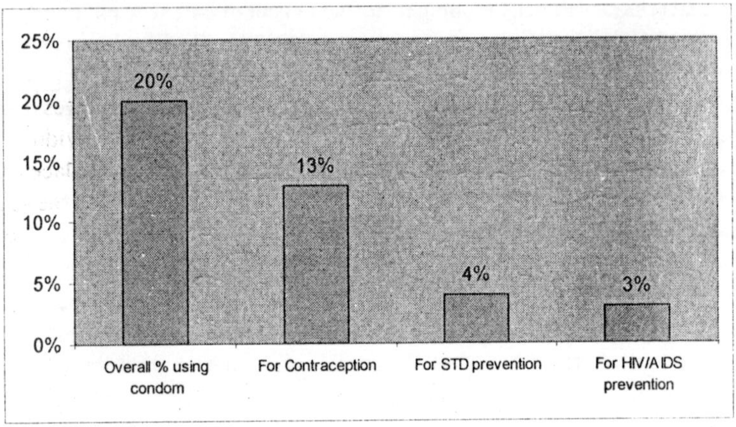

Base : Male sample indulging in PMS/EMS (N = 42).

Fig. 3.49: Reasons for Using a Condom.

Out of a total of 20 per cent of men using condoms for pre-marital/extra-marital sexual relations, 13 per cent said that they used condoms primarily for contraceptive purposes, 4 per cent stated to be using condoms for STD prevention and only 3 per cent said that they used condoms for HIV/AIDS prevention. Thus, the data clearly highlights the fact that firstly condom usage among people practicing pre-marital/extra-marital sex (i.e., high risk behaviour) was significantly low and secondly even those using condoms, used it primarily for contraception or STD prevention. HIV/AIDS prevention by condom usage was not known to the majority of the male sample.

The study further revealed that condom usage among the users was not consistent and varied greatly in their sexual transactions. For instance, 33 per cent of the men who reported condom usage said that they used a condom only "sometimes" during their pre/extramarital sexual transactions, 50 per cent reported to be using a condom "most of the times" and only 17 per cent of the men said that they "always" used a condom during their pre/extramarital sexual transactions.

Although consistent condom usage (i.e., using a condom for each and every sexual transaction) is one of the pre-requisites for HIV/AIDS prevention amongst people practicing high-risk behaviour yet, many of them were not adhering to consistent condom usage behaviour. The finding is substantiated by the latest Operation Research Group's survey which noted that the percentage of people using condoms consistently with all non-regular partners within a specific period of time that was past twelve months for the survey, was very low (*Indian Express*, April 4, 2002).

Contrary to the male sample, 80 per cent of the commercial sex workers reported consistent condom usage with their clients as a preventive measure against AIDS. The rest 20 per cent cited reasons such as non-availability of compliant customers and lean business periods for compromising with clients to have sexual transactions without using a condom. Here, it is important to note that only old sex workers aged 35 years and above, reported sexual transactions without using a condom. The basic reason cited by these sex workers for their indulgence in unprotected sex at times was their growing age, which led to fewer customers turning to them. This limited number of customers could be further curtailed if the sex workers did not yield to their demand of having sex without a condom. Thus, indulging in unprotected sex was an economic necessity for most of these sex workers in order to earn their livelihood. One of the brothel owners on being advised about the risks posed to sex workers by having unprotected sex had defensively remarked "*Bhook ek aisee chiz hai, joh maut ko bhi nahin dekhti.*" meaning "Hunger is one thing that does not care even for death (a synonym used for AIDS)." Unfortunately, so widespread is the onslaught of hunger that it may not be wiped out before the year 2200 (Human Development Report cited in *Times of India*, Dec.12, 2003).

It is further important to observe that although majority of the sex workers reported consistent condom usage yet, the presence of STD among them suggested that all of them were not using a condom for every sexual transaction. Further, non-consistent condom usage among the sex workers was also verified by some (40 per cent) of the truck drivers and rickshaw pullers who visited the brothels at the G. B. Road. They reported that condom usage pre-condition by the sex workers could be waived off by paying them a tip of Rs. 20 or so.

Thus, cross verification of self-reported data was made possible by studying the service provider (i.e., the commercial sex workers) and the service user (i.e., the clients like truck drivers and rickshaw pullers) communities simultaneously. This helped greatly in making corrective efforts at both the levels in an effective manner.

Various reasons were given by the sample for not using a condom at all or for not having consistent condom usage during premarital and extramarital sexual relations. The major reasons cited by 72 per cent of the men indulging in premarital/extramarital sex was that since they had sexual relations with steady partner/s, whom they knew well, there was no need to use a condom with them. According to Stayanoff et al. (1996) a steady partner has been defined as that with whom a person has sexual contact for at least three or more times. Having a steady partner usually applies to having sexual relations with one sexual partner over a period of time. But in the present study, it is interesting to note that 38 per cent of the men indulging in pre/extramarital sex had more than one sexual partner at a given time whom they treated as steady partners. This aspect needs to be delved into seriously since having regular sexual contact with many partners at the same time does not imply that all sexual partners can be treated as steady partners.

Thus, the study sample having more than one sexual partner at a given time was under the wrong impression of treating all or most of their sexual partners as steady partners. This misinformation was enhancing their vulnerability to HIV exposure. Apart from the notion that condom use was not required in case of steady partner/s, other reasons such as condom acts as a barrier and prevents body-to-body contact (67 per cent) were also generally cited by the male sample. Similar reasons justifying non-condom usage by people practicing high-risk behaviour have also been reported by NACO (2001).

Thus, it can be concluded from the above findings that the concept of having a steady partner needs to be redefined and that condom usage with all non-regular partners irrespective of any factor needs to be promoted vigorously amongst the communities under study.

Further, carrying a condom with them at all times, while going in for pre/extra-marital sexual transactions was also studied among the sample. It was found that 76 per cent of the men indulging in pre/extramarital sex never carried a condom with them while going in for such sexual transactions. On the contrary, a study has shown that commercial sex workers whose customers frequently brought condoms with them reported a high rate of condom usage (Ravelo, et al., 1996). Thus, in order to increase condom usage among the clients as well as the sex workers, HIV/AIDS prevention campaigns should stress on the need to carry a condom at all times while going in for pre/extramarital sexual transactions.

In the present study, out of 24 per cent of the male sample who reported to be carrying a condom with them while going in for pre/extra-marital sexual transactions, 10 per cent admitted carrying a condom only "sometimes" while 9 per cent reported to be carrying a condom "most of the time". As little as 5 per cent of such sample said that they "always" carried a condom while going in for pre/extra-marital sexual transactions.

The data suggests that the pre-condition of carrying a condom must be inculcated and reinforced among those practicing high-risk behaviour. The sex workers reported that although they always kept a ready supply of condoms for their clients yet, some of them brought their own condoms. This was due to the prevalent opinion that the condoms supplied to commercial sex workers by various NGOs were of poor quality and thus, the customers did not like using them.

Condom usage negotiation skill was another vital aspect that was studied in the present research. The use of a condom can be greatly increased if people are able to negotiate condom usage prior to a sexual act/transaction. But contrary to this, various studies have shown that lack of negotiation skills regarding condom use have resulted in condom usage failure (Wolf and Dejong, 1996; Rosensnard & Campbell, 1996). It means that many people were not able to use condoms because they found it difficult to discuss condom usage with their sexual partners. This is substantiated by the finding in the present study in which 76 per cent of the male sample indulging in pre/extramarital sex said that they never initiated condom use negotiation with their sexual partner/s because negotiating such acts was not easy and they felt embarrassed to do so. Further out of 24 per cent of the men who admitted negotiating condom use, 14 per cent said that they felt shy while discussing condom use with their partner whereas only 10 per cent of the individuals said that they felt normal/comfortable while making such negotiations. None of the individuals reported to be confident in negotiating condom use with their sexual partners.

Further, the frequency of such negotiations was found to be very low among the negotiators as shown in Fig. 3.50.

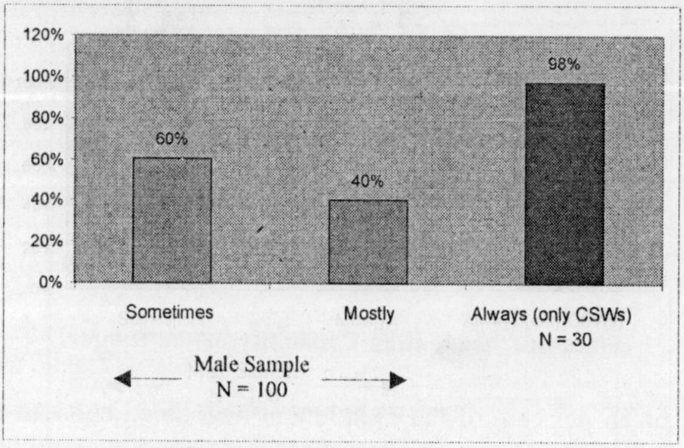

Base Sample negotiating condom use with their non-regular sexual partner/s (N = 40).

Fig. 3.50: Frequency of Condom use Negotiations.

Sixty per cent of the male sample negotiating condom use said that they negotiated condom use "sometimes" and only 40 per cent reported negotiating condom use "mostly" with their sexual partners. Contrary to this, nearly all the sex workers (98 per cent) reported 'always' negotiating condom use with their clients. Higher and consistent negotiating rates were noted among the commercial sex workers again because of their exposure to the ongoing condom promotion programmes in their area. Further, 67 per cent of the sex workers negotiating condom use said that they felt comfortable and 33 per cent of them stated to be confident while making such negotiations.

Here, it is important to observe that overall, out of 80 per cent of the sample (including all the commercial sex workers) that had ever indulged in pre/extramarital sex, only 56 per cent negotiated condom use and just 41 per cent (comprising only the commercial sex workers) admitted negotiating condom use "always" with their clients. The "always" negotiating aspect was totally missing among the truck drivers and rickshaw pullers. Hence, there lies the need to develop condom negotiation skills among these communities.

The success in condom use negotiations was also assessed by the condom usage scale in order to assess the potential of the sample as good negotiators. Fig. 3.51 shows the relative percentage of the sample in accordance to their negotiating capability.

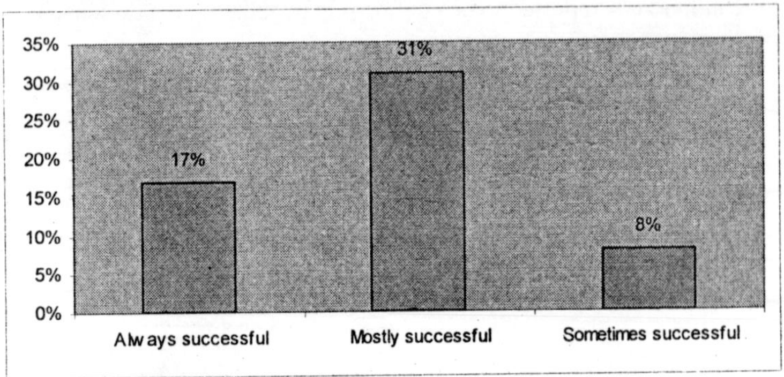

Base: Sample negotiating condom use with their non-regular sexual partner/s (N = 40).

Fig. 3.51: Negotiating Capability of the Sample.

Out of 56 per cent of the sample that negotiated condom use with their non-regular sexual partner/s, only 17 per cent of them said that they were "always" successful in such negotiations. Thirty-one per cent of the individuals reported to be successful " most of the time" and 8 per cent admitted to be successful only "sometimes". These findings reveal that effective condom negotiation skills were lacking among majority of the sample. The ability to negotiate such terms needs to be developed on a high priority basis among the masses especially those practicing high-risk behaviour with the view of preventing new HIV infections from taking place.

The sample's skill to practice condom use correctly was another major area that was studied in the present research. Studies have shown that many people using condoms are not doing so in a correct manner (Susan, et al., 1996; Toppich & Christiansen, 1996; Pott, et al., 1996) thus rendering them ineffective against the protection from HIV/AIDS. In the present study, although 84 per cent of the entire sample was confident that they knew the correct method of using a condom yet, on being asked to describe the same, only 38 per cent were able to do so, 31 per cent of them described the incorrect method while 15 per cent chose not to reply. Overall, 16 per cent of the sample was not at all aware about condoms and thus their usage skills. In the Indian context, while discussing the issue of undisputed faith being placed on condom alone for the prevention of HIV, Chhabra (2003) rightly questions, "Can a largely illiterate, hygiene - lacking populace be expected to learn and practice consistent, correct use of a condom?"

Further, 71 per cent of the entire sample was not aware about correct condom disposal procedure after use. Correct condom disposal after use has been recognized as vital in containing the HIV infection, as the semen of an infected individual is known to contain the HIV virus and the same can act as a potential source of HIV through accidental/casual contact. Majority of the sample (62 per cent) using a condom was found to be disposing used condoms simply after wrapping them in a paper or a piece of cloth. The procedure advocated by the health authorities to dispose the used condom after tying a knot was not known to them. Tying a condom is advised to ensure that there is no spillage of infected body fluids.

All these findings suggest that condom advertising alone cannot be an effective method of controlling the spread of HIV/AIDS. The protective skills such as condom negotiation, correct condom usage and correct condom disposal need to be developed, promoted and supported among the masses. Mere advocacy, urging people to use condoms for protection against HIV/AIDS will not help till people are taught the skills of using a condom correctly.

Further, easy availability of condoms especially to people who need them the most is a major factor determining condom usage. Formative research suggests that unavailability of condoms is one of the primary barriers to consistent condom use (Dawson, et al., 1996; Maticka-Tyndale, et al., 1996). Studies continue to show that factors such as price as well as access to condoms determine the levels of their usage (Dahl, et al., 1996; Schechter, et al., 1996). Thus, many people are not using condoms because they find them to be either expensive or not freely accessible to them.

In the present study, out of 51 per cent of the sample that had ever used a condom either with their spouse or with non-regular partner/s, 30 per cent of them felt that though condoms were easily available in the market but they found them to be expensive. Seventy-five per cent of the truck drivers and rickshaw pullers using a condom were found to be purchasing them from the market. Most of them said that they were paying Rs. 20 for a box of condom containing 5 pieces. Although government hospitals and dispensaries are supposed to be providing condoms to poor people free of cost yet, majority of the sample was not able to avail these facilities. Thirty-eight per cent of the male sample using a condom said that since government hospitals and dispensaries were far away from their place of residence in rural areas and secondly, as there were long queues in those establishments for availing these facilities, thus due to shortage of time they were not in a position to avail such free services. Thirteen per cent of such sample also pointed out that during most of the times, free condom supply in government health facilities was out of stock. Out of the entire 35 per cent of the male sample using condoms, only one rickshaw puller was found to be visiting a government hospital in Delhi and getting the free condom supply from there to be taken to his native village for usage with his wife.

As far as the commercial sex workers were concerned, all of them agreed that there was no shortage of free supply of condoms being provided to them by various NGOs. But 47 per cent of the sex workers also pointed out that condoms supplied to them were non-lubricated and of inferior quality resulting in more condom burst outs as well as rejection to use by many customers.

Overall, 52 per cent of the sample that had ever used a condom was of the opinion that good quality condoms should be made available to them at cheaper prices. Similarly, 87 per cent of the commercial sex workers desperately wanted female condoms to be promoted in a female-friendly environment. This was important for them in order to gain some control in issues related to condom usage, which could in turn increase consistent condom usage by the CSWs without depending upon the wishes of their male clients.

Another important aspect studied during the pre-intervention period was the condom usage by the sample during their last pre/extramarital sexual transaction. Out of 70 per cent of the truck drivers and rickshaw pullers having pre/extramarital sexual relations, only 19 per cent of these reported having used a condom the last time they had such a sexual transaction. As far as the commercial sex workers were concerned, all of them reported having used a condom during their last sexual transaction.

However, consistent condom usage as reported by the sample was verified by asking the approximate number of condoms purchased or used by the sample in a week's/month's time. The number of condoms thus used was matched with the number of sexual transactions taking place within a week or a month's time as reported by the sample. The closer the tally the more consistent was the condom usage. During the pre-intervention period, consistent condom usage could be reasonably justified only in 28 per cent of the respondents having pre/extramarital sex.

Further, the intention of the sample to use a condom in future while indulging in pre/extramarital sex with a non-regular partner was also gauged by the condom usage behaviour scale. The evaluation of the intention to use a condom was important in order to assess the chances of a condom being used in future pre/extramarital sexual transactions which in turn could help in motivating the sample to do so. Fig. 3.52 shows the relative percentage of the sample along with their intention to use a condom for pre/extra-marital sex.

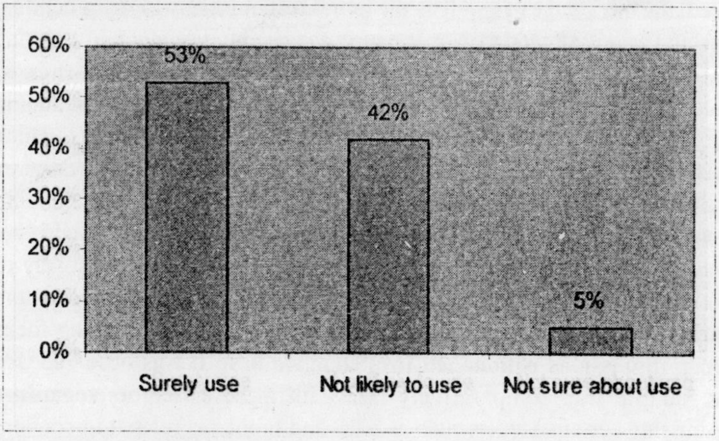

Base : Sample indulging in PMS/EMS (N = 72).

Fig. 3.52: Intention to use a Condom with a Non-regular Partner.

During the pre-intervention period, only 53 per cent of the sample having sex with a non-regular partner reported that they were "sure" to use a condom while having sex, 42 per cent of such sample said they were "not likely" to use one, while 5 per cent of them were "not sure" if they would use a condom while indulging in pre/extramarital sex.

Women's right to assert their partner for condom usage was another area, which showed vast gender-based variation. For instance, 74 per cent of the men who were aware about condoms were of the opinion that women do not have any right to ask their partners for condom usage, whereas contrary to this 80 per cent of the women were of the opinion that women should have the right to assert their partners to use a condom. The advocacy for women's right to assert for condom usage was found to be inversely related to men's indulgence in pre/extramarital sex. This means that men having pre/extramarital sex were less likely (19 per cent v/s 22 per cent) to endorse women's right to assert for condom usage as compared to those men who did not indulge in such acts. The most probable explanation for this finding is the fact that most of the men having sex with non-regular partner/s wanted their wife to remain submissive to them especially in matters related to sex and sexuality irrespective of their own marital infidelity.

The Intervention – *a review*

Condom usage as an effective method of HIV prevention among the sample was promoted through the use of audio-visual aids developed during the course of study. The photo-script elaborately discussed the need, the advantages as well as the moral responsibility to use a condom during various situations. For instance, the need to use a condom during sexual transactions with non-regular partner/s was repeatedly stressed along with the moral responsibility of condom usage with spouse too, in case of an individual being HIV positive. Similarly, the pamphlet, which was developed keeping in mind the needs of the sex workers, stressed on the importance of consistent condom usage along with correct condom usage and disposal skills. It was emphasized at times and again that practicing safe sex was in everybody's interest and also the best way of preventing HIV/AIDS through sexual contact. Further, the peer educators played a crucial role in promoting condom usage by conducting focus group discussions within their own communities. It was observed that the sample was comparatively free with these educators regarding discussing certain aspects such as STD and problems related to condom usage. Hence, this aspect was fully harnessed by utilizing peer educators' support to mobilize the sample communities in favour of safe sex.

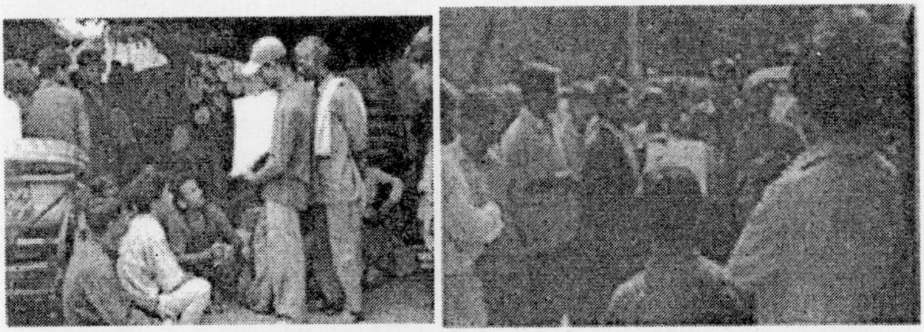

Picture 21: Peer Educators Promoting Condom use for HIV/AIDS Prevention.

Condom Usage Behaviour Assessment : Post-intervention

Significant changes were observed pertaining to knowledge about condoms as well as their usage during the post-intervention period on the condom usage behaviour assessment scale. Fig. 3.53 portrays the marked difference in the pre- and post-intervention scores on condom usage behaviour assessment scale, amongst the three different groups.

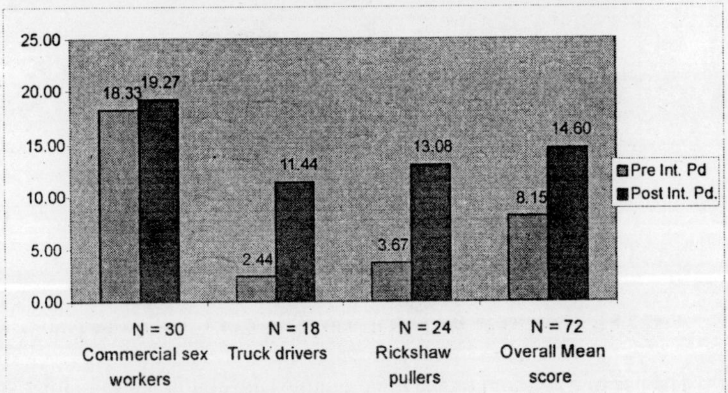

Base: Sample indulging in pre-marital or extra-marital sex.

Fig. 3.53: Mean Scores on Condom Usage Behaviour Scale.

The mean score rose from 18.33 to 19.27 among the commercial sex workers, from 2.44 to 11.44 among the truck drivers and from 3.67 to 13.08 among the rickshaw pullers out of a total of 20 during the pre- to post-intervention period. The overall mean score for the entire base sample registered an increase from 8.15 to 14.60 out of a total of 20 during the course of intervention. The commercial sex workers registered a higher score as compared to the truck drivers and rickshaw pullers because their base level itself during the pre-intervention period was high as a result of the on-going HIV/AIDS prevention programmes going on in the red light area which promoted condom usage.

Major changes were observed in the following areas subsequent to the intervention:

The condom use with spouse rose from 14 per cent during the pre-intervention period to 47 per cent in the post-intervention period among the male sample. This gain was primarily achieved because of the increase in knowledge amongst the sample regarding condom and it's use.

The advantage/s of using a condom were known to 100 per cent of the sample as compared to only 84 per cent during the pre-intervention period. Likewise, the knowledge amongst the entire sample that condoms could protect oneself from HIV/AIDS rose from 38 per cent in the pre-intervention period to 98 per cent during the post-intervention period as shown in Fig. 3.54.

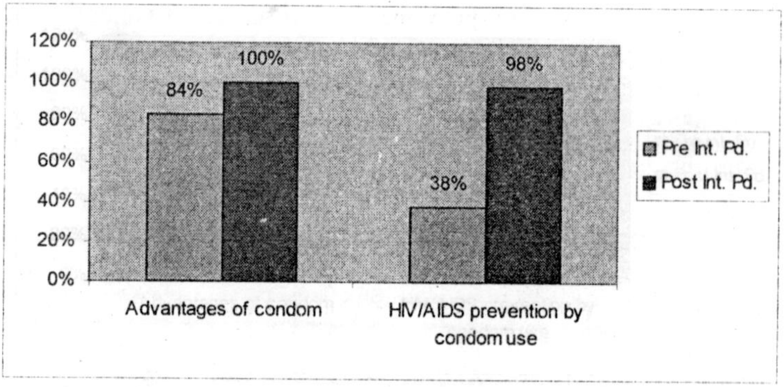

Fig. 3.54: Knowledge Regarding Advantages of Using a Condom (N = 90).

The use of a condom by the male sample who continued to indulge in pre/extramarital sexual transactions during the course of study rose from 38 per cent in the pre-intervention period to 63 per cent in the post-intervention period. Similarly, the percentage of sex workers who reported "always" using a condom during sexual transactions with their clients registered an increase from 80 per cent to 87 per cent during the course of intervention. Further, the concept of carrying a condom at all times while going in for sex with a non-regular partner was also generated amongst the sample. A skit was enacted by two peer educators in which a truck driver practicing high risk behaviour was advised by a friend to carry a condom at all times while going in for sex with a non-regular partner. This concept was generated with the aim of increasing condom usage among sample practicing high-risk behaviour. As a result, 50 per cent of the male sample having sex with non regular partner/s during the post-intervention period reported to be carrying a condom with them while going in for pre/extramarital sex as compared to only 25 per cent of such sample during the pre-intervention period.

It was encouraging to observe that 11 per cent of the sample continuing to indulge in sex with non-regular partner/s reported to have refused unprotected sex with their partner/s. This aspect was also used as one of the indicators to measure the impact of the intervention on the sample. As bringing about behavioural change is a difficult and protracted process, the gain may seem to be subtle yet, was a step towards desired change.

The increase in condom usage was further substantiated by the finding that the cumulative incidence of STD among the sample decreased significantly during the course of intervention. Fig. 3.55 shows the changes in levels of STD prevalence as well as awareness regarding their causes and symptoms during the pre- and post-intervention period.

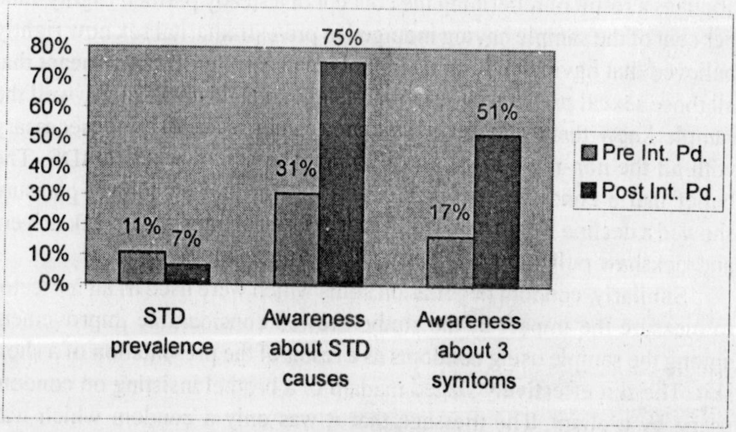

Fig. 3.55: Changes in STD Prevalence and Related Aspects (N = 90).

The self-reported prevalence of STD showed a decline from 11 per cent to 7 per cent during the period of intervention. Further, the level of awareness amongst the sample regarding STD also increased significantly. For instance, the cause/s of STD were known to 75 per cent of the sample in the post-intervention period as compared to only 31 per cent prior to the intervention. Similarly, the awareness regarding three commonly observed symptoms of STD increased from 17 per cent to 51 per cent during the period of intervention. The sample greatly appreciated the manner in which the information regarding STD and their symptoms was presented in the audio-visual aids. For instance, majority of sample especially the CSWs was not aware that lower abdominal pain could be a symptom of sexually transmitted infection and thus did not take any care for that. But after the presentation of the audio-visual aids, many of them had reportedly started considering such an occurrence seriously and resorted to taking of medical treatment. Moreover the treatment seeking behaviour for STD and various other ailments also registered qualitative as well as quantitative changes. For instance, the proportion of sample seeking treatment for various ailments including STD from qualified medical practitioners increased from 58 per cent to 69 per cent.

The barriers to condom usage also showed a sharp decline in the post-intervention period as the sample's perception to HIV/AIDS vulnerability increased. Sixty-seven per cent of the sample having indulged in sex with non-regular partners perceived themselves to be at risk of HIV/AIDS during the post-intervention period as compared to only 33 per cent during the pre-intervention period. This change in perception was brought about as a result of redefining the concept of a steady partner. Eighty-nine per cent of the sample having indulged in pre/extramarital sex now rightly believed that having more than one sexual partner at one time meant that all those sexual partners were not steady partners, no matter how well the sample knew them. Thus, condom use was now considered necessary with all the non-regular partners for protection against HIV/AIDS. The belief that a condom acted as a barrier and decreased sexual pleasure showed a decline from 61 per cent to 25 per cent amongst the truck drivers and rickshaw pullers during the pre- to post-intervention period.

Similarly, condom negotiation skills which were used as an indicator to measure the impact of the study, showed considerable improvement among the sample using condoms as a result of the presentation of a short skit. The skit effectively staged madam of a brothel insisting on condom usage by a client. The message that it was only a condom which was required to protect one-self from ever fatal HIV/AIDS was simply yet, effectively conveyed through the skit to the sample. It also led to shedding of various inhibitions by the sample in negotiating condom usage.

The base sample in the proceeding findings may vary at places due to the fact that some of the sample had indulged in pre/extra-marital sex prior to the pre-intervention phase or sometime during the pre-intervention period but the same behaviour had been given up in the post-intervention period. Thus, such sample has been included as base sample wherever required and possible while for some other pre- to post-comparative aspects such sample could not be included as the base.

The improvement in condom negotiation skills brought about as a result of the intervention is shown in Fig. 3.56.

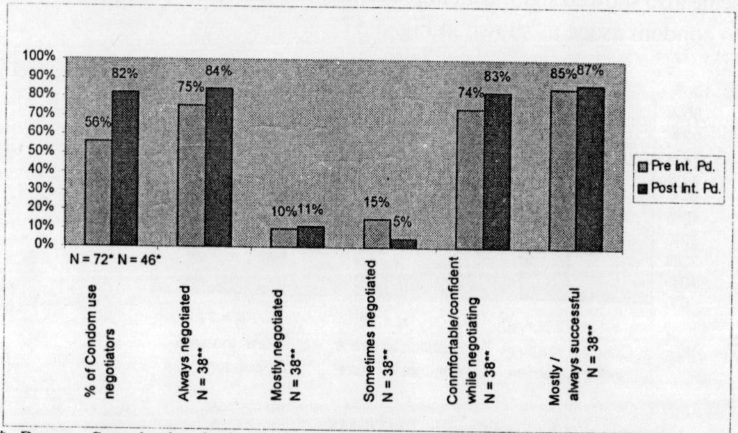

* Base : Sample that had ever indulged in sex with non-regular partner/s.
**Base : Sample continuing to indulge in sex with non-regular sexual partner/s during the pre- as well as post-intervention period and negotiating condom use with them.

Fig. 3.56: Improvement in Condom Usage Negotiation Skill.

The percentage of sample negotiating condom use with their sexual partner/s rose from 56 per cent in the pre-intervention period to 82 per cent amongst the sample who continued to indulge in sex with non-regular partner/s during the post-intervention period. Further, 84 per cent of the negotiators reported negotiating condom use in "all" of their sexual transactions as against 75 per cent during the pre-intervention period, while 11 per cent of the negotiators said that they negotiated condom use in " most" of their sexual transactions as compared to 10 per cent prior to the intervention. The percentage of respondents who negotiated condom use only "sometimes" was registered to be 5 per cent showing a decline of 10 per cent from the pre-intervention period. This decline was due to the desired increase in the number of individuals who negotiated condom use "always/mostly" during their sexual transactions. Besides, 83 per cent of the respondents negotiating condom use during the post-intervention period as compared to 74 per cent in the pre-intervention period said that they did not feel shy or embarrassed but felt comfortable/confident while negotiating condom use. Similarly, the number of "successful" condom use negotiations rose during the intervention period. Eighty-seven percent of the negotiators in the post-intervention period as compared to 85 per cent prior to the intervention said that they were "mostly/always successful" in such negotiations.

The trends obtained on the condom usage behaviour assessment scale also showed significant improvements in various other aspects related to condom usage as shown in Fig. 3.57.

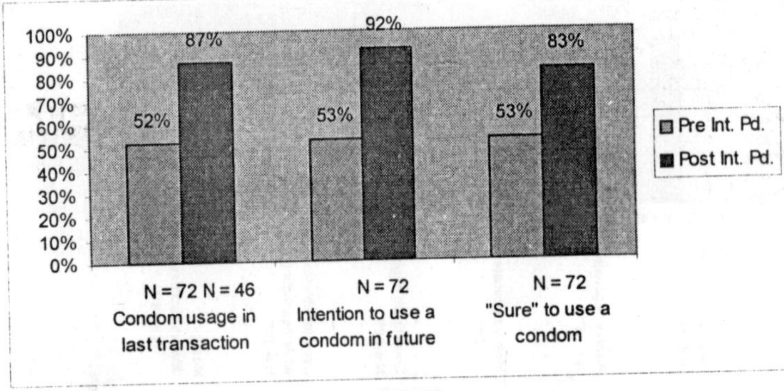

Base : Sample that had indulged in PMS/EMS.

Fig. 3.57: Condom Use with Non-regular Partner/s.

The proportion of respondents who reported using a condom in their last sexual transaction with a non-regular partner significantly increased from 52 per cent to 87 per cent. The sample size varied for this aspect during the pre- and post-intervention period because of the decline in the percentage of sample having sex with a non-regular partner in the post-intervention phase. Likewise, the intention to use a condom in future sexual transactions amongst the sample who ever had sex with a non-regular partner registered a rise from 53 per cent to 92 per cent. Further, in the post-intervention period 83 per cent of the sample as compared to a mere 53 per cent prior to the intervention said that they were "sure" to use a condom with a non-regular partner in future.

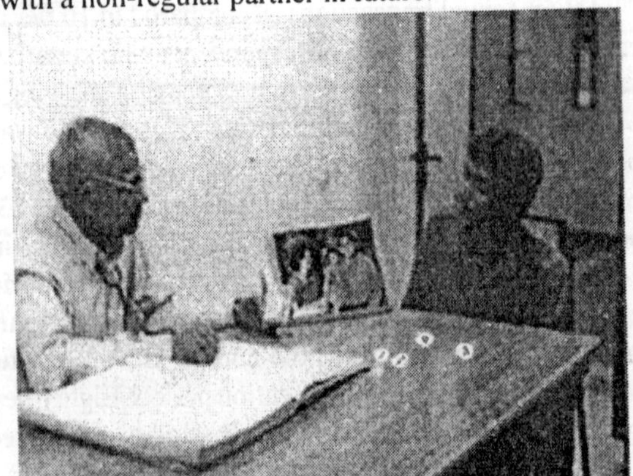

Picture 22: 'Condom Use with Non-regular Sexual Partner/s – A Must' a Skit.

Lastly, but most importantly major improvements were seen in condom usage as well as condom disposal skills amongst the sample. The correct method of using a condom was known to 69 per cent of the sample in the post-intervention period as compared to 38 per cent prior to the intervention. This gain in skill subsequently resulted in a decline in condom failure reporting by the sample such as condom burst-outs and other related failures. Considerable improvements were also noted in the condom disposal skill. Correct condom disposal skill showed a rise of 27 per cent from the pre- to post-intervention level.

At the end of the intervention 80 per cent of the sample as compared to 40 per cent prior to the intervention agreed that women should have a right to assert their partner for condom use. The increase reflects a deep attitudinal change among the sample brought about as a result of the intervention.

Practices Assessment – Pre-intervention

A broad range of unsafe practices as assessed by the condom usage behaviour and practices assessment scale (Appendix X) was observed among the sample, which was found to be enhancing their exposure to HIV. Ignorance about HIV/AIDS was the primary reason responsible for the samples' regular indulgence in these practices. Thus, an acute need was realized to assess and effectively modify such high-risk practices in order to decrease the vulnerability of the sample to HIV/AIDS. Some of the high-risk practices observed in the communities under study have been elaborated as follows:

Overall 49 per cent of the sample reported to be "frequently" injected for various medical reasons, whereas 35 per cent said that they were injected "sometimes" due to various illnesses. The remaining 16 per cent of the sample said that they remembered being rarely injected only during their childhood years. Besides, out of 84 per cent of the sample who reported to be "frequently/sometimes" injected, 29 per cent of these pointed out that in their native villages, doctors injected them with previously used needles after cleaning them with water, 32 per cent of them were not aware if new or used needles were used to inject them and only 39 per cent of these individuals could confirm that they were injected with new needles. The high proportion of the respondents reporting to be injected with used needles by doctors in rural areas sounds alarming. Although, the needles were reportedly washed by the doctors, still the efficacy of such cleaning methods remains highly questionable. Similar findings regarding the high percentage of doctors reusing needle and syringes for their patients have been reported by other researchers too.

Bansal et al. (1994) in their study highlighting the abysmally poor knowledge, attitude, behaviour and practices (KABP) of 100 indigenous as well as registered medical practitioners (RMPs) revealed that as many as 64 per cent of them were reusing disposable needles and syringes for injecting their patients. Similarly in another study, 51 per cent of the doctors "sometimes or never" used disposable syringes and needles for injecting drugs. The most commonly stated reason for non-use or irregular use of disposable injecting equipment was the inadequate supply (Benjamin & Zachairah, 1997).

India has a large number of medical practitioners from various systems of medicine. Although some studies have focused on the assessment/ enhancement of knowledge, attitude, behaviour and practices of allopathic medical practioners yet, a large number of practitioners from other systems of medicine including traditional healers have mostly remained untouched by various HIV prevention strategies. Thus, there lies an urgent need to cover these practitioners under various ongoing HIV/AIDS prevention programmes in order to stop the HIV from proliferating.

Further, the practice of being tattooed was also observed among 11 per cent of the study participants who too were not sure whether new needles had been used on them for tattooing purpose. The risks of getting tattooed by a shared needle have been clearly shown by Bansal and Arya (1993) in their study in which they observed that no aseptic measures were observed during the tattooing procedure and that the tattooist did not change needles between clients nor disinfected any part of the tattoo equipment. Their study revealed that the risk of transmission and contraction of the HIV infection by the tattooing procedure was unacceptably high due to the absolute absence of any aseptic measures. Similarly, in the present research 36 per cent of the sample had gone through ears and/nose piercing procedure and none of them was aware whether new or used piercing equipment/needles had been used on them for piercing purpose. Thus, such ignorant communities exposed to frequent injecting/ tattooing/piercing episodes need to be educated about the needle sharing risks. A recently published report has indicated that the proportion of population aware of the potential risk of HIV infection through unsafe injections in India was only 19 per cent in 1999 (*Hindustan Times*, Nov.8, 2003). Thus, the study strongly suggests that besides general population, tattoo artists as well as ear and nose piercing professionals should be covered by the ongoing HIV/AIDS prevention programmes in order to educate them about the safety of the above mentioned procedures.

Thirty-six per cent of the sample reported that they shared items of personal-use such as shaving blades and razors with their friends. Similarly, 20 per cent of the male sample observed that their barbers were using one single blade for shaving 2-3 customers. Razors were also being re-used in a similar manner. No in-between cleaning of shaving and hair cutting equipment was done except wiping them with a piece of cloth. All these sharing practices with no appropriate cleaning in-between raise serious concerns about the spread of the HIV.

The findings of the study are corroborated by similar findings by Bansal (1994), who in his study on barbers observed that the lowest standards of safer practices were observed by the road-side barbers who were forced to minimize their expenditure on account of paltry sums charged from their customers. The study further revealed that none of such barbers had any inkling of the risk of HIV transmission via infected instruments, hence they did not even observe the simple procedure of thoroughly washing their instruments between clients and usually rinsed them in a small water container. Similarly, another study by Wanjpe and Akarte (1997) showed that 21 per cent of the barbers used one single blade for three or more customers thus enhancing the risk of HIV transmission amongst customers. Various ongoing programmes have somehow overlooked the sharing practices prevalent among the poor and ignorant communities as well as amongst the barbers catering to the needs of such masses. These unsafe practices have been scientifically confirmed to increase the HIV vulnerability of people. Thus, immediate steps need to be taken to educate the vulnerable communities regarding the risks involved in sharing of shaving and hair cutting equipment. Targeted interventions aiming to create HIV/AIDS awareness among barbers are also urgently required to stop the chances of HIV transmission through unsafe shaving procedures.

Further, a broad range of sexual practices enhancing HIV risk was also found to be prevalent among the sample. Fig. 3.58 shows the prevalence of pre/extramarital sex among the three sample groups.

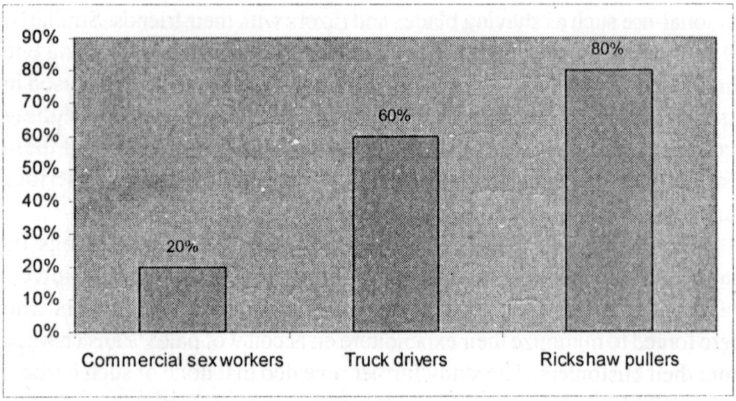

(* For CSWs prior to practicing of sex trade)

Fig. 3.58: Prevalence of PMS/EMS* among the Three Groups (N = 90).

Twenty per cent of the sex workers prior to their entry into the sex trade, 60 per cent of the truck drivers and 80 per cent of the rickshaw pullers reported to have indulged in pre-marital and/extra-marital sexual relationships. Further, the sexual orientation of such sample was found to be diverse and showed vast gender-based variation as shown in Figure 3.59.

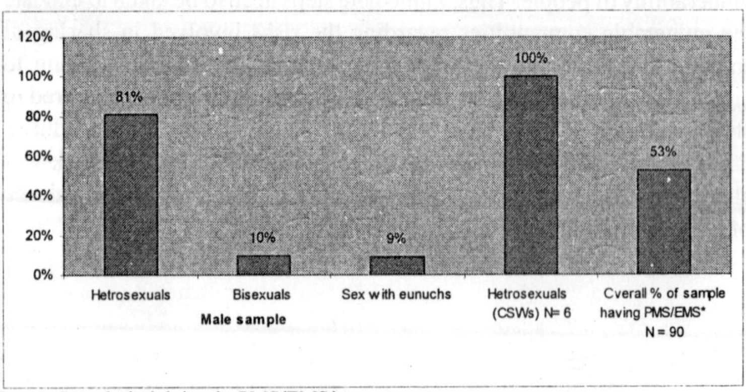

Base : Sample indulging in PMS/EMS*

(* For CSWs prior to their entry into sex trade).

Fig. 3.59 : Sexual Orientation of the Sample Indulging in PMS/EMS

Eighty-one per cent of the men having sex with non-regular partner/s reported to be heterosexuals and had sexual transactions either with paid or casual female partners. The paid partners have been recognized as mainly the commercial sex workers whereas the casual partners are the neighbours, relatives, friends, etc. (APAC-VHS, 2000) who are usually paid in kind for their services. Further, 10 per cent of the men having sex with non-regular partner/s were found to be bisexual, i.e., they had sexual relationships with both men and women, while 9 per cent of the men admitted having sexual relationships with eunuchs.

Contrary to this, all the CSWs that had sex with non-regular partners prior to their entry in the sex trade reported to have indulged only in heterosexual relationships. The overall high proportion of respondents (53 per cent) indulging in pre/extramarital sex shows that values attached to abstinence before marriage and fidelity after marriage are on a decline. Thus, there is an urgent need to address issues related to safe sex rather than insisting only on abstinence and fidelity factors.

The criterion to choose a sexual partner for indulging in pre/extramarital sex is another area, which needs to be explored at length. Various misconceptions were found to be prevalent amongst the sample regarding the same. For example, 47 per cent of the entire sample thought that if a sexual partner appeared healthy looks-wise then there were no chances of being infected with any disease through that partner. Infections such as HIV/AIDS and STD do not usually show up looks-wise but may still be very much present in a healthy looking sexual partner is a concept that people need to be aware of. The survey by NACO (2001) also revealed that awareness level of the fact that a healthy looking person could be suffering from HIV was low amongst people practicing high-risk behaviour.

Further, 33 per cent of the male sample in the present study indulging in pre/extramarital sex with CSWs was found to be placing a lot of importance on the age of their sexual partner/s. It was generally believed by them that young commercial sex workers were disease free since they had been exposed to sex work for comparatively less period of time as compared to the old sex workers. Thus, according to them the chances of young sex workers being HIV infected were negligible in comparison to the old sex workers. Misconceptions like these need to be assessed and addressed for effective control of HIV/AIDS and STD.

The prevalence of multi-partnerism was also found to be very high among the sample indulging in pre/extramarital sex. Fig. 3.60 shows the relative percentage of the sample along with the number of non-regular sexual partner/s they had at any given time.

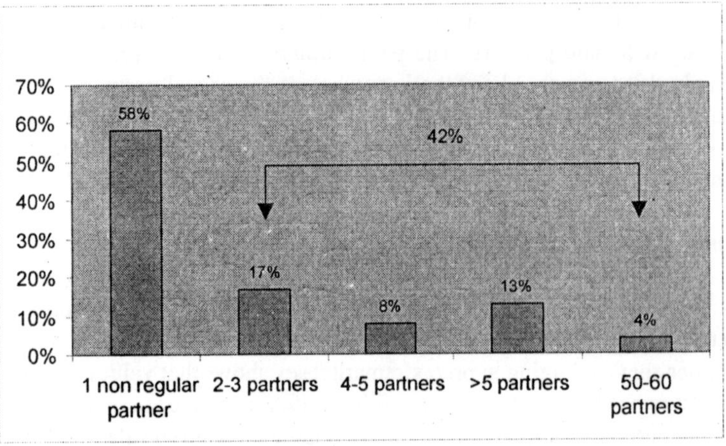

Fig. 3.60: Number of Non-regular Partner/s of Sample Indulging in PMS/EMS*(N=48).

(* For CSWs prior to their entry into sex trade).

Overall, 58 per cent of the sample having sex with non-regular partners was found to be having only one non-regular sexual partner, 17 per cent of such sample had 2-3 sexual partners, 8 per cent had 4-5 partners and 13 per cent were found to be having more than 5 non-regular partners. Amazingly, 4 per cent of the sample indulging in pre/extramarital sex reported to have as many as 50-60 sexual partners spread over a couple of years.

Here, it is important to clarify that in the case of commercial sex workers, the prevalence of multi-partnerism was taken as the number of non-regular sexual partners they had prior to their entry into the sex trade. The prevalence of multi-partnerism in sex trade was not taken into account because firstly it was an occupational necessity and not a matter of personal choice unlike the case of the truck drivers and the rickshaw pullers and secondly, it was not feasible for the CSWs to keep a track of the entire number of sexual partners they ever had during their course of occupation.

Overall, 42 per cent of the sample indulging in pre/extramarital sex had more than one sexual partner at any given time. To make matters worse, the majority of such sample (60 per cent) treated all of their sexual partners as steady partners since they had sexual transactions with them on a continued basis over a period of time. This misconception of treating all sexual partners as steady partners was leading to enhanced high-risk behaviour amongst the concerned sample in terms that the sample was not using a condom with these non-regular sexual partners. Practicing unsafe sex with such partners was a result of the complacency feeling developed among the sample that sexual partners known over a period of time could not pose to be a risk for HIV transmission. Further, it is important to observe that 38 per cent of the men indulging in pre/extramarital sex were having sexual transactions with CSWs (i.e., paid partners) as well as local women of their native villages (i.e., casual partners). Thus, these men were acting as bridges and raising the probability of passing the HIV infection from the vulnerable population (CSWs) to the general population (i.e., local village women).

The study also revealed that the sample was indulging in a vast range of unprotected sexual practices and that the range of these practices varied with the type of sexual partner. For instance, out of 43 per cent of the married male sample having pre-marital and/extra-marital sex, 69 per cent of these reported to be practicing only vaginal sex with their spouses in contrast to the paid or casual partners with whom they practiced all types of sexual practices including the unprotected ones. The different types of unprotected sexual practices practiced with non-regular partners as reported by the sample were – vaginal sex, anal sex, oral sex and deep/ French kissing. Similar tendency to indulge in different types of unprotected sexual acts for the want of sexual adventurism has also been shown in their study by Rompa et al. (1996).

It was further observed that out of 64 per cent of the sample practicing anal/oral sex with their non-regular partners, 57 per cent of these was not using a condom while doing so. They believed that HIV/AIDS could be transmitted only by vaginal sex and not through anal and oral sex. Similarly, the study revealed that although homosexuality was common among 17 per cent of the male sample yet, not a single man out of these was using a condom for homosexual acts. All of them believed that having sex with men was safe and that HIV could be acquired only through heterosexual contact with CSWs. Similar finding depicting a low proportion of condom use by men while indulging in homosexual acts has also been reported by the Operation Research Group's high-risk behavioural surveillance survey (NACO, 2001). The study highlights on the need to recognize homosexuality, which is otherwise viewed as a crime in India Under section 377 of the Indian Penal Code (IPC), (*Times of India*, Sept.22, 2003), as a prevalent factor in our society. Sexual minorities such as homosexuals need to be addressed rather than being penalized/discriminated against on the basis of their sexual orientation, for effective control of HIV to take place. Although targeted interventions for men having sex with men are being implemented at various high-risk sites yet, low condom usage among them suggests that such interventions are lacking substance somewhere. The challenge remains for ongoing HIV/AIDS prevention programmes to adequately expand and upgrade their response in accordance to the needs of the homosexuals.

In essence, the study data clearly portrays a wide and diverse range of sexual practices and the misconceptions related to them, which may potentiate HIV & STD transmission. It has been rightly observed that diversity of sexual practices among sexual partners seems to be much more widespread than is generally appreciated (Morais de Sa'c, et al., 1996). Thus, there lies an urgent need to acknowledge these diversities in context of their ability to enhance HIV transmission and address the same while designing effective HIV/AIDS prevention interventions.

The rate of disclosure to spouse regarding indulgence in pre-marital/ extra-marital sexual relationships was found to be abysmally low. Fig. 3.61 shows the percentage of disclosure by the sample to their spouse regarding their pre- and/extra-marital sexual relations.

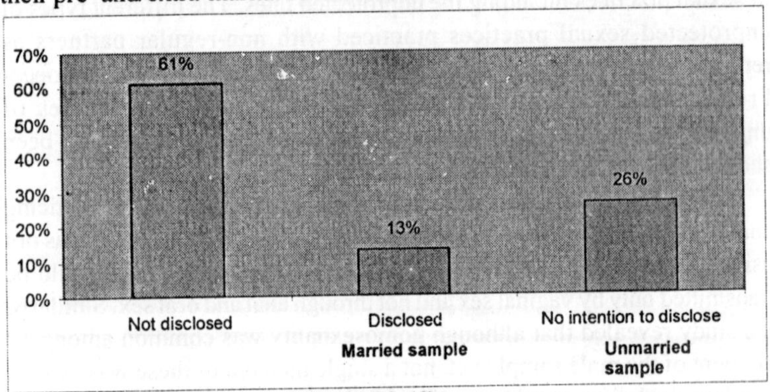

Base : Sample indulging in PMS/EMS* (N=48).
(For CSWs prior to their entry into sex trade).*

Fig. 3.61: Disclosure to Spouse.

Sixty-one per cent of the married sample who had sex with non-regular partner/s had not disclosed about their pre-marital and/extra-marital sexual relations to their spouse, 13 per cent of the married sample admitted that they had disclosed about such relationships to their spouse whereas 26 per cent of the sample (unmarried) said that they did not intend to reveal about such relationships to their would-be spouse before or after marriage. Further, 71 per cent of the men having pre-marital and /extra-marital sexual relations opined that it was not necessary for men to divulge such information to their wives due to the fact that having such relationships was common and acceptable for men in the society. Contrary to this, 50 per cent of the married women who ever had premarital sexual relations (including coerced ones) said that they had not told their spouse about such relationships due to the fear of desertion by them.

Further, it was found that pre/extramarital sexual relationships were not brief but were usually maintained over a long period of time, thus enhancing the risk of HIV transmission by the sheer virtue of the long time spent by the individual in practicing high-risk behaviour. Fig. 3.62 shows the relative percentage of the sample along with their time-wise length of maintaining pre- and/ extra-marital sexual contacts.

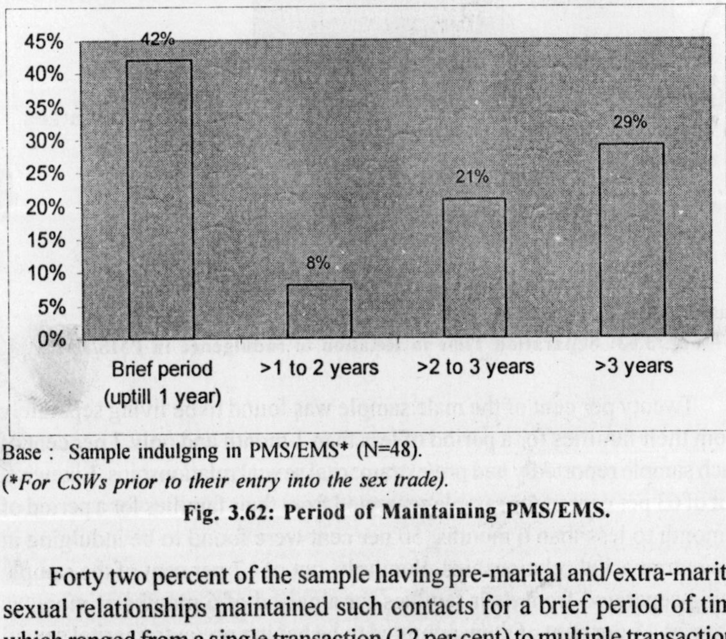

Base : Sample indulging in PMS/EMS* (N=48).
(*For CSWs prior to their entry into the sex trade).

Fig. 3.62: Period of Maintaining PMS/EMS.

Forty two percent of the sample having pre-marital and/extra-marital sexual relationships maintained such contacts for a brief period of time which ranged from a single transaction (12 per cent) to multiple transactions (30 per cent) with in a time-period of up till 1 year. Eight per cent of such sample maintained multiple premarital or extramarital sexual transactions for a period of more than 1-2 years, 21 per cent of them had such relations for more than 2-3 years and 29 per cent of the sample had been having such contacts for more than 3 years. The indulgence of the sample in multiple pre/extramarital sexual transactions over a long period of time suggests that the sample had become habitual of having such sexual relationships and thus giving up of the same in the near future was a distant possibility.

It was further observed that the tendency to indulge in pre/extramarital sex was directly related to the separation period of the sample from their families. The data reveals that men who stayed away from their families for longer durations of time were more likely to indulge in pre/extramarital sexual relationships as compared to their counterparts who were separated only for short durations. Fig. 3.63 depicts the separation time of the male sample from their families along with the relative percentage indulging in pre/extra-marital sex.

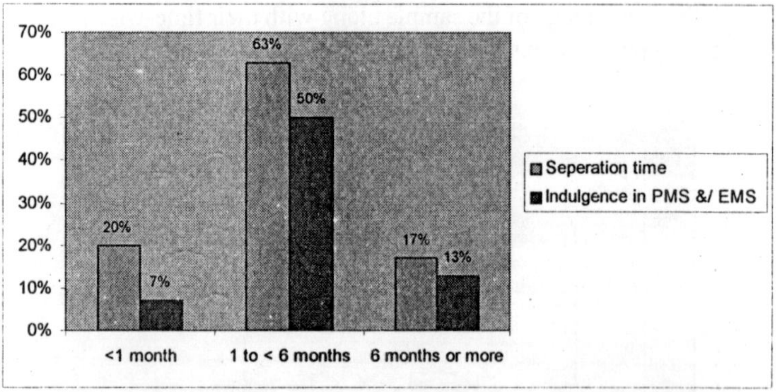

Base : Male sample (N=60).

Fig. 3.63: Separation Time in Relation to Indulgence in PMS/EMS.

Twenty per cent of the male sample was found to be living separately from their families for a period of less than 1 month and only 7 per cent of such sample reportedly had pre/extramarital sexual relationships. Likewise, out of 63 per cent of the sample separated from their families for a period of 1 month to less than 6 months, 50 per cent were found to be indulging in pre/extramarital relationships. Similarly, out of 17 per cent of the sample being separated from their families for a period of 6 months or more, as many as 13 per cent of them admitted to be having pre/extramarital sexual relations.

The familial separation factor in relation to the tendency to indulge in pre/extramarital sex was not applied in the case of CSWs because the sex workers were indulging in such sexual activity due to occupational reasons and not merely to overcome the separation factor.

Further, majority of the sample (71 per cent) indulging in pre/extramarital sex stated that most of the time such sexual transactions were planned before hand, thereby implying, that their unprotected sexual contacts were not a result of an impulsive act. The sample went in for pre/extramarital sex in a planned manner and yet, did not find it necessary to carry a condom with them. This finding reinforces the need of setting the use of a condom as a personal standard especially for those for whom pre/extramarital sex is not a distant possibility. Condoms have to be promoted in a way, which convinces people that using condoms coincides with community norms (Adrien, et al., 1996).

As far as the monetary expenditure incurred by the sample on each of their pre/extramarital sexual transaction was concerned, it was found that the cost for every such sexual transaction ranged anywhere between Rs.30 to Rs.150 depending upon the earning potential of the sample. Fig. 3.64 depicts the average monthly expenditure incurred by the male sample for indulging in pre/extra-marital sex.

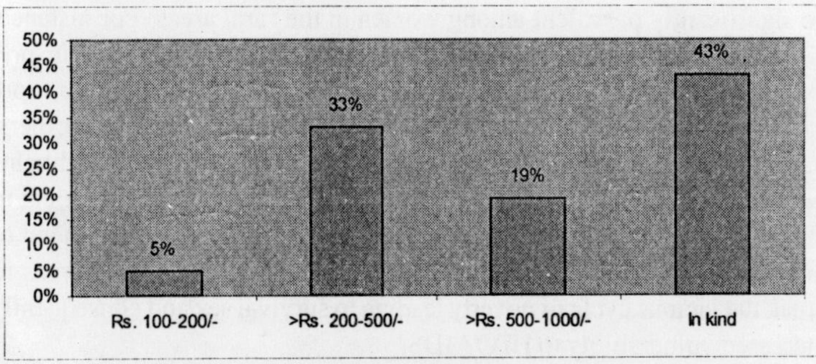

Base : Male sample indulging in PMS/EMS (N=42).

Fig. 3.64: Average Monthly Expenditure on PMS/EMS.

As far as the monthly expenditure was concerned, 5 per cent of the male sample indulging in sex with non-regular partner/s was found to be spending Rs.100 to 200 per month on such sexual transactions, 33 per cent were spending anywhere between more than Rs. 200 to 500 per month, while 19 per cent reported to be spending more than Rs. 500 to 1000 per month. On being asked if the expenditure incurred on pre/extramarital sexual transactions was felt to be taxing, 71 per cent of the sample replied in negative. Fifty-seven per cent of them even thought that it was essential for them, as it kept their spirits high and they were able to earn better for their families.

The expenditure pattern detailed above shows that although the sample was found to be spending a reasonable amount of their earnings on pre/extra-marital sexual transactions yet, 19 per cent of them felt that condoms were expensive and found it hard to spend an additional Rs. 3 to

Rs. 5 (i.e., the purchasing cost of a condom) for each of their sexual transaction.

This finding substantiates the fact that the price factor may not really be a barrier to condom usage for some of the sample as reported earlier by them. Rather, it was the lack of responsibility to practice safe sex that was a major reason for no condom usage. The findings strongly suggest that it is vitally important to create an understanding of responsibility pertaining to sexual matters. Various modes that help in transmitting information related to sex and sexuality from one generation to another should also stress on the need to practice sex safely. Safe sex has to become a universal norm in order to contain the spread of the HIV.

Another crucial finding of the study was that "survival sex" i.e., exchanging sex for services in kind such as food and clothing seemed to be significantly prevalent among women in the rural areas. For instance, 43 per cent of the male sample in the present study indulging in pre/extramarital sex was found to be paying in kind (i.e., items such as food, clothes and household commodities) to their rural female sexual partners. Such high percentage of women practicing survival sex ironically highlights the extreme poverty in rural areas as well as the resultant need leading to the selling of sex solely for survival basis. There lies an urgent need to improve the economic condition of women especially in rural areas to break the vicious cycle of poverty leading to survival sex and consequently increased vulnerability to HIV/AIDS.

The Intervention – *a review*

Based on the assessment of practices as observed by the sample during the pre-intervention period, group discussions and demonstrations were mainly used as tools in conjunction with the audio-visual aids to change the same in a desired way during the intervention period. Discussions focusing on the risks involved in sharing of needles, syringes, blades etc. were conducted with the sample. The sample was accordingly counselled. Further, the practice to indulge in drinking alcohol, subsequently leading to practicing of unsafe behaviour was portrayed and challenged by the photo-script. Similarly, the tendency to indulge in PMS/EMS was questioned through the photo-script. The sample was related instances through the use of these audio-visual aids where they had chances to introspect into their own behaviour and practices enhancing their vulnerability to HIV/AIDS.

Demonstrations proved to be very effective in teaching the sample on how to disinfect used needles by boiling them in water for twenty minutes. Likewise, demonstrations on conducting a few easy exercises with the goal of living a healthy life were considered to be unique and beneficial by the sample. The communities under the study participated in these activities by acting as human resource.

Practices Assessment - Post-intervention

A positive impact of the intervention on the sample was reflected in the form of various changes observed by them in their day-to-day practices. Overall, the sample was found to switch over to various general as well as sexual practices, which were safe with regards to HIV transmission. The significant changes recorded from the pre- to post-intervention period in certain practices as followed by the sample have been discussed as follows:

Fig. 3.65 shows the level of awareness amongst the sample regarding use of new or disinfected needles for injecting purpose.

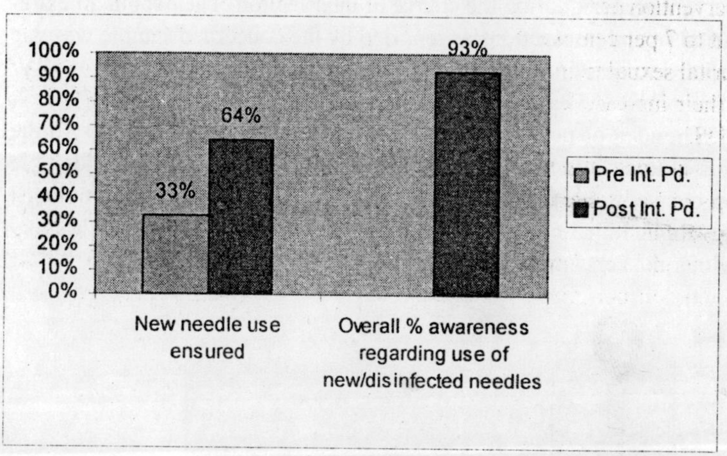

Fig. 3.65: Awareness Regarding use of New/disinfected Needles (N = 90).

Sixty-four per cent of the entire sample in the post-intervention period as against 33 per cent in the pre-intervention period now reportedly ensured that they were injected with a new needle and syringe whenever required by a doctor, for their medical ailments. Similarly, 16 per cent of the sample that had not been injected in the recent past said they would ensure in future that a new needle and syringe is used for the injecting purpose. Overall, 93 per cent of the sample was now aware that new or disinfected needles should be used for injecting, ear piercing and tattooing purposes.

There was a tremendous decline in the practice of sharing of items of personal-use such as blades and razors among the sample as reported by them. The proportion of respondents who shared these items declined from 36 per cent to 7 per cent during the intervention period. Most importantly, out of 20 per cent of the male sample that during the pre-intervention period had reported that their barbers were using a single blade or razor for shaving 2-3 customers, 17 per cent of them in the post-intervention period said they ensured that their barbers used a new blade for shaving them, 13 per cent of them also said that they asked their barbers to clean the razors thoroughly prior to any reuse.

A slight but crucial decrease was recorded in the percentage of truck drivers and rickshaw pullers indulging in extra-marital sex during the post intervention period. The percentage of such sample decreased from 13 per cent to 7 per cent during the course of intervention. The decline in extra-marital sexual transactions as reported by the concerned sample was due to their increase in knowledge regarding high-risk behaviour and HIV/AIDS.

The idea of perceived vulnerability to HIV/AIDS and STD on the basis of looks and age of the sexual partner/s also showed considerable improvements as a result of dispelling of various misconceptions amongst the sample. Fig. 3.66 depicts the decline in percentage of sample holding various misconceptions.

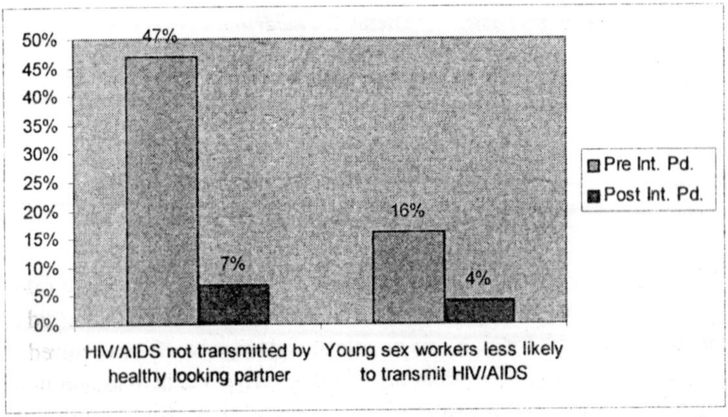

Fig. 3.66: Percentage Decline in Various Misconceptions amongst the Sample (N=90).

As compared to 47 per cent of the sample who during the pre-intervention period wrongly believed that a healthy looking sexual partner could not transmit HIV/AIDS, only 7 per cent of the sample in the post-intervention period thought it to be correct. Similarly, only 4 per cent of the sample in the post-intervention phase as against 16 per cent prior to the intervention felt that young sex workers were less likely to transmit HIV/AIDS as compared to the old sex workers. The decline in these ratios confirms the dispelling of myths and misconceptions of the sample related to HIV/AIDS transmission.

Further, the prevalence of multi-partnerism decreased during the period of intervention. Fig. 3.67 shows the quantitative changes in the prevalence of multi-partnerism during the pre- and post-intervention period.

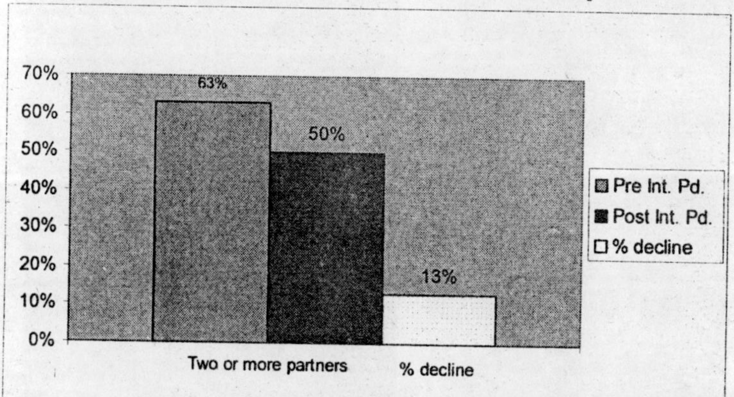

Base : Male sample continuing to indulge in PMS/EMS during pre- and post-intervention period (N=16).

Fig. 3.67: Changes in Prevalence of Multi-partnerism.

The sample showed a decline in the number of sexual partners they had at a given time. For instance, the proportion of male sample that continued to indulged in premarital and/extramarital sex and had two or more sexual partners at any given time during the course of intervention decreased from 63 per cent to 50 per cent. It was encouraging to observe that the decrease in the number of sexual partners was a result of the understanding inculcated amongst the sample that having more than one sexual partner at any given time meant that they were not steady partners and thus posed a high-risk of HIV transmission. The concept of steady versus non-steady partner/s had started becoming clearer among the sample groups.

Although the range of sexual practices observed by the sample did not show any quantitative change in the post-intervention period yet, the manner in which they were practiced showed positive qualitative changes. For instance, though the proportion of sample practicing anal and/oral sex remained the same at 64 per cent during the pre- and post-intervention periods, yet the percentage of sample practicing these acts without a condom decreased from 57 per cent to 26 per cent. The role of peer educators in convincing the sample to indulge in sexual activities (especially with non-regular partners) in a safe manner was appreciable as they were able to motivate the sample to practice safe sex.

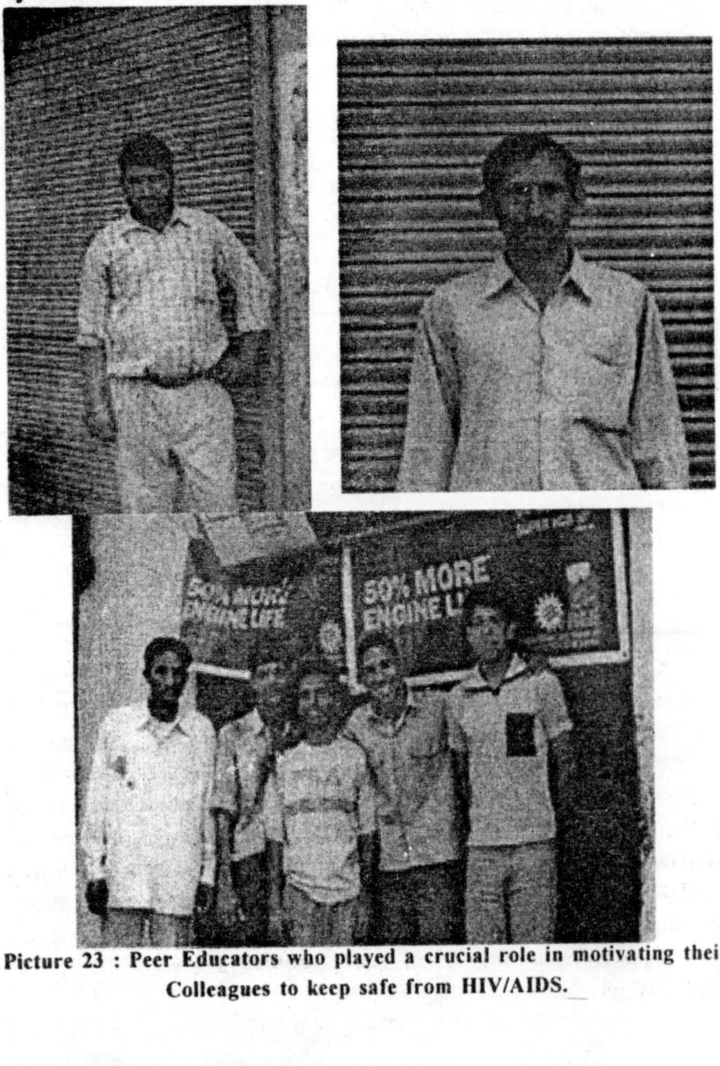

Picture 23 : Peer Educators who played a crucial role in motivating their Colleagues to keep safe from HIV/AIDS.

Likewise, the enactment of a skit in which two homosexual individuals were seen negotiating safe sex, was crucial in making the sample realize that safe sex was to be practiced in all relationships, be it hetero/homo sex or sex with eunuchs. Subsequently, the percentage of men using a condom for homosexual acts increased from zero to 50 per cent amongst the homosexual sample during the course of intervention. These changes depicted behavioural change amongst the sample in terms of their refusal to practice unsafe sex at all times. This aspect was used as one of the indicators to evaluate the study.

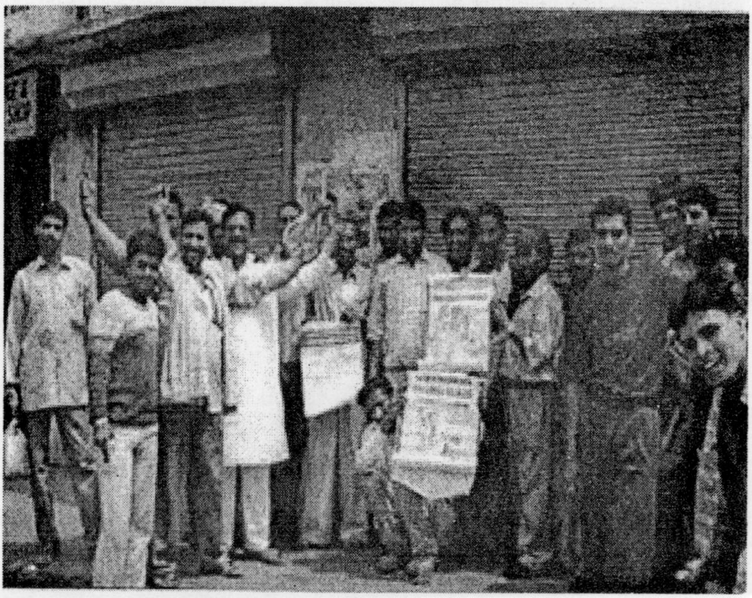

Picture 24: Sample seen in a Jubilant Mood during one of the Presentations in their Neighbourhood.

To summarize, the trend to practice safe anal, oral and homosexual behaviour by the sample marked a beginning of the realization amongst them that practicing safe sex was in their interest, which was ultimately the desired aim of the research.

Overall Changes in the KABP of the Sample from the Pre- to Post-intervention Period

The findings of the present study show that the intervention was effective in bringing about desirable changes in KABP of the sample in context of HIV/AIDS.

The comparison between the pre- and post-intervention data showed a substantial gain in the overall mean scores of the sample on the KABP scale. In order to see whether the gain was significant 't-test' was applied to the pre- and post-intervention scores of the sample. Table 3.2 depicts the overall changes in the mean scores of the sample groups on each scale (knowledge, attitude, behaviour and practices) during the pre- and post-intervention period along with the computed t-test values.

As is evident from the table, the scores of the sample in the post-intervention period showed an appreciable gain in all aspects i.e., knowledge, attitude, behaviour and practices. The comparison between the three groups in terms of their mean KABP scores showed that the commercial sex workers scored a fairly high score in all the aspects during the pre-intervention period as compared to the truck drivers and the rickshaw pullers. This was evidently due to their exposure to various ongoing HIV/AIDS prevention programmes in the red light area. Similar trends were observed in the post-intervention period with the commercial sex workers faring better than the other two groups due to their comparatively high base level. Such trends were expected due to the fact that improvisation in the scores took place reasonably in accordance to their pre-intervention values.

The t-test provided a statistical base to the data obtained and since the absolute values of t-calculated > t-tabulated values for knowledge, attitude, behaviour and practices scale, the hypothesis that, "There is no change in knowledge, attitude, behaviour and practices (KABP) of the sample due to the intervention is rejected." Hence, proving the significance of the intervention.

In order to have some tangible outcomes of the research "AIDS Awareness Through Community Participation - An Action Research", a modest attempt was made to develop a set of communication aids. These aids comprised of a photo-script, a pamphlet and a poster. From concept to completion, the community was involved in their development. Keeping in mind the expertise and resource availability, the presentation of the material is simple, candid and easy to comprehend even without an interpreter. Moreover, these aids can be easily replicated for further use. The proceeding section highlights the need to develop, the characteristics as well as the field-testing results of these audio-visual aids.

Table 3. 2 : Mean KABP Scores during the Pre – and Post– intervention Period with t-test values

	Knowledge Assessment Scale Mean Scores		*t-test Values*		*Attitude Assessment Scale Means Scores*		*t-test Values*		*Condom Use Behaviour and Practices Assessment Scale Mean Scores*		*t-test Values*	
Max. Score	**20**				**9**				**20**			
Sample groups	Pre	**Post**	N	**t calculated* & t tabulated****	Pre	**Post**	**N**	**t calculated* & t tabulated****	Pre	**Post**	**N**	**t calculated* & t tabulated****
Commercial sex workers	8.07	**13.67**	30	**-16.93*** **± 2.04 ****	5.73	**7.87**	30	**-16.00*** **± 2.04 ****	18.33	**19.27**	30	**-7.39*** **± 2.04 ****
Truck drivers	7.13	**13.60**	30	**-21.96*** **± 2.04 ****	2.67	**6.40**	30	**-12.47*** **± 2.04 ****	2.44	**11.44**	18	**-13.90*** **± 2.11 ****
Rickshaw pullers	1.40	**11.53**	30	**-25.32*** **± 2.04 ****	2.27	**6.80**	30	**-22.16*** **± 2.04 ****	3.67	**13.08**	24	**-10.07*** **± 2.06 ****
Overall mean score (For the three sample groups)	**5.53**	**12.93**			**3.56**	**7.02**			**8.15**	**14.60**		

Development and Field-Testing of the Audio-Visual Aids — A Community Participated Action

The Need to Develop Audio-Visual Aids During the Course of Study

Audio-visual aids were developed and used in the present study to create AIDS awareness among the sample communities. The need to use audio-visual aids arose from the fact that 64 per cent of the study sample was illiterate and thus creating AIDS awareness through the distribution of print material such as brochures and pamphlets was not feasible. The study further revealed that mass media channels such as T.V. and radio had not been very helpful in imparting AIDS awareness, as 42 per cent of the sample did not have an access to these media. Even those who had an access to these channels had not been reasonably exposed to AIDS awareness information messages.

Moreover, 62 per cent of the sample was found to be harbouring various forms of myths and misconceptions regarding HIV/AIDS as well as STD. It was realized that various existing audio-visual aids developed by NACO and other organizations had not been very effective in dispelling the same due to certain reasons which have been elaborately discussed in the proceeding section related to the evaluation of existing audio-visual aids. Thus, a need to develop audio-visual aids based on the needs of the communities with regards to their knowledge level, attitudes, behaviour and practices was acutely felt.

Evaluation of a Few Existing Audio Visual Aids Used with the Sample

Some of the audio-visual aids developed by NACO, Drishtikone, Maharashtra network for positive people (MNP+) and other organizations (as listed in Appendix XI) were initially used with the sample for creating AIDS awareness and also for need assessment basis. The use and subsequent evaluation of these audio-visual aids revealed that some of them required specific improvisations in order to increase their accessibility and to make them community-appropriate. The findings pertaining to the evaluation of some of the audio-visual aids along with a few suggested improvisations have been discussed as follows:

Firstly, it was observed that many of the visual aids in the form of hoardings, posters and banners were put up at places such as outside big hospitals, railway stations, cinema halls and by road sides in cities and on highways.

The placement of these messages on such points relied heavily on the assumption that people will have an access to these places and that they will read and understand the AIDS awareness messages put up there. Contrary to this, there lies an urgent need to reach the masses without relying on the targeted groups to reach such locations. For instance, in the present study 38 per cent of the people had not seen any of the public display AIDS awareness messages due to reasons such as illiteracy, lack of interest and limited mobility as in the case of commercial sex workers.

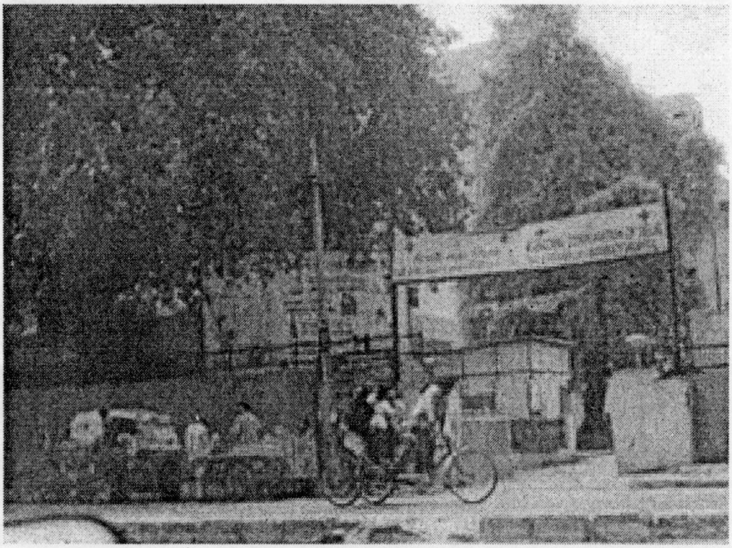

Picture 25 : A Partially Visible Hoarding showing Modes of HIV Transmission Outside a Hospital in Delhi.

The coverage of AIDS awareness programmes needs to be greatly increased by adopting proactive measures, which aim at reaching people before the infection reaches them and not just depending upon people to seek such life-saving information.

Secondly, it was noticed that these public display messages were crafted with the assumption that people would be able to read as well as comprehend them in a correct manner. In a sense, the display messages catered only to the needs of the literate population as exemplified by picture 26. In contrast, 64 per cent of the study sample was found to be illiterate and thus AIDS awareness messages in the form of written text material were not suitable for them. Hence, there was a need to develop audio-visual aids, which could cater to the needs of the illiterate sample.

Thirdly, it was also experienced that many of the existing aids conveyed only partial information and did not equip people with the practical skills that were essential to implement their new knowledge. For instance, the brochure developed by NACO as shown in Fig. 3.68 advices people to use a condom to protect themselves from AIDS but it does not give any information about the correct method of using a condom.

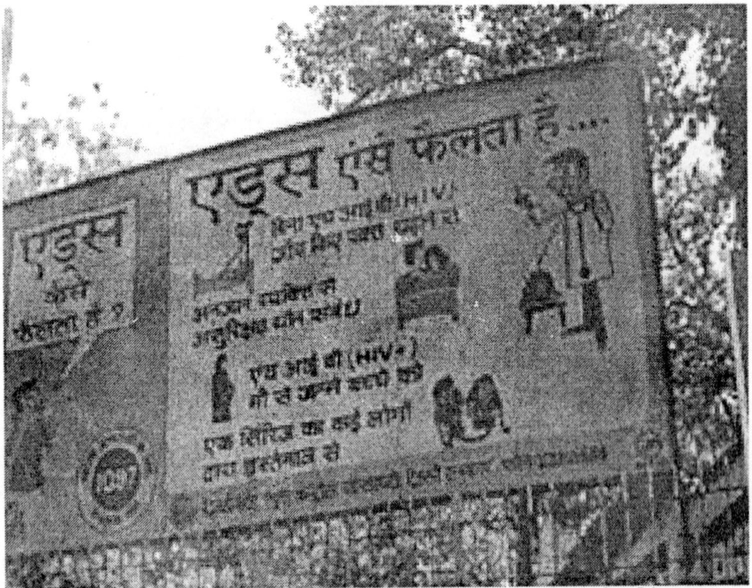

Picture 26: A Hoarding on HIV/AIDS Awareness - Only for Literate Population.

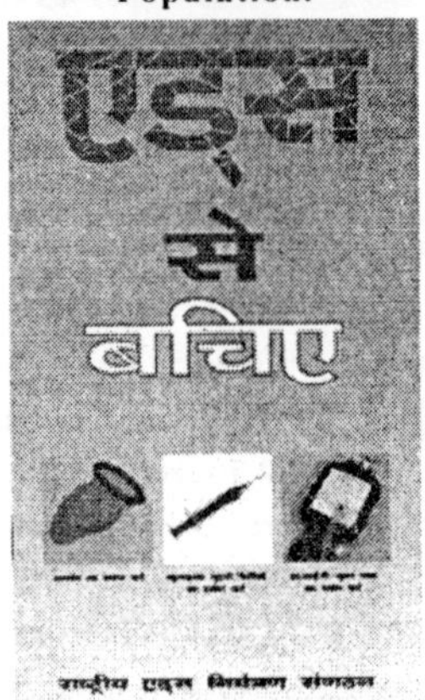

Fig. 3.68 : **A Brochure by NACO Advising People for usage of Condom and Sterilized Needles and Syringes as Protection against HIV/AIDS.**

Similarly, this aid also suggests people to use sterilized needles and syringes as protection against AIDS but no information is given regarding ways to sterilize a needle and syringe in the absence of new equipment. Thus, imparting mere theoretical information is not going to help in containing spread of the virus. There is a massive need to integrate preventive skills along with AIDS information.

Further, some of the visual aids were found to be ambiguous by the study sample. For example, a poster developed by NACO shown in Fig. 3.69 was meant to convey to the masses that having sex with a non-regular partner could be an invitation to STD (including AIDS), however, 64 per cent of the study sample because of their illiteracy/ignorance and lack of awareness regarding HIV/AIDS were unable to comprehend this message. Instead, 58 per cent of such sample thought that the poster advised people to walk carefully on the road, while 42 per cent of the sample was of the opinion that the poster suggested to the masses to follow traffic signals properly.

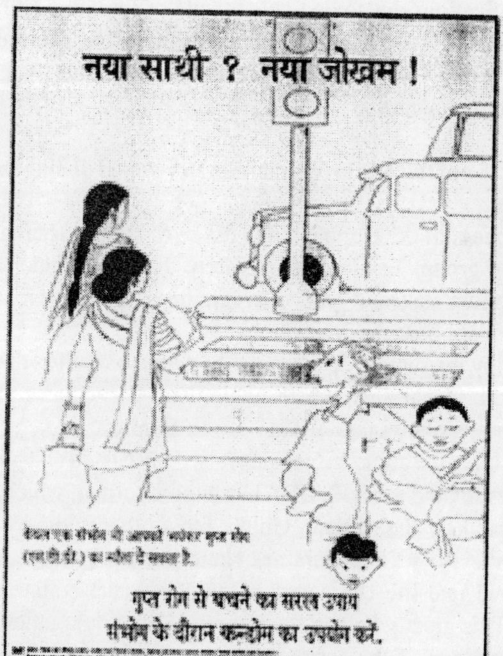

Fig. 3.69: A Poster Developed by NACO that Conveyed Ambiguous Meaning to the Sample because of the their Illiteracy.

Thus, the findings confirm that the comprehending ability of the people may vary in accordance to their perception as well as literacy status. In order to overcome subjective ambiguity, emphasis should be placed on having AIDS awareness programmes that rely more on interpersonal communication than on mere visualization. Lastly, but most importantly it was observed that even participants who had been exposed to AIDS awareness messages through media such as T.V., newspaper or road side hoardings were not fully aware about the entire aspects of the disease. For instance, 74 per cent of the individuals who has even seen/heard an AIDS awareness message reported that they had not been able to understand the symptoms of the disease, 61 per cent said that they had confusion regarding modes and preventive aspects of AIDS.

Overall, 78 per cent of the sample exposed to any AIDS awareness message reported that they had not fully understood the entire contents of the message and some doubt/s regarding AIDS still persisted. The major reason cited for the lack of complete understanding was the inability to seek clarifications due to one-sided mode of communication.

Therefore, a good strategy for creating AIDS awareness should incorporate interactive mode of communication rather than relying on one-sided communication.

Characteristics of the Audio-Visual Aids Developed during the Course of Intervention

The process of development and usage of audio-visual aids with the three sample groups has been elaborately discussed under the heading "Implementation stages of HIV intervention in the present study" in the chapter on methodology.

The following section details out the features as well as the advantages of these audio-visual aids, which made them particularly effective and attractive amongst the sample. They are as follows:

1. The script of the audio-visual aids raised, discussed and gave solutions to issues related to HIV/AIDS in a simple format, which was easy to understand by the sample. Unlike most other audio-visual aids, in which the story characters are sketched, the present audio-visual aids used real-life characters belonging to the communities under study. This greatly helped the sample in identifying themselves with the characters of the script and also in introspection of their own behaviour. Many participants said that they too could be in similar situations in their real lives as the characters of the script.

2. The usage of the audio-visual aids helped as a powerful tool in breaking down the literacy and socio-cultural barriers. People who were illiterate and could not be reached by other modes of HIV prevention information were most benefited. Similarly, some of the socio-cultural issues such as recognition of rights of CSWs and curbing the usage of alcohol were effectively addressed in the audio-visual aids.
3. The audio-visual aids were also innovative with the following features incorporated into them:
   (a) **Fast** – The audio-visual aids proved to be a fast way of creating AIDS awareness as many people could be reached within a short period of time. No intensive training of any sort such as learning of dialogues or staging of performances was required on the part of the implementer. Only a single person (who could be a peer educator) was required to read out the script and explain it to the sample.
   (b) **Focused** - The audio visual aids focused on the needs of the community. The script of these aids was designed on the basis of a through understanding of the target population; its knowledge, myths and misconceptions, attitudes and practices. The contents were localized keeping in mind the cultural context and emphasized on how HIV really affects one's life rather than just imparting impersonal knowledge about HIV/AIDS.
   (c) **Integrated** – The audio-visual aids were integrated in the sense that they were comprehensive and touched almost all aspects related to HIV/AIDS. For instance, these aids not only provided information about HIV/AIDS but also stressed on the need to have positive attitudes, a sense of self-esteem, self-affirmation and above all a sense of responsibility towards others. Most importantly, communicative skills stressing on condom negotiation and practical skills like correct condom usage and disposal were emphasized. Further, concrete actions that needed to be taken for HIV prevention/management like practicing safe behaviour and leading a healthy life style were adequately stressed upon.
   (d) **Cost-effective** – The audio-visual aids were very economical to use as they were developed and implemented by using community resources. Some of the community members acted as role models in the development of these audio-visual aids while, few others helped as peer educators in using these audio-visual aids amongst their communities. In all, nine peer educators (i.e., three from

each of the sample groups) were trained to carry out the outreach activities. This was done with the aim of sustaining the preventive efforts even after the present intervention was over, which further enhanced cost-effectiveness of the programme. Further, no infrastructure or electronic media was required to operate these aids. Only an individual was required to read out the contents. The cost-effectiveness was also enhanced by the fact that these aids are easily replicable by merely photocopying them and thus can be used in similar sites with similar populations.

Overall, the audio-visual aids proved to be an innovative means of reaching the targeted population with crucial information and motivated them for safe practices. The ability to interact with the audience while presenting these aids helped in adding a human touch to the otherwise raw and general information.

The three audio-visual aids developed during the course of study formed to be a part of the dependent variable. This can be best explained by considering the fact that each audio-visual aid reflected the inter-group differences in terms of their message content. For example, the photo script was specifically developed keeping in mind the needs of the rickshaw pullers with regards to HIV information. This implies that on the basis of the pre-intervention KABP assessment of the three groups, it was observed that the rickshaw pullers constituted to be the most uninformed/unaware group in context to HIV/AIDS information primarily due to their illiteracy as well as non-exposure to HIV prevention programmes. Thus, a comprehensive audio-visual aid, detailing out each and every aspect related to HIV/AIDS was required to create awareness amongst them. Hence, an elaborate photo-script in which a few rickshaw pullers enacted different roles was evolved.

Similarly, while assessing KABP of the truck drivers, it was realized that although the truck drivers had a fairly reasonable knowledge regarding various aspects of AIDS yet, they had developed a sense of complacency towards the disease believing that they could not be affected by it and thus many of them were found to be practicing high-risk behaviour. Hence, it was imperative to intervene and stress on the fact that nobody was immune to AIDS and that prevention was of prime importance. Thus, a poster stressing on prevention from AIDS as a way to happiness was designed with a few truck drivers acting as role models.

As far as the commercial sex workers were concerned, it came into light while carrying out the intervention that they had developed a sense of lack of self-esteem/worthiness. Majority of them thought that their work was demeaning and thus they had no right as workers. Exploitation as a way of life had been ultimately, accepted by them. Many of these workers had been so demoralized that prevention from HIV/AIDS in order to live long was not what they valued. Thus, efforts were made to revive their value system by designing a pamphlet for them, which incorporated their rights as sex workers. The need for these workers to live a HIV/AIDS free life was also stressed for the sake of their children.

Although these audio-visual aids were designed depending on the needs of each sample group yet, all of them contained some information about HIV/AIDS, which could be commonly imparted to all the three groups. Hence, all the three aids were cross-used with each group. Another advantage of cross-using these aids amongst the sample was that each group came to know something about the lives, problems as well as experiences of other groups. This led to a better understanding amongst them resulting in some mutual respect/recognition. For instance, the truck drivers and the rickshaw pullers after viewing the pamphlet (designed for the sex workers) were able to realize that sex work too was work like their own and thus, sex workers too had certain basic rights just like them.

Field-Testing Results of the Audio-Visual Aids

The audio-visual aids developed during the course of study were field tested with a group of 15 individuals (i.e., 5 individuals from each community of commercial sex workers, truck drivers and rickshaw pullers). These participants were selected through purposive sampling method and were not a part of the earlier intervention. The three audio-visual aids were used consecutively with the sample groups as a package starting with the presentation of the poster through which it was conveyed that the audience too could be happy as the characters in the poster if the audience had some vital awareness regarding HIV/AIDS. This was followed by narration of the photo-script which gave information regarding all the crucial aspects of the disease and finally, the pamphlet was presented which apart from providing important information regarding AIDS also stressed upon the rights of commercial sex workers as well as the feeling of empowerment realized through AIDS awareness.

The detailed procedure entailing the process of field-testing has been discussed in the chapter on methodology under the heading "Field testing of the audio-visual aids". The following section deals with the comparison of the pre- and post-audio-visual aids field-testing results that reflect the changes brought about in the KABP of the sample as a result of the application of these audio-visual aids.

The mean age of the CSWs that represented the sample for field-testing of audio-visual aids was 29 years, for the truck drivers it was 27 years and for the rickshaw pullers 21 years. The median age of the respondents ranged between 21 to 27 years. The changes registered subsequent to the audio-visual aids field-testing have been discussed as follows:

Knowledge Assessment – Pre to Post-Field-Testing

The knowledge regarding AIDS showed considerable improvement amongst the sample as was assessed by the knowledge assessment scale (Appendix VIII). Overall, 27 per cent of the sample was not aware about HIV/AIDS prior to the field-testing of these audio-visual aids. However, in the post field-testing stage 100 per cent of the sample knew that AIDS was a fatal disease. Besides, various myths such as AIDS was a God's way of punishing people for their wrong doings and that AIDS could be cured by traditional healers registered a decline of 13 per cent, i.e., from 20 per cent to 7 per cent amongst the sample.

The knowledge regarding ways in which HIV is transmitted from one person to another showed an increase from 67 per cent to 100 per cent in the post-field-testing stage. Further, 87 per cent of the sample as compared to 20 per cent prior to the field-testing was now aware about other modes of HIV transmission too, apart from sex as shown in Fig. 3.70.

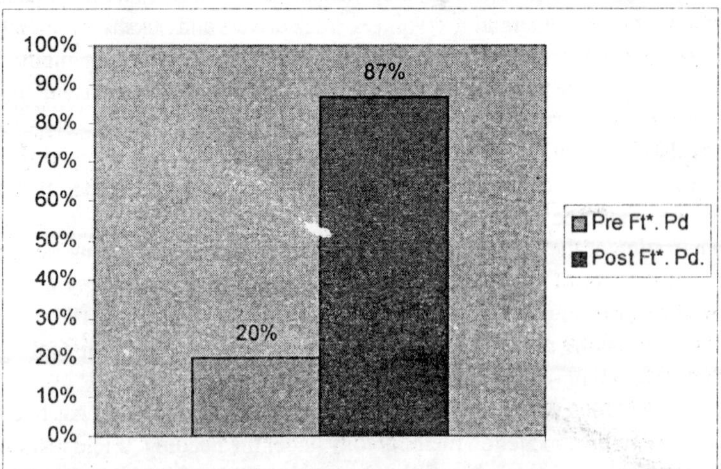

* Field-testing

Fig. 3.70 : Awareness Regarding other Modes of HIV Transmission apart from Sex (N = 15).

It is also important to note that misconceptions like AIDS could be acquired by casual contact, by sitting next to an infected person or by sharing food and water showed a significant decline of 20 per cent, i.e., initially from 33 per cent to 13 per cent in the post-field-testing period. Further, 73 per cent of the sample was able to enlist at least one of the symptoms of HIV/AIDS in the post-field-testing stage as compared to a mere 7 per cent during the pre-field-testing stage as shown in Fig. 3.71.

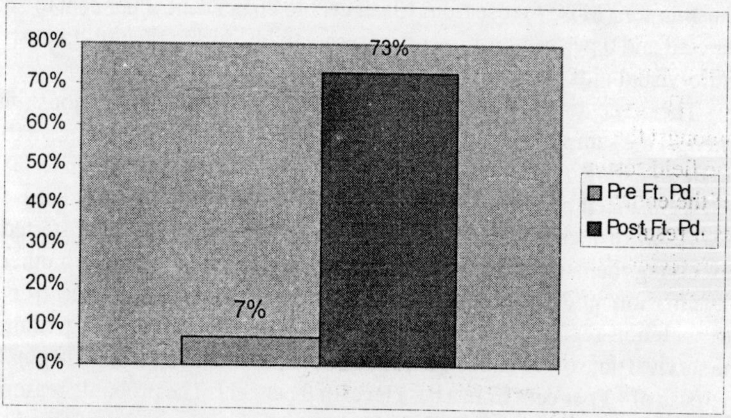

Fig. 3.71 : Awareness Regarding Symptoms of HIV/AIDS (N = 15).

Similarly, the knowledge regarding HIV/AIDS testing through blood tests and the availability of such facilities rose from 20 per cent to 93 per cent during the course of field-testing. The concept of fatality of the disease registered an increase of 54 per cent amongst the sample. Most importantly, the gain in knowledge regarding ways of preventing HIV/AIDS was significant. Fig. 3.72 shows the relative increase in awareness level of the sample regarding various modes of HIV/AIDS prevention during the pre- and post-audio-visual aids field-testing stages.

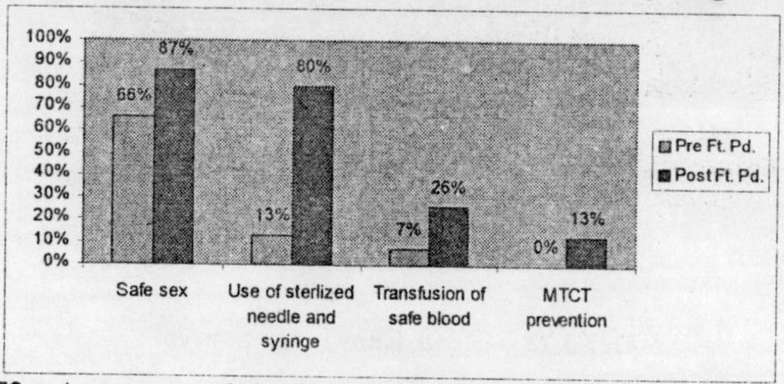

Fig. 3.72 : Awareness of the Sample Regarding various Methods of HIV/AIDS Prevention (N = 15).

Eighty-seven per cent of the sample in the post-audio-visual aids field-testing stage was aware about the importance of practicing safe sex as a mode of HIV/AIDS prevention as against only 66 per cent in the pre-field-testing stage. Similarly, the level of awareness regarding three other modes of HIV/AIDS prevention, which are the use of sterilized needle and syringe for injecting purpose, transfusion of safe blood when required and adherence to prophylactic measures to reduce mother to child transmission (MTCT) rose from 13 per cent to 80 per cent, 7 per cent to 26 per cent and 0 per cent to 13 per cent respectively during the pre- to post-audio-visual aids field testing stage.

The perception of risk of contracting HIV/AIDS showed a major shift amongst the sample and rose from 13 per cent to 40 per cent subsequent to the field-testing of the audio-visual aids. The rise was significant in terms of the enhanced perceived self-vulnerability of the sample to the disease as a result of increase in AIDS awareness. The sample had now started perceiving themselves to be at risk of acquiring HIV/AIDS due to other transmission modes too, such as sharing of needles and blades apart from sex with non-regular partner/s. Further, the level of awareness regarding the survival time of HIV and AIDS infected people registered only a marginal increase of 13 per cent from a base level of 0 per cent. The probable reason for registering only a small rise here was the complexity experienced by the sample in differentiating between HIV and AIDS.

The changes observed in the mean scores of the sample during the pre- and post-audio-visual aids field-testing periods are shown in Fig. 3.73.

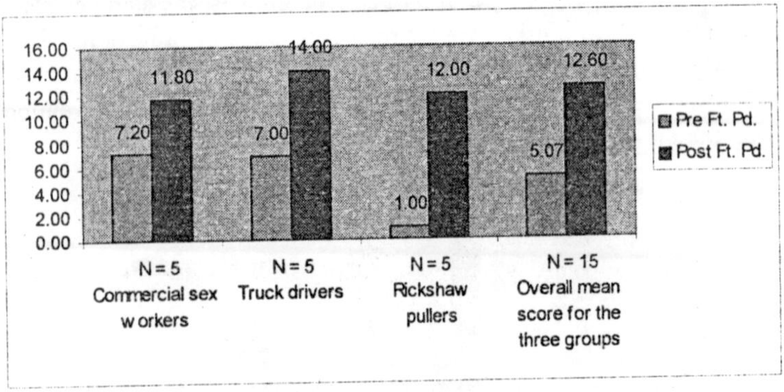

Fig. 3.73 : Mean Knowledge Scores.

The mean score for the CSWs increased from 7.20 to 11.80, for the truck drivers it increased from 7.00 to 14.00 and for the rickshaw pullers it rose from 1.00 to 12.00 out of a total score of 20. The overall mean score for the entire sample increased from 5.07 to 12.60 out of a total of 20 during the pre- to post-audio-visual aids field-testing period.

Attitude Assessment – Pre- to Post-Field-Testing

The comparison between the pre- and post-audio-visual aids, field-testing data showed marked differences in the attitude of the sample regarding HIV/AIDS and issues related to it, as assessed by the attitude assessment scale (concise form-Appendix XII). Positive changes were documented in the attitudes of the sample towards issues related to sexuality, vulnerability of people to STD, HIV/AIDS, rights of PWHA and the intention to get HIV tested.

Hundred per cent of the sample in the post-field-testing stage was convinced that education regarding sex, STD and HIV/AIDS should be given to the general population including appropriately aged children in schools. Prior to their exposure to the audio-visual aids, only 87 per cent of the sample approved of such an idea. Further, the concept of perceived vulnerability to STD, HIV/AIDS became much clearer as well as less stigmatized amongst the sample. For instance, 60 per cent of the sample prior to their viewing of these audio-visual aids believed that only commercial sex workers and people having unsafe sexual relations with them were vulnerable to STD and HIV/AIDS. But after their exposure to the audio-visual aids the proportion of such respondents decreased to a mere 33 per cent. This was due to the fact that other modes of HIV transmission such as contaminated needle, transfusion by infected blood and mother to child transmission were also seen as HIV vulnerability enhancers.

The attitude towards people living with HIV/AIDS (PWHA) also showed a significant difference as shown in Fig. 3.74.

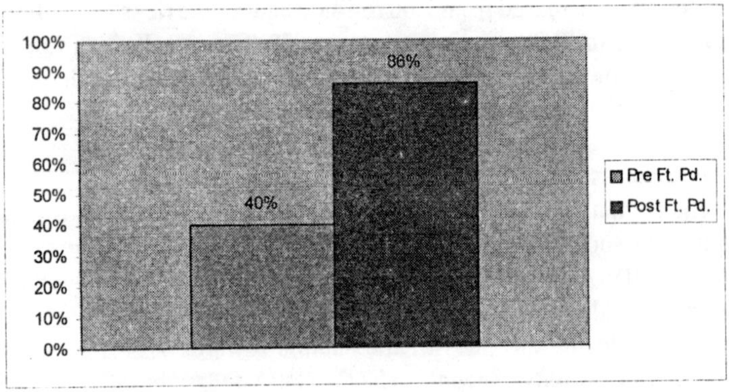

Fig. 3.74 : Attitude towards PWHA (N = 15).

The percentage of sample believing in equal rights of PWHA increased from 40 per cent to 86 per cent. In line with this change, was the shift registered in the attitude of the sample regarding treatment to be meted out to a HIV positive spouse. Fig. 3.75 shows the change in attitude of the sample towards a HIV positive spouse.

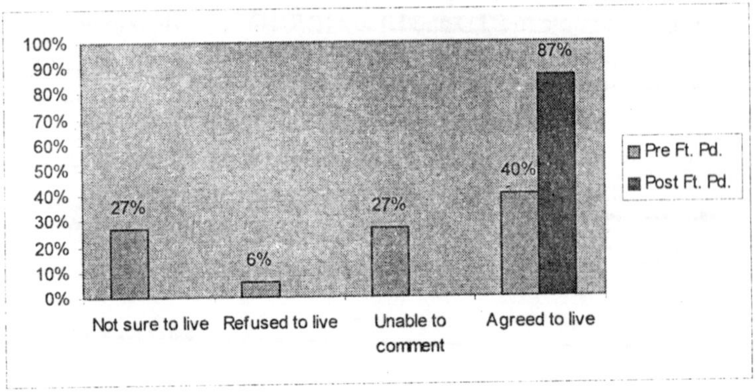

Fig. 3.75 : Attitude of the Sample towards a HIV Positive Spouse (N = 15).

Whereas, 27 per cent of the participants during the pre-field-testing stage were not sure if they would live with and take care of their spouse in case he/she got HIV infected, 6 per cent of them flatly refused to live with a HIV positive spouse. Twenty-seven per cent of the sample was not able to comment on the issue due to their lack of awareness about the disease. Only 40 per cent of the sample said that if their spouse tested HIV positive, they would still continue to live with them and take care of them. However, after the field-testing as high as 87 per cent of the sample stated that if during the course of time their spouse got HIV infected they would still continue to live with him/her.

The intention to get oneself tested for HIV increased significantly from 13 per cent to 33 per cent. Although the rise was not very big in terms of the numerical value owing to the shorter duration of the programme however, major gains are expected as has been previously shown through the intervention in the present study, when the programme is run on a continued basis. To summarize, the sample showed significant changes in their attitude towards various aspects related to HIV/AIDS. Fig. 3.76 shows the changes from the pre- to post-audio-visual field-testing period.

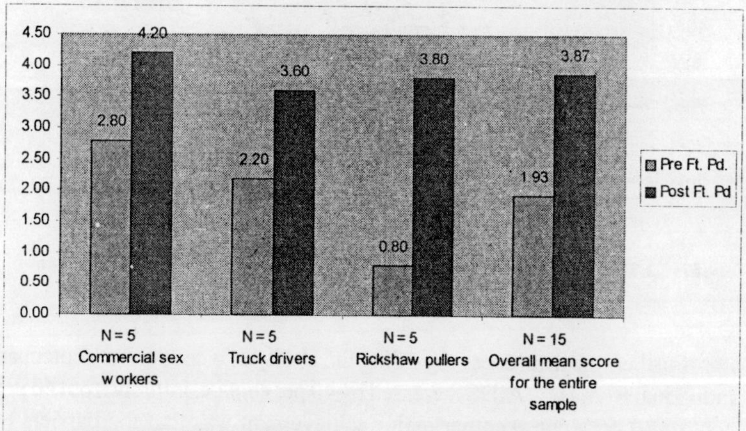

Fig. 3.76: Mean Scores on the Attitude Assessment Scale.

The mean score for the CSWs rose from 2.80 to 4.20, for the truck drivers it increased from 2.20 to 3.60 while for the rickshaw pullers it registered an increase from 0.80 to 3.80 out of a total score of 5. The overall mean score of the positive attitudes held by the sample on attitude assessment scale registered a rise from 1.93 to 3.87 out of a total of 5.

Condom Usage Behaviour and Practices Assessment – Pre- to Post-Field-Testing

The perception of the sample towards condom usage showed considerable improvement subsequent to the presentation of the audio-visual aids as was shown by the condom usage behaviour and practices assessment scale (concise form-Appendix XIII). The scores on this scale showed that 73 per cent of the sample in the post-field-testing phase was aware about at least two advantages of using a condom as compared to only 20 per cent prior to the field-testing period as shown in Fig. 3.77.

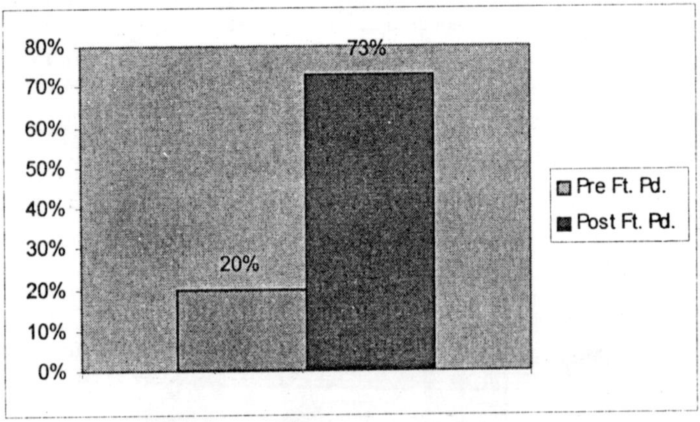

Fig. 3.77 : Awareness Regarding Two Advantages of using a Condom (N = 15).

Further, the awareness regarding the ability of a condom to protect an individual from HIV/AIDS increased by 40 per cent i.e. initially from 40 per cent to 80 per cent. Another major achievement was that the barriers to condom usage declined amongst 13 per cent of the sample, i.e., from 33 per cent to 20 per cent as a result of dispelling of misconceptions such as condoms were uncomfortable to use or that condoms acted as a barrier to sexual pleasure. Consequently, 44 per cent of the sample who had never used a condom with their non-regular partner/s said in the post-field-testing phase, that they will try using one in future.

Most importantly, it was encouraging to observe that the condom usage skills showed refinement in terms of correct method of using and disposing a condom as shown below in Fig. 3.78.

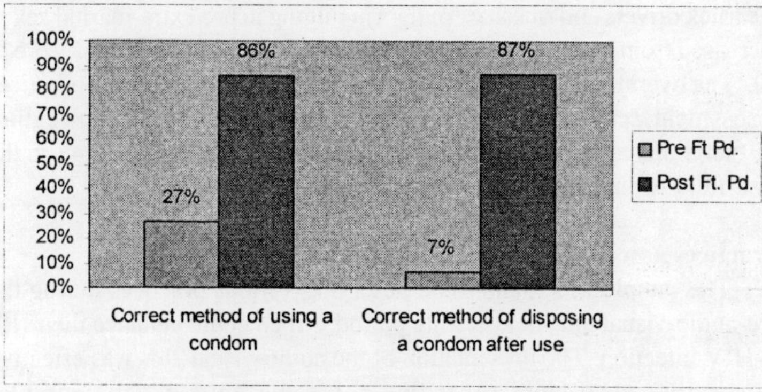

Fig. 3.78 : Refinement in Condom usage Skills (N = 15).

Eighty-six per cent of the sample was able to describe the correct method of using a condom as compared to only 27 per cent prior to the presentation of the audio-visual aids. Similarly, the skill regarding the right method of disposing a condom after use, registered an increase of 80 per cent, i.e., from 7 per cent to 87 per cent amongst the sample. Further, the ability to overcome various inhibitions and initiate condom use negotiations with non-regular sexual partner/s in future, recorded an increase of 40 per cent amongst the sample indulging in pre/extra-marital sex.

Overall, significant improvements were observed on the condom usage assessment scale as shown in Fig. 3.79.

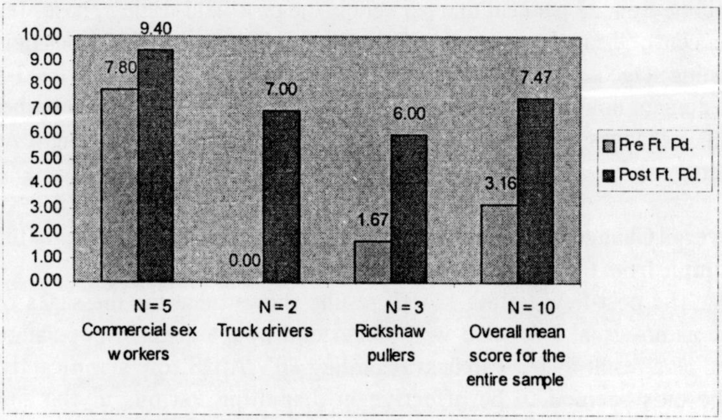

Base : Sample indulging in sex with non-regular partner/s.

Fig. 3.79 : Mean Scores on Condom Usage Assessment Scale.

The mean score for the CSWs increased from 7.80 to 9.40, whereas for the truck drivers and rickshaw pullers indulging in pre/extra-marital sex, it increased from 0 to 7.00 and 1.67 to 6.00 respectively out of a total score of 10. The overall mean score on the condom usage behaviour and practices assessment scale for the sample indulging in sex with non-regular partner/s increased from 3.16 in the pre-field-testing stage to 7.47 in the post-field-testing period out of a total of 10.

Practices Assessment - Pre- to Post-Field-Testing

The sample was found to be observing various practices during the pre-audio-visual aids field-testing period, which could enhance their risk to HIV infection. The presentation of the audio-visual aids was effective in creating awareness regarding the same amongst the sample. Subsequently, majority of them showed a tendency to curtail these practices in the post-audio-visual field-testing period as is shown by the evaluation on the concise condom usage behaviour and practices assessment scale (Appendix XIII).

Prior to field-testing of the audio-visual aids, 20 per cent of the sample who had been injected for some or the other reason said that they had been at times injected with previously used needles, while 40 per cent of the sample was not aware if a new needle and syringe had been used for them for injecting purposes. However, subsequent to the presentation of the audio-visual aids, 93 per cent of the sample said that they would ensure in future that a new needle and syringe is used for injecting purposes whenever required. Further, the intention to practice the sharing of personal use items such as blades and razors registered a self-reported decline from 27 per cent to 0 per cent in the post-field-testing phase. Ten per cent of the male sample who had during the pre-audio-visual aids field testing stage said that their barbers used the same blade for shaving 3-4 customers now stated that they would ensure in future that the barber either changes or cleans the equipment thoroughly before reusing it on them.

Overall Changes in Knowledge, Attitude, Behaviour and Practices of the Sample from the Pre- to Post-Field-testing Period

The post-field-testing KABP results showed that the messages of the audio-visual aids were well understood by the targeted population and as a result their awareness regarding HIV/AIDS rose significantly. The aids seemed to be effective in dispelling various myths and misconceptions of the sample related to the disease as was documented by the rise in the post-field-testing KABP scores. The comparison of mean scores of the sample groups on each scale (knowledge, attitude, behaviour and practices) during pre- and post-audio-visual field-testing periods is shown in Table 3.3.

Table 3.3: Mean KABP Scores* during the Pre and Post Field-testing Period.

	Knowledge Assessment Scale			*Attitude Assessment Scale*			*Condom Use Behaviour and Practices Assessment Scale*		
Sample groups	N	pre	Post	N	Pre	Post	N	Pre	Post
CSWs	5	7.20	**11.80**	5	2.80	**4.20**	5	7.80	**9.40**
Truck Drivers	5	7.00	**14.00**	5	2.20	**3.60**	2	0	**7.00**
Rickshaw Pullers	5	1.00	**12.00**	5	0.80	**3.80**	3	1.67	**6.00**
Overall mean Score (For the Three sample groups		**5.07**	**12.60**		**1.93**	**3.87**		**3.16**	**7.47**

(For supplementary information please refer to appendix XIV).*

The comparative analysis of mean scores during the pre- and post-intervention period reflected a significant gain for all the three sample groups on the KABP scale. The overall mean score for the entire sample on knowledge assessment scale increased from 5.07 to 12.60 out of 20, on attitude assessment scale it increased from 1.93 to 3.87 out of 5 and on condom usage behaviour scale from 3.16 to 7.47 out of 10.

The comparison between the pre- and post-field-testing results of the three groups showed that the CSWs scored a higher score in all aspects during the pre-field-testing phase. This was again as mentioned earlier due to their exposure to various HIV/AIDS prevention programmes going on in their area. Further, these trends were followed during the post-field-testing period depicting a proportionate rise in the scores, with the CSWs leading in almost all the aspects (barring the knowledge score). The sex workers scored a little lower than the truck drivers and the rickshaw pullers in the post-field-testing knowledge assessment score apparently due to high level of illiteracy (80 per cent) among them as compared to the truck drivers (0 per cent) and the rickshaw pullers (60 per cent) that led to a limited rise in their knowledge level.

However, it is worth mentioning here that this aspect did not hold true for the sex workers during the course of the main intervention where they scored comparatively a little higher than the truck drivers and the rickshaw pullers on the knowledge scale irrespective of their illiteracy. The basic reason for this was the continuity of the intervention for a reasonably long period of time (i.e., approximately 12 months time for creating HIV/AIDS awareness and reinforcing the same information). The time factor bridged the gap between their illiteracy and the gain in knowledge. This shows that long-term programmes have the potential to erase the illiteracy barrier and lead to a substantial gain in knowledge. Hence, sustainability of HIV prevention efforts becomes imperative.

As is evident from the comparison of pre and post field-testing mean scores on each scale viz. knowledge, attitude, behaviour and practices, the gain seems to be substantial. To summarize, the exposure of the sample to audio-visual aids produced tangible results in terms of positive changes in their KABP in context to HIV/AIDS.

Evaluation of the ongoing HIV/AIDS Prevention Programmes at the G.B. Road – An Overview

During the period of study, it was observed that eight NGOs were functioning at the G.B. Road with a common goal of improving the lives of the commercial sex workers living here. The organizations were found to be providing educational and medical facilities to the sex workers as well as their children. Few also provided mid-day meals to the children attending their make-shift schools.

The NGOs found to be functioning in the G.B. Road area during the course of intervention were:

1. AIDS Awareness Group (AAG)
2. Joint Women's Programme (JWP)
3. Shakti Vahini
4. Sharan
5. STOP (Stop Trafficking, Oppression and Prostitution of Children and Women)
6. Nari Raksha Samati Sanghthan
7. Sawera
8. Modi Foundation

According to the CSWs who constituted the sample, the quality of services rendered by these NGOs needed some critical changes, which could vastly improve their reach and effectiveness. For instance, it was observed that although two NGOs were operating mobile vans in the G.B.

Road area with the aim of delivering free supplies of condoms and medicines to the CSWs yet, the majority of sex workers were not availing these facilities. The main reason cited for non-availment of these services was that since these mobile vans were parked and delivering services by the main roadside, majority of the CSWs felt embarrassed to seek these services. Procuring condoms from these vans in the presence of roadside passers-by was experienced as humiliating by many sex workers. Another important revelation made by a social worker working with these sex workers was that most of the brothel owners did not allow/approve the idea of sex workers going out of their brothels due to the presumed fear of runaways. Thus, accessibility to such services was critically curtailed. Most of the ongoing HIV prevention programmes have overlooked this aspect of accessibility of services to sex workers. Programme planners while implementing delivery of HIV/AIDS prevention services need to ensure that the targeted populations have an easy access to such services.

It was also observed that many NGOs focused heavily on distribution of materialistic services such as condoms and medicines rather than imparting skill-building services such as correct condom usage and negotiation skills. The present study confirmed a major lack of such skills amongst the sample. Similar findings showing a lack of condom usage skills amongst the sex workers have also been reported by Bhave et al. (1997). There lies an urgent need to shift the focus of ongoing programmes from being distribution-oriented to be skill-building oriented. The environment in which the services were being delivered also created a lot of difference in their receptivity. For instance, most of the sex workers pointed out that one of the NGOs was trying to promote condoms by giving demonstrations about correct condom usage on the road itself. Since these programmes were targeted at the commercial sex workers, the sex workers felt stigmatized and found it indecent to watch these demonstrations. Hence, the reception to these demonstrations was curtailed. In order to enhance the effectiveness of such practical efforts, the surrounding environment should be appropriate and as user-friendly as possible.

Another major revelation of the study was the sub-humane conditions in which the children of these sex workers were kept. During the period of intervention, the researcher had a chance to visit a day-care center run by a NGO in the red light area. It was observed that the center had only too small rooms for keeping the children of sex workers. It was further noted that there was no provision of an electric fan in one of the rooms, which aggravated the heat condition during the summer time. The mid-day meal served to the children attending the center was found to be sub-standard in terms of hygiene and palatability.

Most ironically, it was noticed that small children in the crawling stages were prevented from moving out of these rooms in a cruel manner. The sketch below (Fig. 3.80) portrays the method in which the mobility of small children was severely curtailed.

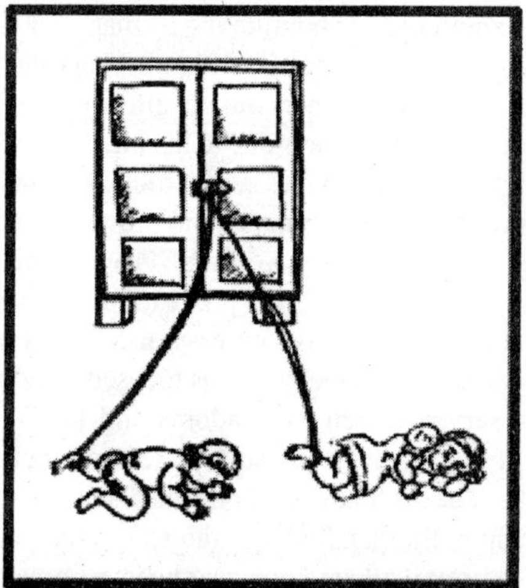

Fig. 3.80: Plight of Sex Workers' Children as Observed in a Day-care Center.

One of the feet of small children in the crawling stages was tied with a rope, which in turn was tied to the handle of a cupboard kept nearby. Thus, such children had no other option accept to remain tied near the cupboard. During the researcher's visit, two children aged approximately 8 months and 16 months were found to be tied in such a manner. In fact, the younger infant was found to be crying bitterly due to the lack of mobility. On being asked the reason for tying children in such a way, one of the staff members explained that there was a scarcity of staff, which was further aggravated if children were allowed to roam here and there. In essence, if children were tied, no continuous supervision was required in contrast to the crawling children who had to be followed at all times.

A few pictures showing the above-mentioned details were photographed by the researcher but the same were taken away by the NGO's management with the help of local police personnel. In crux, the plight of sex workers' children was pathetic and needed immediate corrective actions. The prevailing conditions highlight the fact that NGOs need to work in a more humane and transparent manner to serve the communities effectively.

Lastly, a sense of mistrust towards some NGOs working in the area was found to be building up amongst the brothel owners as well as the sex workers. The major grudge harboured by these people was the apathetic attitude held by a few NGOs towards the plight of sex workers. Majority of them felt that NGOs had vested interests and thus were not fully committed towards their welfare. Some brothel owners pointed out that during certain police raids when many sex workers had been wrongfully taken into custody, none of the NGOs came to their rescue. Similarly, many sex workers stated that NGOs were delivering services only at the superficial level and nothing was being done to improve their living and work conditions or to rehabilitate them.

Rehabilitation - A Missing Factor

During the course of study, it was realized that most of the CSWs and brothel owners who were interviewed, harboured a feeling of deep anguish over the critically missing rehabilitation factor concerning them. Many sex workers pointed out that even if they genuinely wanted to give up the sex trade, they were unable to do so because of the lack of opportunities to earn for their survival. Further, many of the sex workers from their personal experiences critically questioned the efficacy of the so-called rehabilitation programmes run by the state Government. It was reported that the state Government rehabilitation programme was not effective in providing any kind of relief to the sex workers who were sent over there from the police custody. As per policy matter related to the functioning of the rehabilitation programme it was observed that minor girls (aged less than 18 years) rescued from the sex trade were lodged at "Nirmal Chayya" a welfare home run by the Delhi state government, whereas major sex workers (aged 18 and up) were kept in Nari Niketans. Once the court proceedings against them were over, minors were reunited with their parents or sent to remand homes in their home states, whereas girls aged 18 and above were sent back to their homes if they desired so or allowed to leave as such. But this stand was contradicted by the sex workers who reported that many major sex workers had been forcefully sent back to their homes in their native villages along with police personnel. The police personnel had ruined the chances of acceptance of these sex workers by their respective families due to the exposure of their highly stigmatized profession.

Further, the sex workers who have nowhere to go choose to stay back in these homes where they are taught skills such as embroidery, stitching and crochet as a part of the rehabilitation programme. But, not many of these women have been able to get integrated into the mainstream of our society. For instance, in the past five years only 2 out of a total of 215 inmates housed in these remand homes have been rehabilitated (*Times of India*, Aug. 26, 2001). Alarmed by the low rehabilitation statistics, in August 2001, the Delhi High Court asked the Delhi Commission for Women (DCW) to take up the rehabilitation of sex workers effectively, with the goal of providing alternative means of earning a livelihood. Yet, this directive still remains to be transformed into real action.

Evaluation of the Study

Quantitative as well as qualitative parameters were used to evaluate the impact of the present study or rather the result of several interactions and community-involved interventions. The quantitative indicators were based on the WHO guidelines (as reported in NACO, 1996) and are as follows:

1. Knowledge about HIV/AIDS prevention practices
2. Condom usage practices
3. Incidence of STD.

Two other indicators based on the work of Chan et al. (1996) were also adopted which are as follows:

(a) Negotiating skills related to condom usage such as, frequency of condom use negotiations and success in these negotiations.

(b) Behaviour change as measured by the percentage of sample refusing unprotected sex at all times.

Apart from these indicators, other parameters as assessed by the KABP scale devised for the study were also used for the purpose. All these quantitative indicators showed major favourable changes from the pre- to post-intervention period. In addition to these, other indicators an assessed by the KABP scale also showed significant changes. These changes have been elaborately analyzed and discussed in their respective post-intervention KABP assessment scores. Besides these, the qualitative parameters relied on vital components such as community involvement, mobilization and participation. Most importantly community satisfaction formed an important part of the evaluation process. These indicators have been effectively used to assess the community based prevention programmes by various researchers (Rugg, et al., 1996).

The research demonstrates that involving the concerned communities is an easy, cost-effective and reliable strategy to carry out targeted interventions. In the present research, the communities under study were involved and mobilized to support the intervention and provide infrastructural as well as informational inputs in developing a culturally appropriate programme. The inputs provided by the community members not only increased the programme relevance but also generated a greater acceptance for the same.

Many studies continue to emphasize the fact that beliefs, values and socio-psychological frameworks of the targeted communities need to be incorporated into HIV/AIDS prevention programme. According to Fabian et al. (1996) prevention and educational campaigns need to consider the value framework and belief system of the people and social groups affected by the epidemic. Likewise, in the present study the incorporation of community perspectives while planning, developing and implementing the present intervention helped a long way in increasing the reach and credibility of the programme.

Further, the grass-root participation of members from the three communities proved invaluable in the development of the audio-visual aids. Similarly, the crucial role-played by the peer educators in conducting educational and counselling outreach activities helped in fostering ownership as well as sustainability of the programme. Another crucial factor contributing to the success of the intervention was that the study was based on community-needs' assessment. Various factors such as socio-cultural, psychological, economical and occupational were taken into account while planning and implementing the intervention. The study was tailored to meet the specific needs of the sample and was thus, by and large a community-appropriate intervention.

The sample satisfaction with regards to the present intervention was quiet high. Ninety-five per cent of the sample at the end of the intervention opined that the programme was useful and wanted it to be continued on a regular basis. Besides, apart from the study sample approximately 250 people from the same sample communities participated in the HIV/AIDS awareness meetings on a casual-basis as listeners. A total of nine peer educators were trained during the course of intervention.

The participants appreciated the community specific language used in the interview schedules and the audio-visual aids. On the completion of the intervention, 87 per cent of the sample said that they now felt empowered to take safe decisions. The empowerment according to them was a result of their increased awareness regarding HIV/AIDS, which was the ultimate aim of the study.

Utility of the Study

1. The study has generated a large database on a wide range of myths and misconceptions reflecting low levels of AIDS awareness,

harbouring of adverse attitudes, practicing high-risk behaviours and practices that increase the vulnerability of certain communities to HIV infection. The data provides much needed information on socio-cultural, psychological, economical as well as legal aspects that tend to limit an individual's capacity to protect oneself from HIV/AIDS. All this information can help a long way in effectively planning and implementing sound strategies to combat HIV/AIDS effectively.

2. Some of the findings of the study have consequently paved way for a limited evaluation of the ongoing HIV prevention efforts targeted towards commercial sex workers at the G.B. Road (Delhi). These evaluations can help to a significant extent in bringing about some of the desired changes as proposed by the sample and thus, enhancing the effectiveness of the ongoing HIV/AIDS prevention programmes. Similarly, few of the audio-visual aids developed by NACO and other NGOs have been evaluated as a part of the study. These findings too can be helpful in modifying and making these audio-visual aids more community- appropriate.
3. The audio-visual aids developed in the present study, on the basis of needs assessment of the communities under study can be further used and promoted in similar sites with similar populations for HIV/AIDS awareness generation programmes.
4. Areas requiring further research have been identified through the study. The findings/results of the present study may be used by HIV prevention policy-makers to develop and implement coherent policies related to HIV prevention.
5. Lastly, the study has prepared a recommendation document, which if implemented effectively, can definitely help in checking the further spread of the HIV infection among the commercial sex workers, truck drivers and rickshaw pullers representing the vulnerable sections of the society.

Limitations of the Study

1. In view of the sensitive and intimate nature of the study, there may be some under or over reporting of certain behaviours especially those related to sexual matters. Although, the evaluation indicators used to assess the impact of the study were in strict accordance to the parameters laid down by the WHO, yet reporting biases to a limited extent cannot be ruled out.
2. Since professional help and financial resources were limited during the course of the study, therefore certain components that could

have supplemented the intervention efforts could not be fully incorporated into the programme. For example, individuals suffering from STD were referred to nearby government hospitals for treatment purposes instead of calling a doctor to give them on-site treatment that could have saved the sample's time as well as efforts and increased the comprehensiveness of the intervention.

3. A few suggestions proposed by the study participants could not be implemented due to financial, infrastructural and legal constraints. For instance, the rickshaw pullers suggestion to have a hand pump installed near their place of residing could not be implemented. Although availability of water is of prime importance in helping them to keep themselves free of diseases and infections yet, some legal constraints did not permit the installation of a hand pump at this site.

Case Studies

In order to have an insight into the lives of the sample groups, a case study from each of the three sample groups was done. The case profiles cover information regarding the forces and circumstances that have shaped the lives of these individuals. Factors such as poverty leading to exploitation and mobility, lack of awareness giving rise to high-risk behaviour and complacency and finally frustration resulting in disintegration of basic human values, were found to be elevating the spread of HIV/AIDS among such communities.

Three individuals who were earlier a part of the intervention sample were selected for the purpose of making these case profiles. In order to make the sample statistically representative, one individual was picked up from each of the three sample groups. The criterion for choosing these three individuals was their willingness to share personal details and sometime to spare. Information was gathered in their natural living and/ work environment by interview and observation methods. Since the researcher was well known to the sample by then there was the unquestionable trust and confidence in the researcher. Real life experiences were narrated without any fear or inhibitions.

The lives of these three individuals by and large represent the lives of other individuals belonging to the same occupational groups. The names of the three individuals whose case profiles are given below have been changed in order to maintain anonymity. The case profiles are as follows:-

Rani (A Commercial Sex Worker)

Forty years old, Rani earns a livelihood by working as a commercial sex worker in one of the G.B. Road brothels in Delhi. She is five feet and two inches tall and the contours of her body clearly depict her middle age. She has two daughters and a son who live in her husband's native village in Haryana with one of her distant relatives.

Rani qualifies to be a true representative of an uneducated woman braving poverty, exploitation and injustice. She nostalgically remembers her childhood years when she used to live happily in Delhi with her blind mother. Rani never went to school as she was needed to look after her blind mother. Time passed by and Rani entered into her teens. She fell in love with a neighbour and slowly and steadily their relationship turned into physical intimacy. Because of the fear of her mother, Rani eloped with her lover one day. She stayed with him for some time and then after being exploited by the lover she was sold to one of the brothels at the G.B. Road. With nowhere to go and no one to complain, Rani accepted her fate and started practicing sex work in order to survive. Now it has been seventeen long years since Rani took to full-fledged sex trade.

She says that there have been many ups and downs in her life during all these long years. While practicing sex work she again fell in love with one of her clients. The client too had a liking for Rani and finally one day he proposed to marry her. Rani was very happy as she too dreamt of having a happily married life with a home and children of her own. By then, since she was on the verge of entering middle age and did not have many customers thus, the brothel owner did not create any fuss in allowing her to leave the brothel with her would-be husband.

In the preceding few months Rani's so-called married life was filled with joy and happiness although she says that the man never married her openly in public. Over the next few years she had three children born in her questionable wedlock. As time passed by, things started taking a turn for the worse. The attitude of Rani's husband towards her started showing many signs of ill-treatment. Frequent arguments started turning into fights and one day during one of those heated fights, Rani's husband beat her up, abused her and threatened to leave her back at the brothel. Rani with deep anguish and sadness verbalizes what her husband said, "*Tuzh jaise randi ki jagah kothe par hi hoti hai*" meaning "Whores like you only deserve to live in a brothel." Rani was humiliated and equally infuriated at the unjust behavior of her husband towards her. She realized that all the years that she had put into her marriage with this man and all the time that she had given for bringing up her three children from this man had just gone in vain.

So perturbed was Rani with the feeling of worthlessness of her life that she herself returned to the brothel she said good-bye to. But now she was well in her middle age and thus, earning by sex work too was not easy or lucrative for her. Yet, with no other skills or options on hand she held on to her old profession.

As of now, Rani is not able to get more than two–three clients for herself per day. She laments, "*Har grahak choti ladki mangta hai*" meaning "Every customer wants a young girl." Thus, she is frequently seen sitting near the stairs of the brothel and trying to help fellow sex workers who are young in age by fixing up customers for them. If the deal strikes she gets a share of 10–20 per cent from her fellow sex workers for helping them find a client.

Rani is addicted to chewing pan and tobacco. She says she feels good after eating them. She is a doting mother and has not told about her occupation to her children in order to avoid a feeling of low self-esteem amongst them as well as to protect them from social discrimination. She somehow manages to send money to her relative in the village so that her children are able to go to school and get educated. She hopefully says, "*Main Chahti Hoon Mere Bacche Is Dhande Main Na Pare. Woh Padh Likh Kar Kuch Aur Karen*" meaning "I don't want my children to enter into this trade. I wish they get educated and do something else." Rani visits her children once in every one to two years. She sometimes feels sad as she has no contact with her mother at all and doesn't even know if she is alive or dead.

Rani's overall awareness regarding HIV/AIDS was found to be very low prior to the intervention. She was only aware about the sexual mode of HIV transmission and prevention. Further, Rani honestly admits that she is not in a position to insist for condom usage to all of her clients. Most of the time she prevails on her clients to use condoms before sex. The fear of losing her clients due to insistence for condom usage hinders Rani from having consistent condom usage with all of them. When asked if she suffered from any sexually transmitted disease, Rani firmly replied in negative. She said she never had any such disease because she always kept herself clean. But with a little bit of probing, Rani agreed that she sometimes suffered from the problem of itching in genital areas for which she applies medicated cream to get relief. Rani believes that the problem of itching is quite common in other women too, and that it is caused because of excessive heat in the body.

As far as the range of indulgence in unsafe practices is concerned, Rani agrees without much inhibition that due to the insistence of certain clients and because of her economic need to do, she has at times practiced unprotected anal sex. But, in spite of instances of unsafe sex she does not perceive herself to be at risk of HIV/AIDS because she says, she is quite healthy till now and also because she used condoms in most of her sexual transactions.

However, in the post-intervention period Rani was much more informed about other modes of HIV transmission and her perceived vulnerability to HIV/AIDS showed a major shift. Now, she realized that she may have acquired the infection during instances of unsafe sex but still she doesn't seem to be too concerned about it. She plainly defends her complacent attitude by telling, "*Ab kya farak parta hai, jo hai so hai*" meaning "Now how does it matter, whatever has to happen will happen".

Avtaar Singh (A Truck Driver)

Avtaar Singh is a twenty-eight year old truck driver. He is a native of a village in Madhya Pradesh. He is about five feet and six inches tall and well-built. Avtaar Singh is usually seen wearing a printed shirt and a dark coloured pant. He mostly sports a pleasant smile and is willing to talk and be friendly. Avtaar Singh has been married for the last nine years and his wife is 25 years old. He has a joint family and his parents along with his wife and four children live together in their native village. The family owns a piece of land, which is cultivated in order to run the household expenditure. Since the income earned from agriculture is not enough, Avtaar Singh had to search for some other work. Since childhood he was fond of driving and thus, came to Delhi and learnt how to drive a truck. He got a driving license and started working as a truck driver for a transport agency in the Kamla Market area (Delhi). The truck is owned by the owner of the transport agency while Avtaar Singh is paid a monthly salary of Rs. 4500.

Avtaar Singh has to stay away from his home for most of the time due to the nature of his job. Sometimes, when he has to transport goods on a long route he is separated from his family for upto six months or so. On an average, Avtaar Singh remains away from his family for 2 to 3 months at a stretch. Sometimes Avtaar Singh's family has to face crucial problems while he is away from home. To quote one, Avtaar Singh has four small children aged eight years and less. Sometimes if a child falls sick, Avtaar Singh's wife has to rely on neighbours to take the child to a hospital, as Avtaar Singh's father is too old to accompany her. To add up to the problem there is no hospital nearby.

Besides his family, Avtaar Singh too faces living problems because of the nature of his work. For most of the time, while Avtaar Singh is in Delhi waiting for a tour to be fixed up by his transport agency, he has to park his truck in the parking lot of the New Delhi railway station. The parking lot serves as a waiting place for most of the truck drivers. Avtaar Singh laments that sometimes when a suitable tour is not fixed up then he has to wait endlessly in his truck in the parking lot itself. Besides coping up with long and tiring waiting hours during peak summers and chilly winters, he has also to put up with a major lack of basic amenities such as adequate shelter and toilet facilities nearby.

Avtaar Singh says that driving a truck is not an easy task. It needs a lot of stamina and alertness on the part of the driver. He further convinces, "I have to remain awake mostly at nights because driving trucks for the purpose of transporting goods is allowed only during night hours. Most of the time when other people are sleeping, drivers are on the steering wheel driving alertly". He quickly adds, "It is very important to transport goods carefully at the place of destination. If there is a little bit of carelessness on the part of the driver leading to an accident then he may not only lose his job but his life too."

Avtaar Singh has been on the job of driving a truck for the last eight years. He points out – "It has been a long time and during all these years I have experienced and learned many new things – some good ones and some bad too. Apart from smoking *bidi*, I occasionally drink liquor once or twice in a week. On an average, I usually spend Rs. 40 per day for buying cigarettes and sometimes tobacco too. But on days when I buy a liquor bottle for myself, I have to part with Rs. 80 to 100." Avtaar Singh honestly admits that he had pre-marital sex with four local women of his native village. But he is quick enough to justify his acts by saying that such relations are quite normal and acceptable as "love/attachment" during youth. He admits, "I never used any precaution (i.e. condom) while indulging in such acts. I did not feel the need to do so because I knew all my sexual partners well by face. I believed that since all my sexual partners were good looking without showing signs of any disease thus, they were healthy and could not pass on any infection to me." Avtaar Singh also says that he always thought condoms acted as a barrier in deriving sexual pleasure. Thus, after marriage he put the entire responsibility of using a contraceptive (pill) on his wife.

Avtaar Singh shyly admits, "Since I have to stay away from my wife for long periods, visiting commercial sex workers once a while has become a need for me like many other truck drivers".

He reports that at the insistence of some sex workers he sometimes used a condom while having sex with them but the fact remains that consistent condom usage has not been practiced and several unprotected sexual transactions have already taken place. Avtaar Singh has been visiting around three to four different sex workers every month.

Although Avtaar Singh earns only Rs. 4500 per month yet, he spends around Rs. 1500 on his addictions for cigarettes and liquor and Rs. 300 per month for indulging in extra-marital sex with commercial sex workers. Still, he says he doesn't mind spending so much on himself as he needs to relieve himself of stress and strain.

Avtaar Singh has sometimes in the past suffered from STD as concluded by the symptoms reported by him. But he calls the problem of STD as "*garmi ki bimari*" meaning a disease caused by excessive heat in the body. He casually says that these problems are common occurrences and are cured on their own. Thus, he has never felt the need to go to a doctor for treatment purposes. Further, even during the episodes of being infected with a STD, Avtaar Singh has not used a condom, as he is unaware of the fact that sexually transmitted diseases are highly contagious. He also reported to have suffered from a STD in the six months prior to the pre-intervention period of the study.

As far as his knowledge regarding HIV/AIDS is concerned, Avtaar Singh says that prior to the intervention he knew about AIDS as a disease as he had seen an AIDS awareness message being displayed on a public train in Mumbai. But, he humbly admits that he was not able to understand the contents of the message. He could only understand that AIDS was a disease primarily caused by having sex with commercial sex workers and because of needles used for injecting purposes. Other vital aspects of the disease such as HIV transmission modes, symptoms of the disease were not understood by him. He strongly believes that men and women should not have equal rights in matters pertaining to sexuality. He feels strongly that women should not have sexual freedom like men because he feels women are the weaker sex.

The range of unsafe practices followed by Avtaar Singh vary from practicing unprotected sex with four local women in his village as well as commercial sex workers in cities to sharing of shaving blades with his fellow truck drivers. Avtaar Singh says that he has been frequently injected for various medical reasons but he does not know whether new needles were used for the purpose.

After the intervention Avtaar Singh reported that some major changes had set into his life. He knew about all the four HIV transmission modes as well as the procedure and availability of HIV testing facilities. Avtaar Singh also realized that knowing a woman by face is no guarantee of safety in matter of sex. Using a condom is a safeguard that he knows now.

Although he has planned to give up the practice of having extra-marital sex with commercial sex workers and thus, has not visited a sex worker for quite sometime now. He said that if ever he visited a sex worker in future he would surely use a condom. Avtaar Singh now doesn't share shaving blades with his friends any more as he knows that it may be risky. A major change was also observed in the attitude of Avtaar Singh towards people living with HIV/AIDS. For instance, prior to the intervention he was not sure if he would continue to live with his wife in case she got infected with HIV, while in the post-intervention period Avtaar Singh confidently said that he would live with as well as take care of his wife if she ever got infected with the virus. This change in attitude reflects a positive shift in favour of people living with HIV/AIDS.

Iqbal (A Rickshaw Puller)

Nineteen-year-old Iqbal, a rickshaw puller, is an unmarried boy. He is five feet and three inches tall. His native village is in Bihar and he had come to Delhi when he was ten years old. He keeps himself fairly well dressed as compared to other rickshaw pullers since he wants to look good most of the time. Iqbal always wears a shirt and pant. He never wears a '*lungi*' or a '*kurta*' like many others in the same occupation. His hair is well oiled and neatly combed always.

Iqbal's father died when he was still an infant. He had only his mother and an older brother. Though the family had a small piece of land on which some cash crops were grown, his brother did not show interest and soon had to part ways. This was not the end of the family's woes. Iqbal's upper right arm was mildly paralyzed due to polio while he was only five years old. His mother tried several traditional methods of treatment with only a marginal improvement in his status. When Iqbal was ten years old and studying in class V, his mother sent him to Delhi to stay with a relative so that he could get good education in the city. But very soon, the promise of helping Iqbal to get good education was breached by the so-called relative and Iqbal was left to fend for himself. Iqbal tried very hard to find some work for himself so that he could earn for his survival. Since he was partially handicapped people hesitated to employ him. After many efforts, Iqbal was finally able to get work as a washer boy at a fruit-juice shop. Although he toiled hard and washed glasses from morning till night yet, he was not able to earn enough to be able to send some money to his mother back home in the village.

The hope of getting some good work took Iqbal to Mumbai. There, he managed to get the work of a waiter in a small hotel. He worked as a waiter for two years and during these two years he had premarital sex with a commercial sex worker in one of the brothels in Mumbai. Iqbal said that he developed a liking for this girl and used to visit her once a week. He used to pay Rs. 150 per visit. The girl revealed about her past to Iqbal. She told him that she had come from Bengal to Mumbai in search of a job. One "Baba" (meaning a spiritual guru) met her on the Mumbai station and gave her a "*Laddoo*" (traditional Indian sweet) laced with some drug. After eating it, the girl lost her senses and the "Baba" raped her. Thereafter, she was sold at one of the brothels in Mumbai.

Iqbal said that he was in love with this sex worker because of her looks and wanted to marry her. He asked her to run away from the brothel with him but she refused, as she was afraid of running away from the brothel.

Somewhat heart broken, Iqbal came back to Delhi and started looking for a job, but was not successful in getting one. With no money in hand he started living on the pavement of the Chitra Gupta Road in the Pahar Ganj area. There he came in contact with a few rickshaw pullers who too were living on the same pavement. One of them became a friend of Iqbal and offered him help by getting him a cycle rickshaw on rent. Iqbal started pulling the rickshaw but this was not easy for him because of his partially paralyzed arm. Iqbal says that he feels tired very soon and can't pull the cycle rickshaw for long durations.

In spite of his poor financial status, Iqbal visits the brothels at the G. B. Road frequently to enjoy sexual pleasures at the brothels. He treats some of these women as his steady partners.

Iqbal doesn't have access to a T.V. or a radio, as rickshaw is all that he has. He is also not fond of reading a newspaper. He says that he has not seen/heard any AIDS awareness message but he knows that AIDS is a dreadful disease. On being asked as to what causes AIDS Iqbal promptly replied, "People having sex with commercial sex workers only get AIDS". Although Iqbal too had sex with commercial sex workers but he did not perceive himself to be at risk. Iqbal justifies saying that "I have had sexual relations only with three particular sex workers whom I know well. Moreover all these girls have been healthy looking and do not show signs of any illness as such". Iqbal admits that although he has indulged in different types of sexual practices including anal and oral sex and that he has never used a condom. According to him, condom acts as a barrier and kills the pleasure.

Iqbal knows about STD and has suffered in the past. He said he took treatment from a nearby doctor for his ailment. Iqbal had very low level of awareness regarding HIV/AIDS and thought that AIDS could be cured. He also believed that a person with AIDS could live as long as any other normal person if given the required treatment.

However, the post-intervention period saw the dispelling of some of the crucial misconceptions. For example, Iqbal now perceives himself to be at risk of HIV/AIDS due to his indulgence in unprotected sex with sex workers in contrast to his notion prior to the intervention. He now knows that HIV/AIDS is not something, which immediately shows signs of itself. Iqbal has immense regret for his ignorance and his past indulgence for pleasure.

Iqbal is still contemplating to use a condom but his friends assured me that Iqbal would adopt safe ways.

Conclusion

The content analysis of these case profiles concludes with the observation that factors such as illiteracy, poverty, exploitation, mobility and migration were all found to be playing a major role in propelling the sample towards HIV/AIDS vulnerability. Although the sample and their families were found to be facing various major problems on account of migration/mobility yet, the sample had no choice except to stay separated from them for long periods due to compelling economic necessities. Long separation from families coupled with psychological stress were found to be driving the sample into various addictions as well as their practicing sex with non-regular partners.

Pre/extra-marital sex was found to be significantly prevalent amongst the sample evidently showing a decline of the so-called socio-cultural constraints. Further condom usage with non-regular sexual partners was very low partially due to lack of awareness regarding HIV/AIDS as well as because of nurturing of various myths and misconceptions related to the disease. Subsequently, the occurrence of STD was a common phenomena amongst the sample and yet, denial of the condition or non-adherence to treatment were commonly observed amongst them. The overall awareness regarding HIV/AIDS and STD was found to be very low prior to the intervention. Economic compulsions were reported by the sex workers as the primary reason for indulging in sex without using a condom. Further, the disintegration of human values like self-esteem, worthiness, hope and responsibility had left the respondents with a complacent/unconcerned attitude towards the disease.

The intervention was observed to have a positive impact on them in a very subtle yet, significant manner. For instance, the sample was found to be shifting from practices of high-risk behaviour to safe behaviour for various aspects related to transmission of HIV as a result of their enhanced awareness regarding the disease. Similarly, major change was reflected in the attitude of the sample towards PWHA, which turned from being discriminatory to that of care and empathy. More crucially, they had now started perceiving themselves to be at risk of acquiring the infection because of their indulgence in risk behaviour, which subsequently helped them in adopting safe behavioural practices in their lives. Issues such as poverty, illiteracy, migration, exploitation, and devaluation of human lives need to be taken up on a priority basis along with the prevention of HIV/AIDS to make the control of the epidemic a success story.

4

Summary and Conclusion

Creating Awareness about HIV/AIDS

Acquired Immune Deficiency Syndrome (AIDS) is recognized as the most devastating disease humankind has ever faced. The epidemic began in 1981 and by the end of the year 2004, nearly 40 million people across the globe were afflicted by it (UNAIDS/WHO, Dec., 2004). The disease is caused by the Human Immuno Deficiency Virus (HIV), which breaks down the immune system of a body completely to combat infections. The virus remains dormant for 5 to 10 years before the onset of full blown AIDS which is always terminal. Today, AIDS is rapidly wiping out the hard-earned gains of human development in terms of regressing life expectancy, rising child mortality rates and killing the most productive and reproductive population in the prime of their youth. The economic impact of AIDS in terms of costs resulting from treatment and care of people living with HIV/AIDS (PWHA) is magnanimous. In India alone, the overall cost on account of AIDS in the year 2000 was around US $ 11 billion (WHO, 1999).

With the rising spread of HIV/AIDS there has been a growing emphasis on understanding its epidemiology and manifestations. Various factors such as biological, socio-cultural, economic, political and psychosocial have been broadly seen as causing the spread of the virus. Migration, prostitution, machismo behaviour, low literacy level, prevalence of myths and misconceptions further aggravate the rapid spread of the disease. It is seen that the infection is rapidly spilling from populations with high-risk behaviour to the general population and also from urban to rural areas. Since there is no sure cure for the disease, its prevention becomes paramount.

As of now, there are only four well-defined routes by which HIV is known to spread. These are through sexual inter-course with a HIV infected person, by exchange of infected blood and blood products as in transfusion, by sharing of contaminated needles/ syringes and lastly transmission from an HIV infected mother to her child before, during or after childbirth. Although, no culture or community is known to be immune to AIDS yet, certain populations are more vulnerable to the disease because of their high-risk behaviours. These are the commercial sex workers, the truck drivers and the rickshaw pullers. Sex related indulgence is common in these three groups.

There is a global reaction and response to HIV/AIDS advocating the importance of education, awareness generation and also for adopting 'safe practices'. Here 'safe practices' has connotations to safety in sexual acts and medical safety (against sharing of needles and syringes). Many millions know nothing or too little about the virus to protect themselves against it (UNAIDS/WHO, Dec., 2001). Globally, low level of knowledge coupled with myths and misconceptions are driving the disease out of control.

The UNAIDS along with other cosponsors is striving to lead and assist in an expansion of the international response to HIV/AIDS. Various NGOs, along with government bodies, also the private sector are putting in their best efforts to launch "Global Media AIDS Initiative". The initiative aims to activate media organizations to reach the world's people especially youth with information about how to prevent and treat HIV and to help combat AIDS related stigma and discrimination. These include efforts in developing and implementing programmes to bring about changes in knowledge, attitude, behaviour and practices (KABP) of people with regards to HIV/AIDS. In the absence of any cure for HIV presently, creating HIV/ AIDS awareness takes on a significant and life-saving role. Knowledge is seen as power therefore, integrating life-skills education into HIV/AIDS prevention programmes would be the basis for awareness generation and for health-seeking behaviour. "When you are working to combat a disastrous and growing emergency, you should use every tool at your disposal" (Annan, 2004).

In India, various surveillances as well as KABP studies continue to show an overall lack of awareness among the masses about the disease, its prevention especially amongst some of the most vulnerable populations (UNFPA, Sept., 2000; *Times of India*, July 4, 2003). The HIV prevalence in India has risen to alarming levels with 5.1 million people living with the virus by the end of the year 2004 (NACO, 2004). If concerted efforts are not made to contain the virus, a threat to human welfare and social stability is imminent.

Innovative ways to reach masses and provide them with crucial awareness and knowledge about HIV/AIDS by ensuring their participation/

involvement seem to be the ideal methodology. Experience across the globe shows that awareness about the disease brings about desirable changes in people's behaviour. Interventions such as the Sonagachi project in Kolkatta (India), AIDS Euro-peer project (Europe) and the Prevention Marketing Initiative (USA) are some of the success stories in bringing about significant behavioural changes made possible by the HIV/AIDS awareness campaigns. Also, it is true that certain vulnerable populations have remained either untouched or non-responsive to the ongoing prevention efforts. The reasons for this lacuna suggest lacking of coherence in the content, scattered publicity and inappropriate method of messaging. The programmes should address the specific needs of communities keeping in mind their socio-cultural ethos. People are more likely to accept and help sustain a programme if it takes care of their concerns and seeks their wholehearted participation.

Methodology – Making Efforts to Reach the Vulnerable Groups

In the foreground of a great threat to the humanity due to the onslaught of HIV/AIDS, a modest attempt was made for creating AIDS awareness amongst certain communities comprising of commercial sex workers (CSWs), truck drivers and rickshaw pullers known for their high-risk behaviour and the consequent vulnerability to HIV/AIDS. In the awareness building action research, community participation was the key instrument.

Locale – Hubs of Vulnerable Population

The study was conducted in three areas of the National Capital Territory (NCT) of Delhi. These were the G.B. Road area (commonly known as the red light area), the Kamla Market area and the Chitra Gupta Road. These areas housed a high concentration of commercial sex workers, truck drivers and rickshaw pullers respectively. Undoubtedly, these population pockets are well known for their unsafe sexual indulgence outside marriage, with the exception of sex workers who practice the sex trade for a living.

Sampling Strategy – A Process: Overcoming Hindrances

Thirty individuals from each of these groups were selected as sample on the basis of operational definitions conceptualized for the study, bringing the final sample size to 90.

The two communities comprising of truck drivers and rickshaw pullers were approached purely on the basis of personal search and contact as there was no local NGO working with these groups to go through at a time of the study. The real challenge was however faced in contacting the commercial sex workers who because of illegality of their profession were not ready to see or talk to the researcher. The process of gaining an access to this section of the sample was long and entailed making requests to various people as well as a NGO working in the area. After facing considerable threats and rejections, a mutual understanding with two local volunteers helped in gaining an access to the sex workers in the brothels. Since the study entailed information on the personal and intimate front, it was crucial to include as sample only those who showed willingness to cooperate and provide information to the best of their knowledge. As days went by more and more people came forward making up the required sample.

Variables

The three different groups that comprised the sample formed the major independent variables with several intervening ones such as the social, cultural and economic factors. The dependent variables comprised of the awareness level, the myths and misconceptions relating to AIDS, the living and work environment and aspects related to health care of the three sample groups. The communication material developed during the course of study also formed a part of the dependent variable because of the inter-group needs/differences.

Study Objectives – In Line with the Global AIDS Strategy

The present study was undertaken with the following main objectives:

1. To have an insight into the respondents:
   (i) Awareness, myths and misconceptions relating to HIV/AIDS, its manifestations, prevention and control.
   (ii) Living and work environment with special reference to socio-cultural ethos and health care.
2. To review the above, identify areas of action and carry out a suitable intervention for AIDS awareness through community participation.
3. To develop a set of communication material for AIDS awareness through community participation and field-test the same.

Action Research – Incorporating Community Participation as a Vital Component

The research was not merely restricted to data collection but involved substantial action in the form of intervention, that entailed bringing about certain desired changes in knowledge, attitude, behaviour and practices of the communities with regards to HIV/AIDS. Community participation formed a vital part of the study and was ensured in the form of innovative approaches like development of audio-visual aids, conducting improvisational drama and fictional stories with the help of community members as well as sharing of experiences by the sample amongst them. The research design therefore employed both qualitative as well as quantitative techniques for data collection and analysis. The qualitative techniques used were the interview schedules (Appendix I-VII), focus group discussions, participant observations and a few case studies while the quantitative tools comprised of the knowledge, attitude, behaviour and practices (KABP) assessment scales (Appendix VIII-X) developed for the study on the basis of need-assessment of the sample groups. Narrative format was used to describe the living and work environment, myths and misconceptions of the study sample. The validity and reliability of the KABP scale were determined after a pilot study.

Conducting the Study – A Small-scale Intervention

The study was conducted in three phases, which were:

(a) The pre-intervention phase that involved gathering of socio-demographic data, assessment of KABP, myths and misconceptions with regards to HIV/AIDS and identification of gray areas requiring suitable intervention.

(b) The intervention/transition phase which involved creating HIV/AIDS awareness amongst the sample by ensuring community participation in various processes of the intervention such as development of a set of audio-visual aids and training of peer educators. It included showing them some of the existing educational and publicity material prepared by NACO, WHO and various NGOs.

(c) The post-intervention phase, which was an evaluation process whereby, the sample's KABP with regards to HIV/AIDS were re-assessed to measure the impact of the intervention and the audio-visual aids developed during the course of study were field tested to assess their appropriateness and efficacy.

Case Studies – Exploring Trends in Human Behaviour

Three case studies were conducted to have an in-depth understanding regarding the sample's lives with a focus to delve into factors that were increasing their vulnerability to HIV/AIDS. These case studies highlighted the fact that AIDS was not an epidemic fuelled merely by the Human Immuno Deficiency Virus but an offshoot of poverty, illiteracy, gender and sexuality issues. A holistic approach was therefore required to combat the disease. Some crucial changes were brought about as a result of the intervention. These are well documented through the case studies.

Salient Study Findings

Keeping in line with the research objectives the findings of the study are discussed under the following heads:

(a) Socio-demographic profile of the sample was taken up as the base to begin with. It included age, marital status, family composition, literacy and occupational status, monthly income, religious and regional trends of the sample groups.

(b) Living and work environment of the communities delving into their living and work conditions, physical and substance abuse patterns, the media exposure of the sample with regards to HIV/AIDS information and their treatment seeking behaviour with reference to STD.

(c) Assessment of the sample on knowledge, attitude, behaviour and practices (KABP) scale - covering knowledge, attitude, behaviour and practices assessment from the pre- to post-intervention period along with conducting intervention.

(d) As per the last objective, the study culminated in the development of a set of suitable communication material comprising of a photo-script, a pamphlet and a poster (Annexure I, II and III) on HIV/AIDS awareness, which was the thrust of the study. The description of the same has been given under the title "Development and Field-Testing of the Audio-Visual Aids - A Community Participated Action" which includes characteristics as well as field-testing component of these audio-visual aids.

(e) Three case studies have also been documented, for a good insight into the lives of the sample community.

Socio-Demographic Profile of the Sample

The socio-demographic profile of the sample portrayed the following trends-

(a) The sample in general came under the most productive and reproductive age group of 15 to 49 years.

(b) Majority of the sample (77 per cent) consisted of married respondents.

(c) The family composition of the sample was unique as all of them were living away from their families for most of the time.

(d) The overall level of literacy among them was very low (36 per cent), resulting in their low-profile occupations and instability in income earned.

(e) More males (50 per cent) were literate than their female counterparts (7 per cent) reflecting large-scale gender-based inequality in terms of educational accessibility.

(f) Regional trends indicated that there was considerably high migration/ mobility from distant states to Delhi for employment.
(g) Religious conservatism emerged as an influencing factor determining the choice of adoption of a contraceptive method among the sample.

Living and Work Environment

- The living and work environment of the sample in the metropolis was pathetic and to a large extent responsible for increasing their vulnerability to HIV/AIDS. Factors such as poverty, unhygienic and polluting environment, lack of basic amenities like water, adequate shelter coupled with psychological stress were all found to be either directly/indirectly escalating the sample's risk to HIV/AIDS.
- Stigma attached to sex trade, hindered accessibility of basic services such as education and health care facilities to sex workers' children consequently, pushing them into a vicious cycle of illiteracy, exploitation/abuse and enhanced vulnerability to HIV/AIDS.
- Sexual and physical exploitation appeared to have adversely affected the lives of the sample resulting in feelings of insecurity, oppression, loss of self-esteem and immense emotional stress.
- Sexually abused individuals were more likely (71 per cent v/s 50 per cent) to describe indulgence in pre/extra-marital sex as something normal as compared to the non-abused individuals.
- Majority (76 per cent) of the sample was addicted to substances like tobacco, alcohol and drugs; the intake of the latter two was reportedly followed by sexual transactions most of the time.
- Men taking alcohol/drugs reportedly were more likely (100 per cent v/s 63 per cent) to indulge in pre- and/extra-marital sex as compared to those not taking these substances.

Mass Media (In)- accessibility

A significant percentage of the sample (42 per cent) did not have access to a radio or T. V. and thus, lacked exposure to various HIV/AIDS awareness programmes aired in these channels. Similarly, print material messages pertaining to HIV/AIDS prevention were also found to be ineffective due to high level of illiteracy amongst the sample.

- Data pertaining to media-viewership patterns indicated wide inter-group differences with CSWs topping the T.V. viewership rates (93 per cent) followed by truck drivers (46 per cent) and rickshaw pullers trailing these two (13 per cent). These inter-group differences were primarily a reflection of inaccessibility of mass media channels to the truck drivers and rickshaw pullers.

- Most of the sample (62 per cent) that reported to have been exposed to HIV/AIDS prevention message/s through various mass media showed an overall lack of awareness regarding the disease.
- Majority of the sample (64 per cent) had not received any form of inter-personal communication on HIV/AIDS despite, the knowledge that they fell in the category of populations with high-risk behaviour.
- The overall awareness of the sample regarding STD and their linkage to HIV transmission was found to be dismal.
- Various myths and misconceptions like STD are caused due to excessive heat in the body or by salivary and blood infections were found to be prevalent among the sample.
- The sex workers due to the nature of their profession were less forthcoming to admitting the occurrence of STD among them as against the truckers and the rickshaw pullers.
- Lack of time as well as discriminatory attitude of the government hospitals' staff were reported to be the major reasons forcing the sample in seeking treatment from private medical practitioners. Invariably, they ended up spending a lot of money without even getting specialized treatment, as most medical practitioners the sample visited were general physicians.

Assessment on Knowledge, Attitude, Behaviour and Practices Scale – Determining the Vulnerability

With the aim of delving into factors predisposing the sample to HIV/AIDS vulnerability, their myths and misconceptions, knowledge, attitude, behaviour and practices with regards to HIV/AIDS were assessed on the KABP scale. The analysis of these factors showed the following salient findings:

Knowledge Assessment: Pre-intervention

- The level of awareness regarding HIV/AIDS amongst the sex workers was found to be more as compared to the truck drivers and rickshaw pullers due to their exposure to the ongoing HIV prevention programmes in the red light area.
- Majority of the sample (80 per cent) had heard about AIDS as a disease but the awareness regarding its cause (HIV) was dismal. A fairly high proportion of the male sample (71 per cent) that had heard about AIDS was of the opinion that only having sex with commercial sex workers could cause AIDS.
- The level of awareness regarding symptoms of HIV/AIDS was almost nil. On the contrary, a significant proportion of the sample had

misconceptions regarding the same like AIDS manifests itself in the form of sores and pain in private body parts, setting in fatigue and weakness, and affecting the facial looks of a person.

- Similarly, awareness regarding the four modes of HIV transmission was very low. Overall, 31 per cent of the entire sample was found to be completely unaware about any mode of HIV transmission. The possibility of HIV transmission to babies through breast-feeding by HIV infected mothers was not known to anyone.
- Information regarding crucial aspects such as practicing unsafe sex during menstruation and pregnancy as well as the presence of STD could enhance mother-to-child HIV transmission was profoundly lacking among the respondents.
- Awareness regarding prevention and control of HIV/AIDS was considerably low. Overall, 40 per cent of the sample was not aware about any HIV/AIDS preventive method.
- Critically, casual sex partners (sex partners other than CSWs) were not seen as a potential threat of HIV infection by a significant number (23 per cent) of the male sample. According to these, only CSWs could transmit HIV/AIDS, as they were dirty and indulged in immoral acts.
- In contrast to the truck drivers and rickshaw pullers, a high proportion of the CSWs (93 per cent) were aware of condom usage as an HIV prevention method.
- A little over half (53 per cent) of the sample that had heard about AIDS believed that the disease was curable.
- Perceived self-vulnerability to HIV/AIDS was considered low by the sample due to their lack of awareness, the fear of being singled out and the sexual stigma attached to the disease.

All this data including the myths, misconceptions, doubts and lack of awareness regarding HIV/AIDS were the guiding factors for the intervention.

The Intervention Period – Moving from Ignorance to Awareness

Based on the pre-intervention knowledge assessment, an awareness campaign was created for the benefit of the sample. Knowledge with regards to HIV/AIDS was imparted by using various audio-visual aids along with the photo-script developed during the course of intervention. Simple pictures and charts highlighting the modes of HIV transmission, symptoms of HIV infection and prevention from HIV/AIDS were crafted and extensively used in accordance with the needs of the sample. Similarly, short stories and skits related to different aspects of HIV/AIDS were staged before the sample in a simple and easy to understand language, also containing some humour. The poster developed during the study period depicting a few happy-looking truck drivers was effectively used with the sample in order to motivate them to be happy in a similar way after acquiring knowledge regarding HIV/AIDS.

Knowledge Assessment : Post-intervention

The intervention was found to have made a significant impact on the sample. Desirable changes in their knowledge, attitude, behaviour and practices were noticed and largely reported too. Some details of the same are:

- A significant increase was exhibited in knowledge of the sample regarding various aspects of HIV/AIDS. The awareness level regarding AIDS as a disease rose to cent per cent amongst the sample.
- The knowledge regarding modes of HIV transmission improved considerably for all the four different modes. Maximum changes were observed in the knowledge level related to symptoms of HIV/AIDS, which increased from 2 per cent to 62 per cent possibly as a result of role-play presentations before the sample.
- The awareness regarding availability of HIV testing facilities in various hospitals helped the sample in putting aside the fear that HIV testing was a difficult/expensive procedure.
- The enhanced awareness regarding HIV/AIDS removed the misconception that the disease was as curable as other common diseases and AIDS ultimately leads to death was understood by 82 per cent of the sample as against only 33 per cent in the pre-intervention phase.
- HIV prevention methods were most emphasized during the entire period of the intervention resulting in a significant rise in awareness regarding the same.
- Majority of the truck drivers and rickshaw pullers (72 per cent) had started perceiving casual sex partners too, as a source of HIV, which was helpful to them in their self-assessment of perceived vulnerability to HIV.
- The overall mean score for the entire sample on knowledge assessment scale increased from 5.53 to 12.93 out of total of 20 during the intervention period.

Attitude Assessment : Pre-intervention

The attitude of the sample regarding sex, sexuality, people living with HIV/AIDS (PWHA) etc., as assessed on the attitude assessment scale during the pre intervention period showed the following important findings:

- Commercial sex workers scored higher on the attitude assessment scale as compared to the truck drivers and rickshaw pullers. Harbouring negative attitudes would have affected them adversely in their day-to-day lives.
- Majority of the sample (76 per cent) felt that there was a need for disseminating sex education with emphasis on HIV/AIDS and STD irrespective of the gender.
- Individuals who had indulged in sex with non-regular partner/s perceived these relationships as a matter of personal choice and neither unethical nor wrongful acts.
- The responsibility to use a contraceptive was a debatable issue – again on gender lines. Majority of the truck drivers and rickshaw pullers (67 per cent) thought that women should be responsible to use a suitable one, while cent percent of the CSWs thought otherwise.
- Data analysis showed that male and female sample held each other responsible for their vulnerability to diseases like HIV/AIDS and STD. The stigma attached to such diseases was probably the reason for such apathy.
- The influence of socio-cultural ethos on attitudes of the sample was reflected when majority of the male sample (60 per cent) expressed that due to cultural stereotypes, women do (*read should*) not have equal rights as men in matters pertaining to sex and sexuality.
- A significant trend pointing towards discrimination of people and children living or affected with HIV/AIDS was observed among the sample. They were misled by their myths and misconceptions regarding the disease.
- Myths and misconceptions like HIV/AIDS spreads through air (55 per cent), by sitting close to a HIV infected person (45 per cent) and by sharing their utensils, clothes, soap, food and water (40 per cent) were commonly cited in support of isolation of HIV infected individuals.
- A direct relationship was observed between the perceived vulnerability to the disease and the intention to get HIV tested by the sample.

Intervention Period – Questioning the Deeply held Adverse Attitudes

Focus group discussions and group talks were effectively used to bring about desired changes in the attitudes of the sample in context to HIV/AIDS. Similarly, hypothetical questions were raised while presenting short stories/skits (i.e., provocative theatre) to the sample in order to challenge their deeply held attitudes that were found to be promoting gender-based discrimination with reference to HIV/AIDS. For example, the appropriateness of a woman being stoned to death due to her HIV positive status (*TOI*, 2003) was taken up as an issue and duly questioned with the sample. Such thought provoking efforts were crucial in helping the sample realize the futility of irrational attitudes.

Attitude Assessment : Post-intervention

Some of the major changes observed in the attitudes of the sample during the post-intervention period are as follows:

- Majority of the sample that spoke against disseminating HIV/AIDS education to women and children were now looking at the same favourably.
- A significant shift in perception of the sample regarding HIV vulnerability-enhancers was observed. A good majority (88 per cent) recognized various other modes of HIV transmission besides the sexual contact.
- The proportion of sample advocating equality of sexual rights among men and women increased considerably (by 29 per cent).
- Similarly, the percentage of the sample advocating equal rights for people living with HIV/AIDS rose from 27 per cent to 73 per cent. This substantial game was an indicator of dispelling of myths and misconceptions of the sample regarding the disease, which was no more stigmatized and dreaded.
- The intention of the sample to opt for voluntary HIV testing showed a crucial increase with a greater understanding and a sense of responsibility for themselves and their families.
- The overall mean score for the sample on attitude assessment scale increased from 3.56 to 7.02 out of total of 9 during the course of intervention.

Condom-usage Behaviour Assessment : Pre-intervention

Under the behavioural aspect of evaluation, condom usage as well as barriers to its use were assessed. The pre-intervention findings are:

- The condom usage by the married sample with their spouse was very low (14 per cent) due to various reasons.
- The advantage of using a condom as a preventive measure against HIV/AIDS was not known to more than half of the sample.
- The socio-cultural inhibitions and economic dependence were the major factors hindering women's right to ask their husbands to use condoms in spite of their infidelity.
- The percentage of truck drivers and rickshaw pullers having pre/extramarital sex without using a condom was found to be 50 per cent,

in contrast to 80 per cent of the CSWs who reported consistent condom usage with their clients.

- HIV/AIDS prevention by condom usage was not known to the majority of the male sample.
- The misconception of considering many sexual partners as steady partners (i.e., sexually faithful partners) due to familiarity with them and thus, not using a condom with them was enhancing sample's vulnerability to HIV/AIDS.
- Majority of the truck drivers and rickshaw pullers (76 per cent) indulging in sex with non-regular partner/s did not negotiate condom use because they felt rather uneasy/embarrassed to do so. However, significantly high percent (98 per cent) of the CSWs reported negotiating condom use with their clients due to their exposure to various ongoing HIV prevention programmes.
- Correct condom usage and disposal skills were lacking among majority of the sample.
- The study revealed that a crucial percentage of the truck drivers and rickshaw pullers (75 per cent) were not able to avail condoms from the free condom distribution services, be it government hospitals or dispensaries due to various reasons.
- Women's right to assert their partner for condom usage was an aspect that showed vast gender-based variation with men (74 per cent) opposing the idea, while women (80 per cent) insisting on the same.

Intervention Period – Promoting Safe Sexual Behaviour

Condom-usage as an effective method of HIV prevention among the sample was promoted through the use of audio-visual aids developed during the course of study. The photo-script elaborately discussed the need, the advantages as well as the moral responsibility to use a condom during various situations. Similarly, the pamphlet, which was developed keeping in mind the needs of the sex workers, stressed the importance of consistent and correct condom usage and disposal skills. It was emphasized times and again that practicing safe sex was in everybody's interest. The peer educators played a crucial role in convincing and promoting condom usage by conducting focus group discussions within their own communities.

Condom-usage Behaviour Assessment : Post-intervention

The intervention had a significant impact on the sample with regards to their heightened awareness of condoms and their usage. Some of the desirable changes brought about as a result of discussions and deliberations are listed below:

- The knowledge regarding the usefulness of a condom as a great protection measure against HIV increased significantly (from 38 per cent to 98 per cent) amongst the sample.
- As reported the condom use with spouse as well as non-regular partner/s rose substantially among the sample groups.
- The presentation of a skit in which a truck driver is being advised by his friend to carry a condom at all times while going in for sex with a non-regular partner helped in doubling the percentage of sample carrying a condom with them while going in for such sexual transactions.
- The increase in condom usage was substantiated by a decrease in the reported incidence of STD (from 11 per cent to 7 per cent) among the sample. As the pre- and post-intervention data-collection period spanned over 24 months, this behavioural fact could be elicited.
- A high proportion of the sample showed increased awareness regarding causes and symptoms of STD, leading to qualitative as well as quantitative changes in their treatment seeking behaviour. For instance, the proportion of the sample seeking treatment from qualified medical practitioners increased from 58 per cent to 69 per cent during the course of intervention.
- The misconception of treating many sexual partners as steady partners was now seen as a great threat of HIV/AIDS by 89 per cent of sample indulging in such sexual transactions.
- The presentation of a skit showing madam of a brothel insisting on condom-usage by a client was effective in shedding off various inhibitions pertaining to condom usage. Consequently, condom use negotiation skills showed positive changes in terms of reported increase in the percentage of condom use negotiators as well as their being increasingly successful in negotiating skills.
- As reported the condom usage by the sample during their last sexual transaction with a non-regular partner as well as the intention to do so in future registered a significant rise.
- Major improvements were observed in the description of correct condom usage (38 per cent v/s 69 per cent) as well as correct condom disposal (29 per cent v/s 56 per cent) skills from the pre- to post-intervention period. This resulted in less percentage of sample reporting condom failure.

Practices Assessment: Pre-intervention

A wide range of unsafe practices in relation to HIV/AIDS was found to be increasing the sample's vulnerability to HIV. Some of the high-risk practices as assessed on condom usage behaviour and practices scale are:

- About one-third of the sample reported that whenever they received injections for some medical reasons, new needles were not used.
- The practice of sharing personal-use items such as shaving blades and razors was found to be observed in 36 per cent of the sample. In the case of 20 per cent of the sample, their barbers would use the same shaving knifes/blades for their clients.
- Overall, a very high percentage of the sample was found to have indulged in sex with non-regular partner/s (53 per cent), with men showing diverse sexual orientation including bisexuals as well as those having sex with eunuchs.
- Various misconceptions amongst the sample were found to be guiding their choice of non-regular sexual partner/s like if a sexual partner appeared healthy looks-wise then there were no chances of being infected through that partner.
- The prevalence of multi-partnerism was significantly high (42 per cent) along with the misconception of treating many of these partners as steady partners (i.e., sexually faithfully partners).
- A vast range of unprotected sexual practices (like anal and oral sex) was being followed by the sample along with the fact that such relationships were maintained over a long period of time thus, enhancing HIV vulnerability.
- "Survival sex" i.e., exchanging sex for services in kind such as food and clothing seemed to be significantly prevalent among women in the rural areas.

The Intervention – Helping Introspect Day to Day Practices

Group discussions and demonstrations were mainly used as tools in conjunction with the audio-visual aids to change the practices of the sample in a desired way during the intervention period. Discussions focusing on the risks involved in sharing of needles, syringes, blades etc., were conducted with the sample. Drinking alcohol, which subsequently, led to practicing of unsafe behaviour, was portrayed by the photo-script. Similarly, the tendency to indulge in pre/extra-marital sex was also questioned through the photo-script. *A number of instances for greater introspection in context of HIV/AIDS were cited.*

Practices Assessment : Post-intervention

A positive impact of the intervention was seen as majority of the sample switched over to certain safe sexual practices. To mention some of these:

- Majority of the sample (93 per cent) was now aware of the importance of using a new needle and syringe for getting injections/piercing done.
- A significant decline (29 per cent) was reported by the sample in the practice of sharing items of personal-use like blades and razors.
- A slight but crucial decrease (6 per cent) was recorded in the percentage of the male sample indulging in extra-marital sex during the post intervention period as a result of increased HIV/AIDS awareness.
- Various misconceptions related to criteria for choosing non-regular sexual partner/s were dispelled giving way to a new sense of responsibility. This was checked and counter-checked several times.
- The prevalence of multi-partnerism decreased (by 13 per cent) among the male sample as a result of their understanding the difference between steady and non-steady partners.
- The range of sexual practices although showing quantitative resilience in terms of the percentage of sample practicing them, reflected qualitative changes. For instance, the percentage of sample practicing anal/oral sex remained constant but those practicing these acts without a condom decreased significantly.

t-test – Statistically Assessing the Impact of Intervention

The impact of the intervention was statistically assessed by using the "t-test". All data were analyzed at .05 level of significance. The computed 't values' indicated that the changes in knowledge, attitude, behaviour and practices of all the three sample groups on the KABP scale were significant. Thus, providing a statistical basis to the data obtained and also proving the effectiveness of the intervention.

Development and Field-Testing of the Audio-Visual Aids – A Community Participated Action

Since majority of the sample was illiterate, a need to develop a set of suitable audio-visual aids for creating HIV/AIDS awareness was felt. In the beginning some of the existing audio-visual aids developed by NACO and a few other organizations (Appendix XI) were used in the community and the feedback obtained. Based on the feedback and in order to cater to the specific needs of the communities, communication material was developed that included a photo-script, a pamphlet and a poster. These aids served as an effective as well as cost-effective means for generating HIV/AIDS awareness. From concept to completion, the community was involved in their development. A brief description of these aids follows :

I. Photo-script – The theme of the photo script was "*AIDS Ka Gyan – Bachaey Jaan*" meaning "AIDS Information-Saves Life". The *script content* was designed in a way to give HIV prevention information in a generalized manner *emphasizing that safe sex was in public interest.* Few rickshaw pullers were motivated and prepared to take up different roles and act in various skits. This led to the culmination of the photo-script (Annexure I). Simple pictures showing transmission modes, symptoms and preventive methods of HIV were developed and used in the photo-script. These were quite helpful in disseminating HIV/AIDS information in a simple and easy to understand manner. Besides, the role-play process by the pullers helped the larger community in identifying themselves with the characters of the script.

II. Pamphlet – Keeping in mind the specific needs of the commercial sex workers, a pamphlet (Annexure II) was designed. The pamphlet titled *"Mere Bhi Kuch Adhikar Hain"* meaning "I too have some rights" highlighted the rights of the commercial sex workers and the need to practice safe sexual behaviour in the larger interest. *The pamphlet symbolized the awakening of a woman from deep slumber as a result of AIDS awareness.*

III. Poster – A photo session with the truck drivers led to the development of a poster advocating safe behaviour. This poster (Annexure III) was quite helpful in motivating the sample communities to be happy by safeguarding themselves against AIDS. The poster-slogan was *"Hum Khush Hain Kyon ki Hum AIDS Se Surakshit Hain"* meaning "We are Happy because we are safe from AIDS". The participation of the truck drivers as the role models for the poster helped the sample communities to realize that AIDS was not a distant threat but a real disease amongst them.

All these aids have an element of audio-visual and interactive phase like.

(a) **Audio** – in terms of the voice of script-reader/ peer educators.

(b) **Visual** – in terms of the drawings, pictures, photos and logo in the photo-script.

(c) **Interactive mode** – The aids had immense scope for interaction and clarification of myths, misconceptions and doubts regarding AIDS, its manifestation and prevention as panacea.

Since the aim was to sustain awareness programme ever after the research was over, it seemed prudent to use peer educators to continue with the HIV/AIDS awareness efforts.

Field -Testing of the Audio-Visual Aids

The audio-visual aids were field-tested with a group of fifteen individuals (i.e., 5 from each sample group) who were selected through purposive sampling method and were not a part of the earlier intervention. All the three audio-visual aids were presented consecutively in the order of presentation being – the poster followed by the photo-script concluding with the pamphlet presentation. *The results of field-testing showed positive changes in the mean KABP scores of the three sample groups as assessed on knowledge, attitude, behaviour and practices scale developed for the purpose.* The details of the results are given below:

Knowledge Assessment : Pre- to Post-intervention

The knowledge regarding AIDS as a disease, its transmission modes and symptoms showed considerable improvement. The pictures developed and used in the photo-script were quite helpful in imparting awareness regarding these vital aspects in an easy to understand manner.

- *Myths and misconceptions* related to the cause of AIDS, its acquisition modes and the treatment aspect were focused upon in the photo-script, and the same were observed to be dispelled after presentation of the audio-visual aids.
- Similarly, the presentation of the pamphlet was quite helpful in generating awareness that *sexually transmitted infections* may not always show up as visible symptoms but need to be treated soon.
- Majority of the sample showed a significant increase (from 20 per cent to 93 per cent) in their awareness regarding HIV testing through a blood test and the availability of such facilities in certain hospitals.
- A major gain was observed in the knowledge regarding prevention of HIV/AIDS from all the four different transmission modes, which reflected the desired change that the audio-visual aids were designed for.
- The level of awareness regarding the survival time of HIV and AIDS infected people registered only a marginal rise, probably due to the complexity experienced by the sample in differentiating between HIV and AIDS condition.
- The overall mean score for the entire sample on knowledge assessment scale increased from 5.07 to 12.60 out of a total of 20 during the pre- to post-audio-visual aids field-testing period.

Attitude Assessment : Pre- to Post-intervention

Positive changes were documented in the attitudes of the sample towards issues related to sexuality, rights of people living with HIV/AIDS and vulnerability to HIV/AIDS during the post-field-testing period.

- In contrast to the pre-field-testing period, the entire sample in the post-field-testing phase was convinced that education regarding sex, STD and HIV/AIDS should be given to the general population as well as to school children at a suitable age.
- The percentage of sample believing only CSWs and their clients to be vulnerable to STD and HIV/AIDS were reduced to half after the field-testing of audio-visual aids. This decline was a result of *emphasizing other modes of HIV transmission* apart from sex in the photo-script.
- The attitude of the sample regarding rights of people living with HIV/AIDS and treatment towards a HIV positive spouse showed considerable empathy.
- The intention to get tested for HIV showed a reasonable rise (from 13 per cent to 33 per cent) amongst the sample. *The presentation of the poster developed during the study was able to motivate the sample to be happy by ensuring prevention against AIDS.*
- The overall mean score of the positive attitudes held by the sample on attitude assessment scale (concise form) registered a rise from 1.93 to 3.87 out of total of 5.

Condom-usage Behaviour and Practices Assessment: Pre- to Post-intervention

The perception of the sample towards condom-usage showed considerable improvement subsequent to the presentation of audio-visual aids.

- Contrary to the pre-field-testing period, majority of the sample became aware of at least two advantages of using a condom subsequent to the presentation of the audio-visual aids.
- The awareness regarding the ability of a condom to protect a person from HIV/AIDS showed a significant (40 per cent) rise.
- The barriers to condom usage saw a substantial decline (13 per cent) as various misconceptions related to its usage were effectively dispelled. A significant proportion of the sample that had never used a condom with their non-regular partner/s showed *the intention and promise to do so in future.*
- Considerable improvement was observed in the description of correct condom-usage and disposal skills by the sample during the post-field-testing period.
- The ability to overcome inhibitions and initiate condom use negotiation with non-regular sexual partner/s registered a significant (40 per cent) rise.

- The overall mean score on condom-usage behaviour and practices assessment scale (concise form) for the respondents indulging in sex with non-regular partner/s increased from 3.16 to 7.47 in the post field-testing period out of a total of 10.

Analysis of Practices in the Context of HIV/AIDS

- Unlike the pre-field-testing period, nearly the entire sample (93 per cent) during the post-field-testing period said that they would take safety measure while getting any injections. They were convinced that the needle and syringe needed to be disposable.
- The intention not to share items of personal-use like blades and razors registered a significant (27 per cent) self-reported decline.
- The entire male sample who had previously reported the use and re-use of blades by their barbers were now aware of the dangers of doing so.

To conclude, the value of the custom made audio-visual aids was well worth the effort in increasing HIV/AIDS awareness of the respondents.

Evaluation of the ongoing HIV/AIDS Prevention Programmes at the G. B. Road

During the course of study, an evaluation of the efficacy of ongoing HIV/AIDS prevention programmes at the G.B. Road showed that the services rendered by a few NGOs to the sex 0workers was curtailed considerably. The NGOs focused only on the *distribution of materialistic rather than skill-building services*. In the absence of an access to other avenues, the young women were moving in the same direction as their elders, that is to remain in the flesh trade. The plight of the sex workers' children needed special attention too as they were the victims of the circumstances, they had been raised into.

Rehabilitation of the sex workers into mainstream life was easier said than done. Once in the flesh trade, the commercial sex workers have very little option for anything else to earn their livelihood. Moreover, socially speaking there is a huge stigma attached to their profession.

Indicators – Assessing the Impact

The impact of the study was measured by using qualitative as well as quantitative indicators including those based on the WHO guidelines as well as the national behavioural sentinel surveillance (BSS, 2001) core indicators. All these parameters showed major favourable changes in KABP of the sample with regards to HIV/AIDS from the pre- to post-intervention period. *A significant transition followed from a state of unawareness to awareness.* Several hard-core myths and misconceptions related to the disease were removed. A convincing, triangulation method (i.e., combining two methods for data verification) was used to cross-check the information. For instance, a validation of safe sex at all times as reported by the sample was cross-checked by observing the incidence of STD among them. In fact, people were offering more information about others on all fronts. In a way, this was very helpful in verifying the truth. *Community's participation and total involvement was the lifeline in confidence building measures to keep the HIV/AIDS disease at bay.*

The sample satisfaction with regards to the intervention was very high. Majority of the sample felt empowered to take safe decisions on the completion of the intervention, which was the desired goal of the study. Thus, the effort demonstrates that AIDS awareness can be effectively generated with the help of community participation. Some suggestions with a view to bring down HIV prevalence amongst such communities with high-risk behaviour have been framed and sent to NACO, Ministry of Health and Family Welfare, Government of India, for their perusal.

Conclusion

The present study concludes with the proposition that awareness, care and empowerment of communities "(ACE STRATEGY)" is imperative in combating HIV/AIDS. To effectively control the spread of the HIV, it is prudent to delve into and address various issues that make people vulnerable to the disease. Informational HIV/AIDS prevention campaigns may not have all the answers to keep the HIV/AIDS under check. Poverty, illiteracy, exploitation, substance abuse, conservatism are all inseparable parts of the health-care and health seeking behaviour. Dreaded diseases like HIV/AIDS thrive in abysmal living and work environment. People are more prone to such infections when they live under sub-human conditions and this is a disabling environment for right thinking and action. As poverty leads to a feeling of helplessness and apathy towards the disease, its roots need to be trimmed.

As far as mass-media approach to combat AIDS is concerned, innovative need-based strategies that rely on interactive and interpersonal modes of communication should be developed and implemented rather than having one-sided communication from top. The provision of basic health care services to the marginalized groups in a non-discriminating environment becomes a requirement for *a win-win situation*. Trust builds confidence and the latter builds a life of quality.

The prevailing myths and misconceptions of the masses with regards to HIV/AIDS, STD and their manifestations would also disappear in an environment of social equity. Giving people the life-saving and skill-building knowledge is highly desirable for sustainability of any good plan. "Staying in touch" is the cornerstone to success. Referral services need to be made available to people so that they know how to go about for any advice or help. Therefore, a holistic approach integrating HIV/AIDS information along with related referral services would bring about desired behavioural changes. Health care professionals as doctors, nurses, traditional healers and families should work hand-in-hand in dealing with situations to bring about healing. Targeted interventions aimed at generating HIV/AIDS awareness among certain communities such as barbers, traditional healers, ear and nose piercing professionals and tattooists need to be taken up. Apart from sensitizing NGOs towards the needs of CSWs, effective policies aimed at rehabilitating sex workers should be formulated and translated into real action to contain sex trade and subsequently HIV. Finally, community participation as a means of generating HIV/AIDS awareness needs to be fully harnessed as a valuable resource in achieving the "Millennium Achievement Goal", which proposes not only to halt but also to reverse the AIDS epidemic by 2015.

Suggestions

The suggestions evolved during the course of the study are as follows:

1. **Implementation of psycho-educational programmes** - A radical change is urgently required in the socialization process with the aim of putting an end to gender-based differentiation, which continues to be a cause of most HIV infections worldwide. Socio-cultural norms that advocate equal rights and responsibilities of both men and women especially in matters related to sex and sexuality and condom use need to be formulated and implemented at the earliest.

2. **Review of laws related to prostitution** – Many advanced countries legally recognize prostitution as a work and have ensured certain basic rights of the commercial sex workers. For instance, in Philippines sex workers are registered and screened every 2 weeks for the presence of STD with the aim of treating these infections and thereby decreasing the spread of HIV (UNAIDS/WHO, Dec., 1999). Similarly, in Rwanda girls engaged in sex work have their HIV test result certificates with them and their partners can ask to have a look at them (Buysse, et al., 1996). But in India, we are still way back in accepting and ensuring even the basic rights of commercial sex workers. In order to curb the further spread of HIV, we need to review the laws related to prostitution, which are by and large oppressive for commercial sex workers and hinder their ability to protect themselves from HIV. Emphasis should not be solely placed on curbing prostitution since experience shows that this may not be possible in real terms in the near future. Till the time, our government is able to put an end to this social menace; emphasis and efforts should be focused on granting certain basic rights to the commercial sex workers. For example, the right to negotiate for safe sex with clients can prove to be a major milestone in preventing many new HIV infections.

3. **Enforcing innovative mandatory measures-** Experience shows that enforcing specific preventive measures on a mandatory basis can be more effective in implementing public health strategies than solely relying on individuals for behavioural change (ICMR cited in NACO, 1997). Thailand's 100 per cent condom use programme which ensures condom use every time by all commercial sex workers is an example of mandatory measure which has proved to be a success. In India too, commercial sex workers should be screened every fortnight for the presence of STD. Since STD are a marker of unprotected sex, their presence would confirm sex without condom usage among commercial sex workers which can then be dealt with appropriately.

   - Similarly, a mandatory measure requiring each truck driver and rickshaw puller to keep a safety kit comprising of bandage, dettol, cotton and a condom in their vehicles should be enforced. Constant keeping of a condom in their safety kit would definitely increase condom-usage among these communities as they are more likely to use a condom if they have it with them. Secondly, it would also help truck drivers and rickshaw pullers to overcome the inhibitions of buying condoms, as they will have to purchase a new condom each and every time they use the one in the kit. The stocking of a condom in the safety kit may be occasionally checked and ensured by police personnel at check-posts while checking relevant papers of the vehicle.
   - In case of truck drivers and rickshaw pullers, integrating AIDS education into school curriculum may not be very helpful because many truck drivers and rickshaw pullers do not have formal/high school education. Therefore, transport authorities issuing driving licenses to these drivers can help significantly in creating HIV/AIDS awareness amongst them. Every transport authority conducts an exam for each individual before issuing a driver's license to a person. It would be extremely beneficial, if the licensing authority incorporates a few very basic questions related to AIDS in their exam administered to the drivers. This will ensure that all drivers aspiring to get a driving license will have to pass AIDS related basic exam along with their driving exam in order to get a driving license. The transport authority may also help in conducting a few special classes on AIDS awareness for these drivers prior to their AIDS awareness related examination.

- Just like a pollution check certificate, a certificate issued on completion of specific criteria showing that the concerned driver is aware about AIDS may be issued to every driver that needs to be displayed on the vehicle along with the pollution check certificate. These measures will certainly help in creating HIV/AIDS awareness among all the drivers.
- In India, illiteracy rate is as high as 34.6 per cent according to the latest report by Census of India (2001). Majority of the masses do not have adequate schooling and thus are not fully aware about issues such as sex, sexuality, STD, HIV and AIDS. To make matter worse boys and girls are married at early ages especially in rural areas. Therefore, ignorance coupled with lack of negotiating power in sexual relations especially in case of young girls who can't assert themselves for condom use increases their vulnerability to HIV. To overcome this major obstacle from blocking success of HIV prevention efforts, a mandatory policy related to marriage act/procedure needs to be enforced. Each and every individual should be married only after acquiring a certificate from a local health center, which provides awareness and training in HIV/AIDS prevention. This could avert a large number of HIV infections among our youth.

4. **Offering Incentives** – AIDS awareness programme targeting people in the age group of 15-49 years could be organized at the national level on similar lines such as the pulse polio programme. Young masses could be motivated to attend the AIDS awareness programme, held on certain dates at specific centers. In return some incentive in cash or kind could be offered to them. For example, a monetary incentive of even Rs. 10 per individual could attract a large number of poor masses and thus bring about AIDS awareness among them. The cost is negligible in comparison to the huge costs incurred on account of death of young workforce and treatment of HIV/AIDS patients.
5. **Female Condoms** – Development, distribution and marketing of effective female condoms at affordable prices should be stressed on a priority basis. Female condoms can truly be a viable means of giving women the right to practice safe sex as and when they desire.

Appendices

APPENDIX – I

Interview Schedule for the Commercial Sex Workers

Background Information

(a) Name - (optional)
(b) Age -
(c) Education -
(d) Religion -
(e) Native Place -
(f) Marital Status -
(g) No. of children and their ages -
(h) Place of residing - (a) self (b) family
(i) Occupation of self and family members -
(j) Approximate daily/ monthly income -
Self -
Family -

General Information

Q. 1. For how long have you been into this profession?
Q. 2. What was your age at the time you started this work?
Q. 3. How did you get into this work?
Q. 4. Is this the occupation by choice or was their some other reason to enter it?
Q. 5. Do you stay here on rental or commission basis?
Q. 6. How much rent/commission do you pay?
Q. 7. Are there any problems that you have with the premises owner or your employer?

Professional Information

Q. 1. How many clients on an average do you have per day?
Q. 2. What age group do your clients generally belong to?
Q. 3. What is the mode of soliciting these clients?
Q. 4. What type of people mostly visit you in terms of their – marital status, occupation and other such related factors?
Q. 5. Do they treat you well?
Q. 6. Do you ever have any type of problem with your clients? If yes, specify?
Q. 7. Do you know if some of your clients are drug addicts/alcoholics? If yes, how many of your clients take these substances prior to sexual transactions?
Q. 8. Can you tell what type of substances are your clients addicted to; like alcohol, opium, cannabis etc.?
Q. 9. Do you experience any difference in their behaviour towards you as compared to sober clients?
Q. 10. Are you able to negotiate your terms with your clients? Elaborate.
Q. 11. How much money are you paid by each client?
Q. 12. Do you get the entire amount or is it shared by others also?
Q. 13. Are you given some tips by your clients?
Q. 14. Are there any peak or lean periods in your profession? How do you sustain yourselves during such times?

Child Rearing Practices

Q. 1. Do you have children? If yes how many?
Q. 2. Do your children go to school? If so, are they treated like other children?
Q. 3. What alternative care do your children have while you are at work?
Q. 4. Explain the type of interaction your children have with other people/children of the area?
Q. 5. What type of attitude do people have towards you and your children?
Q. 6. Are your children/family aware about the nature of work you undertake?
Q. 7. Do you think that your profession or things related to it are having any effect on the overall development of your children? Elaborate.
Q. 8. What type of life do you plan to have for your children?
Q. 9. Would you wish to continue with the same profession or switch over?

APPENDIX – II

Interview Schedule for Truck Drivers

Background Information

(a) Name -

(b) Age -

(c) Education -

(d) Religion -

(e) Native Place -

(f) Marital Status -

(g) No. of children and their ages -

(h) Place of residing -

(i) Family address -

(j) Occupation of self and family members -

(k) Approximate daily/ monthly income -

Self -

Family -

General Information

Q. 1. For how long have you been in this occupation?

Q. 2. Is this the occupation by choice or chance?

Q. 3. The vehicle you drive is your own or is it a rented one?

Q. 4. If its a rented one then how much rent do you pay for it?

Q. 5. Are there any problems that you have with the vehicle owner or your employer?

Q. 6. How often do you go on tours i.e. on weekly or monthly basis?

Q. 7. On what routes and for how many days do you tour?

Q. 8. On an average, how many days in a week/ month do you stay away from your family?

Q. 9. Are there any problems faced by you and your family when you are away? Elaborate.

Q. 10. Whenever you are on a long tour, where do you halt?

Q. 11. Do you halt at a particular place or at different places each time you tour?

Q. 12. What makes you opt for these places?

Q. 13. What are the facilities that are provided at these places?

(a) Good accommodation

(b) Good food

(c) Basic amenities

(d) Any other

APPENDIX – III

Interview Schedule for Rickshaw Pullers
Background Information

(a) Name -
(b) Age -
(c) Education -
(d) Religion -
(e) Native Place -
(f) Marital Status -
(g) No. of children and their ages -
(h) Place of residing - (a) self (b) family
(i) Occupation of self and family members -
(j) Approximate daily/ monthly income -
Self -
Family -

General Information

Q. 1. For how long have you been staying in Delhi?
Q. 2. What made you come to Delhi?
Q. 3. Why did you leave your family behind?
Q. 4. For how long have you been in your present occupation of rickshaw pulling?
Q. 5. The rickshaw you pull is your own or a rented one? If it's a rented one then how much rent do you pay for it?
Q. 6. Is this the occupation by choice or chance?
Q. 7. Do you have any problems related to your staying over here? Explain.
Q. 8. Do you experience any occupational problems? If yes, elaborate?
Q. 9. Are there some lean periods when you are not able to earn? If yes, when and how do you sustain yourself during that time?
Q. 10. Could you tell something about your daily expenditure?
Q. 11. Do you send some money or goods to your family? If yes, could you elaborate?
Q. 12. How often do you contact your family and by what means?
(a) Through letters
(b) Through friends
(c) By visiting them
(d) Any other means

APPENDIX – IV

Specific Information

Q. 1. Usually how long do you stay away from your family at a stretch?

Q. 2. During the stretches when you are separated by work, do you miss out on your family and vice versa?

Q. 3. Do you feel lonely while staying away from your family? If yes, how do you try to cope up with your loneliness?

Q. 4. Do you try to find some means of entertainment such as – company of friends, playing cards, drinking, any form of substance use of any other means?

Q. 5. Do you have a feeling of missing out your wife/ a partner? If yes, how do you try to manage/overcome this feeling of being with your wife/a partner?

Q. 6. Do you visit a CSW/a partner? If yes, would you like to tell us why?

APPENDIX – V

Assessment of Physical/ Substance abuse Patterns

Q. 1. Do you use/take substances like tobacco, liquor, drugs or any other kind of intoxicating substance? If yes, since when?

Q. 2. When do you feel the need to take these substances? How much quantity do you generally consume at one time?

Q. 3. How does the use of these substances have an impact on your behaviour? (Makes you feel good, takes you out of worries, any other)

Q. 4. Approximately how much money do you spend on these substances in a week/ fortnight/ month?

Q. 5. Do you usually have sexual interactions after the use of these substances?

Q. 6. Have you ever been subjected to any form of physical/sexual abuse in your life? If yes, when? (During childhood/young age)

Q. 7. Would you like to tell if the abuser is/was related to your family in some way?

Q. 8. Has that incident affected you in any way? If yes, how?

Q. 9. Would you like to discuss any of your past/ present stressors in life and their impact on you?

APPENDIX VI

Media Exposure

Q. 1 Do you have a radio or a T.V. at your home/workplace?

Q. 2. How often do you listen to radio or watch T.V. in a day? What are the programmes that you listen to/watch in T.V.?

Q. 3. Are there certain fixed hours when .you find time for these activities? If yes, specify.

Q. 4. Do you also read newspaper or any other print material? If yes, specify.

Q. 5. Have you listened to/seen any public service message/information related to AIDS? If yes, specify the media and elaborate on the contents.

Q. 6. Have you understood the contents and the messages that these advertisements /information campaigns want to convey? Elaborate.

Q. 7. Are there certain components that you have not understood? If yes, why?

Q. 8. What are the types of media that you would prefer for getting HIV/AIDS awareness and why?

APPENDIX – VII

STD Information

Q. 1. Do you understand the meaning of STD?

Q. 2. Are you aware about the symptoms and modes of acquiring STDs?

Q. 3. Have you suffered from any STD in the last six months? If yes, what were the symptoms and are they still persisting?

(Questions from serial no. 4 to 10 to be asked from respondents who reply positive for question 3).

Q. 4. Did you undergo any treatment for that? If not, why?

Q. 5. Where did you get yourself treated from for such ailments? What does the doctor say about it?

Q. 6. Did he ask you to take some precautions? If yes, what and did you comply?

Q. 7. Do you get yourself treated from a particular doctor? If so, why?

Q. 8. Do you feel better/cured after getting the treatment?

Q. 9. Do you regularly report to the doctor for follow up purposes?

Q. 10. How much do you spend on your treatment for such infections in a month?

Q. 11. Do you have any idea if your wife/sex worker/sexual partner suffers from any STD? If yes, how do you know about it?

Q. 12. Are they getting themselves treated? If yes, from whom?

Q. 13. Do you think STDs can be cured? If yes, how?

APPENDIX – VIII

Max. Score = 20 Points

Knowledge Assessment Scale

Q. 1. Have you ever heard anything about HIV/AIDS?

Ans. Yes [1] No [0]

Q. 2. If yes, what is AIDS?

Ans. A disease. [1]

Q. 3. What causes AIDS?

Ans. HIV/A virus/ A disease causing organism. [1]

Q. 4. How does the disease spread from one person to another?

(one mark for every correct mode) [4]

Ans. The disease spreads by following modes:

(a) By sexual contact,
(b) Transfusion by contaminated blood,
(c) Use of contaminated needles and syringes, and
(d) Mother to child transmission.

Q.5. What are the three most commonly observed symptoms associated with the disease?

(one mark for every correct symptom) [3]

Ans. Considerable weight loss (more than 10 per cent of body weight), Diarrhea for more than one month, fever for more than one month, any other symptom correctly reported.

Q. 6. What test can be used to know if a person is suffering from HIV infection/AIDS? [1]

Ans. A blood test.

Q. 7. Where can a person be tested for HIV/AIDS? [1]

Ans. At a hospital or a clinic by a Doctor.

Q. 8. Can AIDS be cured? [1]

Ans. No

Q. 9. How long can a person with HIV/AIDS survive? (one mark for every correct answer) [2]

Ans. Survival time for HIV infected individuals varies between 8 - 10 yrs. and for individuals diagnosed with AIDS approximately 2 yrs.

Q. 10. How can one prevent oneself from acquiring this disease?

(one mark for every correct mode) [4]

Ans. The preventive modes are :

(a) By practicing safe sex,

(b) Using safe blood viz. HIV free for transfusion if required,

(c) Using new/disinfected needles and syringes for injecting, and

(d) By following prophylactic measures during pregnancy in case a woman is HIV positive.

Q. 11. Do you perceive yourself to be at risk of having acquired (in past) /acquiring HIV infection in future? If yes – why? If no – why? [1]

Ans. One mark to be given if the respondent analyses his vulnerability (in relation to indulgence in high-risk behaviour and practices) to HIV correctly.

APPENDIX – IX

Max. Score= 9 positive attitudes

Attitude Assessment Scale

Key [+] = positive attitude, [–] = negative attitude, [0] = No opinion
Score = 1 *Score = -1* *Score = 0*

Q. 1. It is right to talk and give education regarding sex/HIV/AIDS/STD to people including children in the schools.

Ans. Yes [+] No [–] No opinion [0]

Q. 2. It is a woman's responsibility to use a contraceptive in all kinds of sexual relationships.

Ans. Yes [–] No [+] No opinion [0]

Q. 3. Anybody practicing high-risk behaviour is vulnerable to STD/ HIV/ AIDS.

Ans. Yes [+] No [–] No opinion [0]

Q. 4. Men should have more rights than women in sexual relationships.

Ans. Yes [–] No [+] No opinion [0]

Q. 5. People living with or affected by HIV/AIDS should have the same rights as any normal person.

Ans. Yes [+] No [–] No opinion [0]

Q. 6. If an individual tests positive for HIV/AIDS then he/she should be isolated from the family/society.

Ans. Agree [–] Disagree [+] No opinion [0]

Q. 7. Both Husband and wife should take the responsibility to protect the family (i.e., children) from HIV/AIDS.

Ans. Agree [+] Disagree [–] No opinion [0]

Q. 8. There is no need for a person to go in for HIV testing irrespective of any behaviour and practice.

Ans. Agree [–] Disagree [+] No opinion [0]

(Scoring done on the basis of response given in relation to indulgence in high-risk behaviour. For instance, if an individual has indulged in high-risk behaviour and stiil doesn't intend to get tested for HIV then negative scoring done).

Q. 9. Everybody needs to know more about safe sexual behaviour.

Ans. Agree [+] Disagree [–] No opinion [0]

Q. 10. What do you think about having homosexual/premarital/extra-marital relationships?

Ans. Normal/Wrong to have such relations.

Q. 11. What ambitions/goals in life do you have for yourself and your family?

APPENDIX – X

Max. Score = 20 Points

CONDOM USE BEHAVIOUR AND PRACTICES ASSESSMENT SCALE

Condom Usage Behaviour Assessment

Q. 1. What contraceptives are used by you/your wife/your partner?
Ans. Pills/condoms/permanent method/any other/none.
Q. 2. Do you know something about a condom?
Q. 3. What are the advantages of using a condom?
Ans. Acts as a contraceptive, prevents STD/ HIV/AIDS, any other advantage.
Q. 4. Do you use condoms with your spouse? Give reasons for your answer.
Q. 5. Should women have the right to assert their partner to use a condom?
Q. 6. Are condoms easily available or do you experience any problems while accessing/purchasing them? If yes, specify?
Q. 7. Do you think you have the skills to practice condom use correctly or would you like to learn more about them?
Q. 8. After using a condom how do you dispose it off?
(To be administered only to individuals having sexual relations with non-regular partner/s)
Q. 9. During sexual interactions outside marriage how often do you use a condom?
Ans. Always - [3], mostly - [2], sometimes – [1], never – [0].
Q. 10. How often do you carry a condom with you while going in for sex with a non-regular partner?
Ans. At all times - [3], most of the times - [2], sometimes – [1], never – [0] .
Q. 11. During times when you do not use a condom for sexual relations with a non-regular partner what are the reasons for doing so?
Q. 12. How often do you negotiate condom use with your non-regular sexual partner/s?
Ans. Always - [3], mostly - [2], sometimes – [1], never – [0].
Q. 13. How do you feel while negotiating condom use with your such partners?
Ans. Confident - [4], comfortable - [3], shy - [2], embarrassed - [1], no usage- [0].

Q. 14. How often are you successful in these condom use negotiations?

Ans. Always -[3], mostly -[2], sometimes – [1], never –[0].

Q. 15. How many condoms do you buy/distribute (in case of CSWs) in a week /month? (Cross verification question).

Q. 16. Did you use a condom the last time you had a sexual relationship with a non-regular partner?

Ans. Yes -[1], No –[0].

Q. 17. How certain you are that you will use a condom in future for sexual interactions with a non-regular partner?

Ans. Surely use it-[3], will think about it-[2], not sure – [1], no usage–[0].

Q. 18. Would you like to give any suggestions regarding accessibility, quality, or pricing of condoms?

Practices Assessment

Q. 19. Have you ever got your self tattooed or gone through ears/nose piercing? If yes, were new needles used for you for these purposes?

Q. 20. How frequently are/have you been injected and for what purposes?

Q. 21. Are new needles used each time for injecting purpose?

Q. 22. Have you or any of your family members being given blood transfusion? If yes, why and where did the transfusion take place?

Q. 23. From where did you procure the blood and were you aware of /told by the doctor that it was safe from all infections including HIV?

Q. 24. Are there any personal items that you share with others, for example, shaving blades and razors? Give reasons for your answer.

Q. 25. While getting a haircut or being shaved by a barber, do you know if a new blade/clean razor is being used for you?

Sexual Practices

Q. 26. Have you ever indulged in pre-marital/ extra-marital sexual relations? *Following questions to be administered only to individuals having indulged in pre-marital/ extra-marital sex* *.

Q. 27. Are your pre/extra-marital sexual contacts planned or unplanned?

Q. 28. Whom do you have your pre/extra-marital sexual contacts with? (CSWs, men, eunuchs, any other).

Q. 29. How often do you have such contacts in a month?

Q. 30. What are the criteria for choosing a sex worker/partner for sexual services? For example, age, looks, rate of services, health of the partner, etc.

Q.31. Do you have sexual relations with a particular commercial sex worker/partner (steady partner) or different commercial sex workers/partners (non-steady partners)?

Q. 32. What has been the time-wise length of such sexual contacts?

Q.33. How many sexual partners do you have on a weekly/monthly basis?

Q.34. What type of sexual practices do you have with these sex workers/partners?

Q.35. Do you also practice French/deep kissing with your partners?

Q.36. How much money do you pay for each of such contacts/services?

Q.37. On an average how much money do you spend on sexual contacts with non-regular partner/s in a month?

Q.38. Do you ever feel that this type of expenditure is taxing you or your family?

Q.39. Have you told your wife/husband about your pre/extramarital relationship/s? Give reasons for your answer.

Q.40. Do you think these relationships will affect/are affecting your married life in any way?

Q.41. Have you ever faced any sort of problem in these relationships? If yes, kindly elaborate.

* *The tense (i.e., present/past) of these questions may be changed in accordance to the responses from the concerned individuals.*

APPENDIX – XI

List of Audio-visual Aids used with the sample

1. Mamooli Si Jalan Bhi Bhyankar Gupt Rog Ka Sanket Ho Sakti Hai.
   - NACO, December 1995.
2. Naya Saathi? Naya Zokhim.
   - NACO, January 1996.
3. Gupt Angon Ka Swasth Rehna, Swasth Bachchey Ko Janam Deta Hai.
   - NACO, December 1995.
4. Gupt Rogon Ka Ilaaz Hai, Yadi Samay Par Kiya Jai.
   - NACO, 2nd February 2002.
5. Rakt Bachayay Jaan Jab Us Per Ho HIV Mukt Ki Pehchan.
   - NACO, 2nd February 2002.
6. AIDS Se Bachiyey.
   - NACO, 2nd February 2002.
7. AIDS Ek Jaan Leva Rog, Bharat Mein Tezhi Se Faihl Reha Hai.
   - Drishtikon.
8. AIDS Roktham Karna Seekhein.
   -(UTA) – DAVP, March 1993.
9. HIV Aur AIDS Sabhi Ko Kya Jaanana Chaiyey?
   - VHAI.
10. Yon Karmiyon Ke Liye.
    - NACO.
11. Swasth Highway Pehchan Hamari.
    - NACO.
12. AIDS – Wafadari Mein Hi Samazhdari Hai.
    - Drishtikon.
13. Chalo Khatrey Ko Vardaan Banayein – Jawan Aur HIV/AIDS.
    - NACO, UNESCO.
14. Raktdaan Karein – Jeewan Bachayein.
    - NACO, February 2000.
15. Love affection and care key to fuller life – NACO, August 1997.
16. Unprotected sex - invitation to AIDS – NACO, August 1997.
17. Don't just guess, know how AIDS spreads – NACO August 1997.

18. Safe blood starts with me – WHO, 7th April 2000.
19. My friend with HIV is still my friend. He needs my support more than before – Maharashtra Network for positive people.
20. India responds to AIDS – NACO.
21. AIDS – The Challenge – WHO, 1999.
22. AIDS – No Time for Complacency – WHO, 1997.
23. STDs are curable if treated in time – NACO, 2nd March 2000.
24. Anybody can get AIDS – Drishtikon.
25. Should you get tested for HIV? – Synodical Board of Health Services.
26. Stop AIDS – Drishtikon.
27. Protect yourself from AIDS – NACO, September 2000.
28. Vulnerability of women – WHO.
29. AIDS men make a difference – WHO, 1st December 2000.
30. AIDS can be prevented – WHO.
31. Adolescents and youth – WHO.
32. Handbook on AIDS Home Care – WHO, Regional Office for South East Asia, New Delhi, India, 1996.
33. Break the silence - Maharashtra Network for positive people, Mumbai.
34. Let blood bring life not AIDS – NACO, September 2000.
35. Programme of AIDS prevention in Adolescents (PAPA) – Drishtikon.
36. HIV/AIDS at a glance – Church of North India.
37. More about AIDS – Department of Youth Affairs and Sports.

APPENDIX – XII

Max. Score = 5 positive attitudes

Attitude Assessment Scale (Concise Form)

Key [+] = positive attitude, [–] = negative attitude, [0] = No opinion
Score = 1 *Score = -1* *Score = 0*

Q. 1. It is right to talk and give education regarding sex/HIV/AIDS/STD to people including children in the schools.

Ans. Yes [+] No [–] No opinion [0]

Q. 2. Anybody practicing high-risk behaviour is vulnerable to STD/ HIV/ AIDS.

Ans. Yes [+] No [–] No opinion [0]

Q. 3. People living with or affected by HIV/AIDS should have the same rights as any normal person.

Ans. Yes [+] Disagree [–] No opinion [0]

Q. 4. If an individual tests positive for HIV/AIDS then he/she should be isolated from the family/society.

Ans. Agree [–] Disagree [+] No opinion [0]

Q. 5. There is no need for a person to go in for HIV testing irrespective of any behaviour and practice.

Ans. Agree [–] Disagree [+] No opinion [0]

(Scoring done on the basis of response given in relation to indulgence in high-risk behaviour. For instance, if an individual has indulged in high-risk behaviour and still doesn't intend to get tested for HIV then negative scoring done).

APPENDIX – XIII

Max. Score = 10 points

Condom Use Behaviour and Practices Assessment Scale (Concise Form)

Condom Usage Behaviour

Q. 1. Do you know something about a condom?

Q. 2. What are the advantages of using a condom?

Ans. Acts as a contraceptive, prevents STDs and HIV/AIDS.

Q. 3. Do you use condom with your spouse or non-regular partner/s? Give reasons for your answer.

Q. 4. Do you think you have the skills to use a condom correctly as well as dispose it of correctly after use?

Q. 5. During sexual interactions outside marriage how often do you use a condom?

Ans. Always - [3], mostly - [2], sometimes – [1], never – [0]

Q. 6. How often do you negotiate condom use with your non-regular sexual partner/s?

Ans. Always - [3], mostly - [2], sometimes – [1], never – [0]

Q. 7. How do feel while negotiating condom use with your partner?

Ans. Confident [4], comfortable- [3], shy- [2], embarrassed – [1], no usage – [0]

Practices Assessment

Q. 8. Have you ever got yourself tattooed or gone through ear piercing? If yes, were new needles used for each client?

Q. 9. How frequently have you been injected and for what purposes?

Q. 10. Are new needles used for every injecting purpose?

Q. 11. Are there any personal items that you share with others, for example, shaving blades and razors? Give reasons for your answer.

Q. 12. While getting a haircut or being shaved by a barber do you know if a new blade is being used for you?

APPENDIX – XIV

Supplementary Information

The gain in the mean scores scored by the three sample groups on the KABP scale during the post-field-testing stage may seem to be equal or for certain aspects be a bit on the higher side as compared to the gain in the mean scores during the post-intervention period primarily due to the following reasons.

Firstly, the post field-testing assessment of the sample to measure the impact of audio-visual aids was done on a concise KABP scale, which comparatively had fewer and simpler question as compared to the KABP scale used for the post-intervention assessment. The application of a concise KABP tool was neccessry keeping in mind the purpose of the audio-visual aids that aimed to create awareness about HIV/AIDS and vital aspects related to the disease in a relatively short period of time, unlike the main intervention which strived to bring about changes in the KABP of the sample with regards to HIV/AIDS and thus, required an elaborate and a comparatively complex KABP scale to do so resulting in a score-rise comparable to the audio-visual aids post-field-testing phase.

Secondly, the post-field-testing assessment of the audio-visual aids was done on the same day subsequent to their presentation, which enabled the sample to perform better on the KABP scale as the contents of the audio-visual aids were still fresh in their minds, unlike the assessment during the post-intervention period which was conducted after a reasonable period of time (i.e., 6 months) to measure the long-term impact of the intervention.

However, it is worth mentioning here that these reasons have been given only to clarify the resultant gain in scores during the two phases, namely the post-intervention period and the audio-visual aids field-testing period and that the same do not bear any effect on the implementation/efficacy of these two phases.

Annexure I

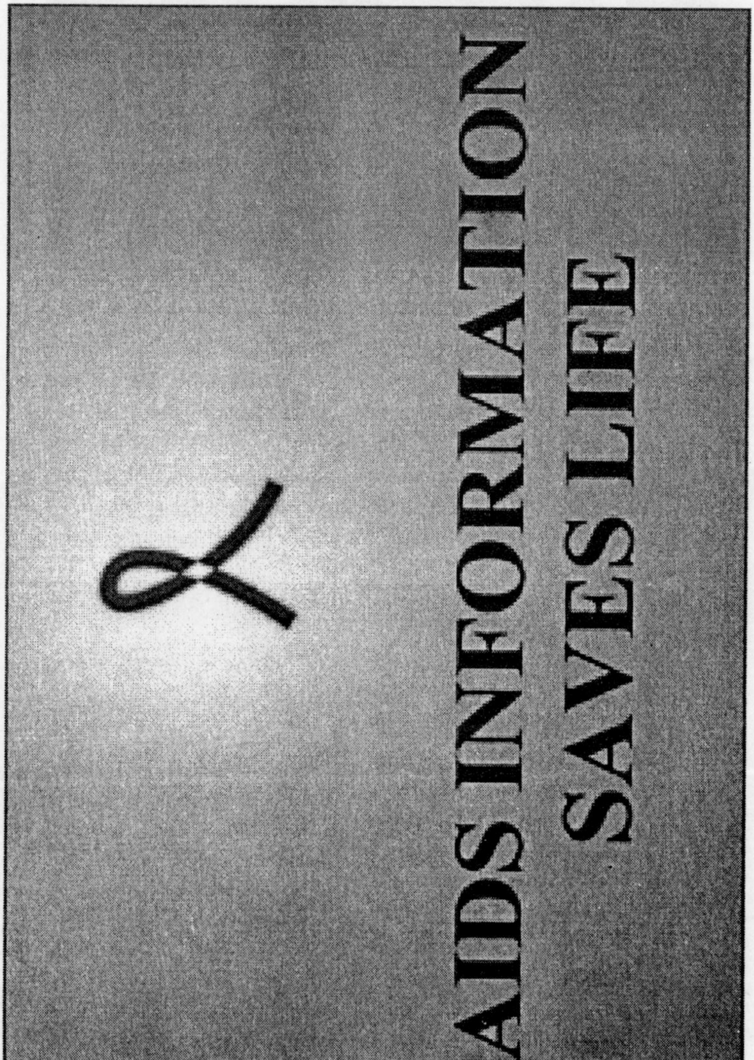

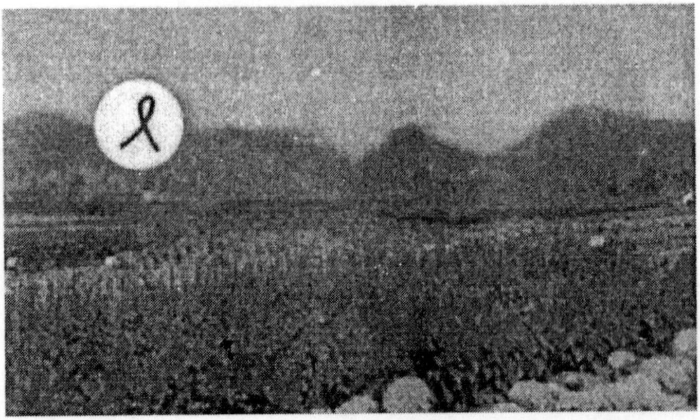

Life is the most precious gift that God gave to mankind. We do a lot of work in our life for ourselves, our children and the society too. Nothing is more important than leading a healthy and prosperous life. But sometimes, due to our ignorance or carelessness we endanger our as well as our near and dear ones' lives. Today, we shall be talking about a person whose unawareness and carelessness transformed his as well as his entire family's happy life. But at the same time we shall also be talking about a very important issue behavioural change and how it can protect us from the fatal disease AIDS.

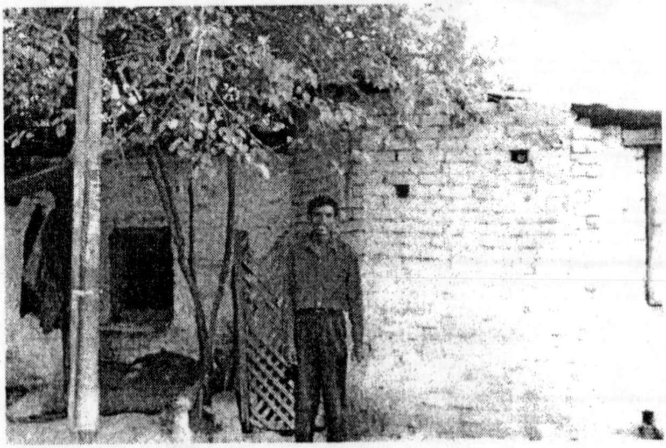

Let us introduce you to the hero of our story — Irfan. Irfan was a simple young man who lived happily with his mother, father and wife in a village. The family owned and cultivated a piece of land which was the sole means of earning their livelihood. Days passed by and after some time Irfan's wife gave birth to a baby girl.

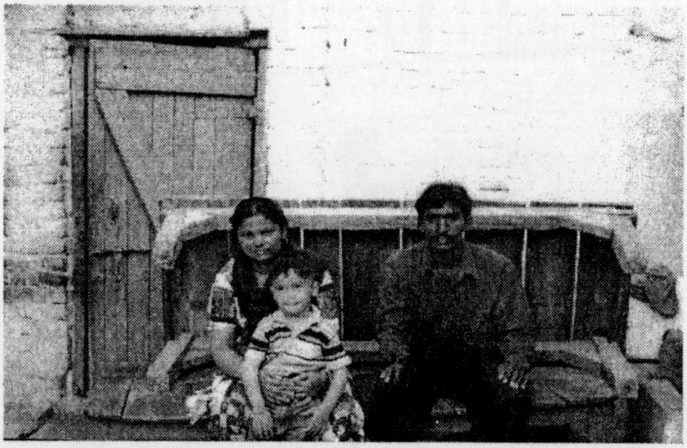

The family was very happy with the arrival of a new born baby. But along with happiness came additional responsibility and expenditure. Slowly, with passage of time the family started realising that income from agriculture was not enough to sustain their livelihood. So to supplement family income, Irfan decided to go to a city and work there. With no other option in hand the family reluctantly accepted his decision.

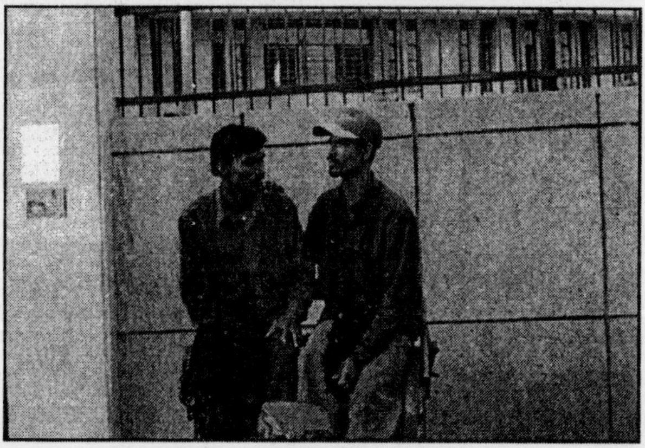

For a couple of days after reaching the city, Irfan was not able to find any job for himself as he was illiterate. One day while sitting idle he met Sakir, a rickshaw puller, who was from his native village. Sakir advised Irfan to take to rickshaw pulling too. He convincingly said "Look Irfan, rickshaw pulling is a work without any tension. We don't need to have a license and neither is any investment required to start it. I will talk to my rickshaw owner to get you a rickshaw on a rent of Rs. 22 per day." So tense was Irfan beacause of his unemployment that he readily accepted Sakir's help. As days passed, Irfan and Sakir became good friends and were seen together during their thick and thin.

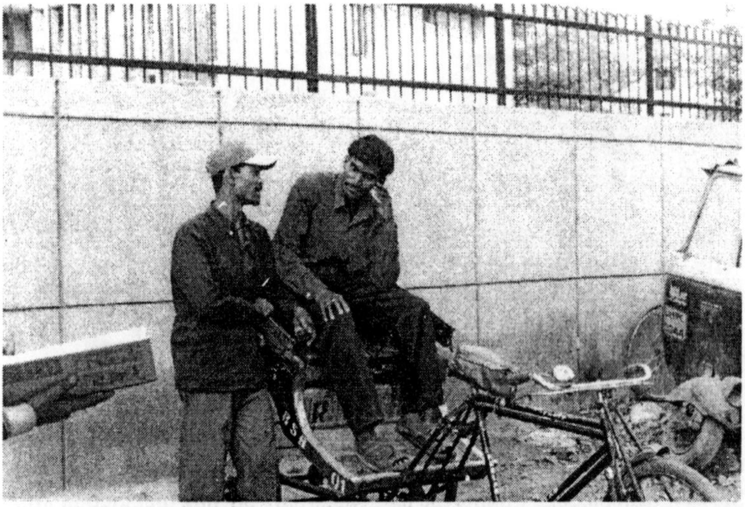

One evening Irfan was sitting quietly. He was feeling very sad and lonely as he was missing out on his family – his mother, father, wife and daughter. It had been six months since he left his home and he had not been able to save enough money so as to afford his visit to meet his family. Suddenly Sakir came and started enquiring about Irfan's well-being. Irfan's slowly responded "Sakir, what should I tell you? I am feeling so lonely. This life is not worth living without a wife and children." Sakir could sense Irfan's loneliness. He nodded and replied "Yes friend. You are right. Poor people like us have lot many worries. Our problem is further compounded due to separation from our family. But you leave aside your worries. Today, I will take you out for some pleasure."

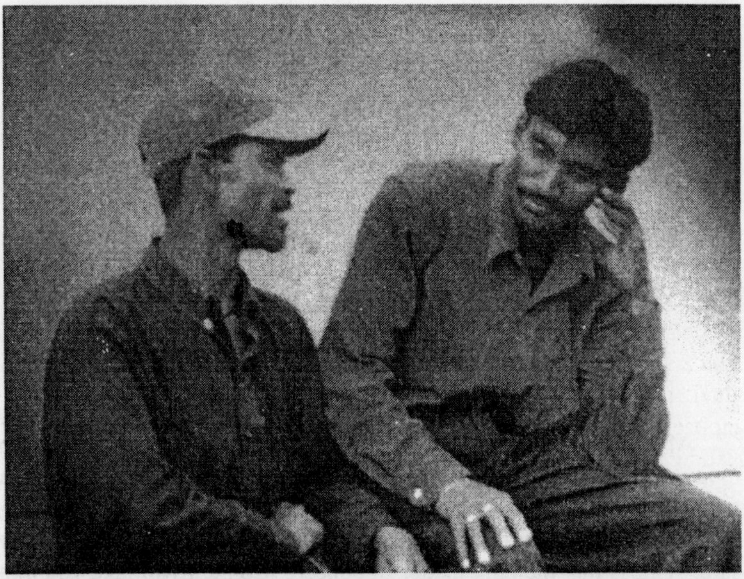

Then Sakir took Irfan to a brothel. Irfan was surprised and questioned "Oh! Sakir, where have you brought me?" Sakir smiled and replied "Dear, this is a place where all tensions are wiped out." Then he took out a liquor bottle from his pant's pocket and drank some liquor from it. He asked Irfan also to drink some of it. Initially, Irfan was hesitant but to overcome his anxiety he drank a little of it. After that Irfan and Sakir had sex with commercial sex workers and after gratifying themselves they came back from the brothel. And from now on visiting a brothel every week became a routine with them.

Here we would like to pose a question to you – Can a person be really happy after getting drunk? Some of you said that such a person can be happy for at least some time as he is away from his worries and problems.

But just think is it right to put our and our families' happiness and future at stake for the sake of such momentary pleasure. Let's see how far this habit of drinking takes Irfan from here.

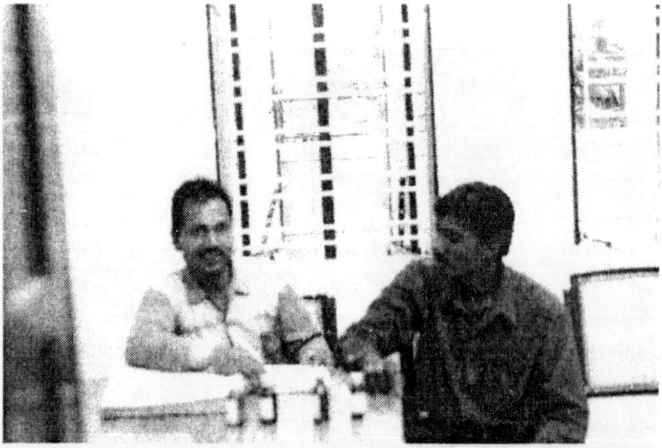

After some days, like every weekend when Sakir came and asked Irfan to accompany him to the brothel, Irfan refused. On Sakir's probing Irfan hesitantly confided "Friend, I don't know how to put it but I am suffering from a disease caused due to excessive heat in my body." Sakir lightly said, "Oh! Is that the only matter of concern. Come, I will take you to a nearby doctor who also hails from our village. He treats me for the same ailment." Irfan went with Sakir to the doctor and took the medicines as prescribed by him. After a few days, Irfan was cured and then he went to the village to meet his family.

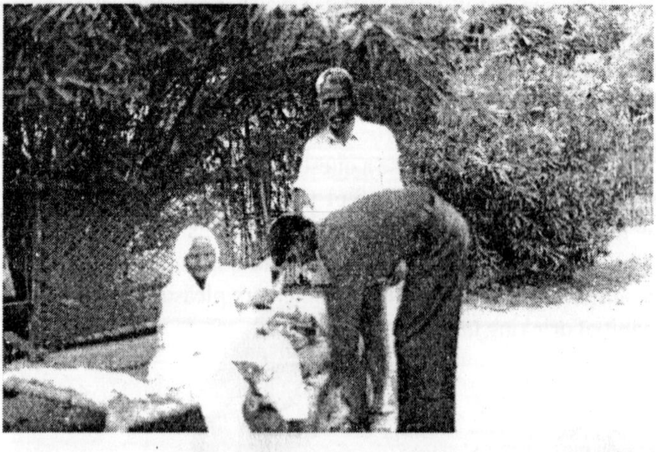

Everybody in the family was happy to see Irfan and a month passed by very quickly. Irfan came back to the city and was soon absorbed with rickshaw pulling, his old routine work.

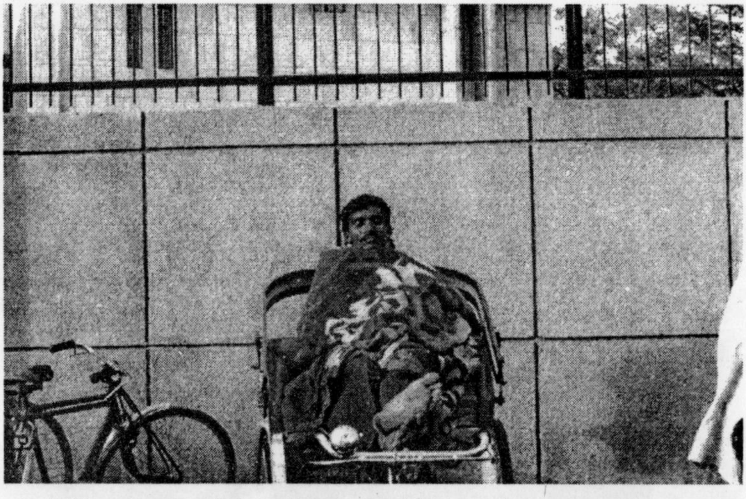

With passage of time, Irfan's health started deteriorating. He was constantly suffering from fever and diarrhoea because of which he lost a lot of weight. Although he was under treatment of his doctor, but still there was no relief. Due to prolonged illness when his daily earnings started getting adversely affected he decided to consult another doctor in a city hospital.

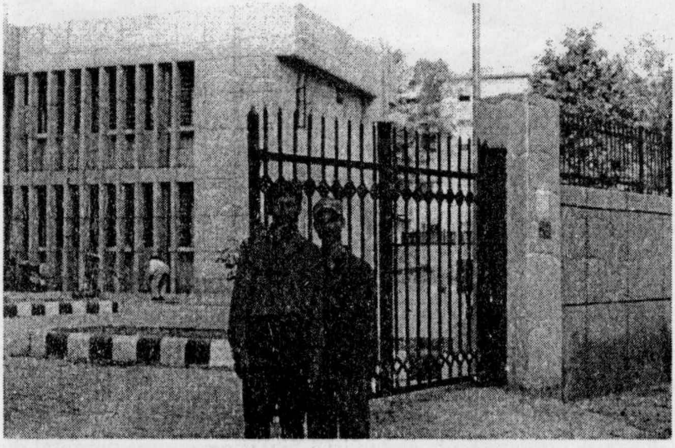

Irfan went along with Sakir to the hospital. There he was attended by a doctor who gave him some medicines to eat. After eating those medicines Irfan felt a little better but now most of the time he felt fatigued and suffered from some or other infection like persistent cough, fever and diarrhoea. Ultimately, one day he was so fed up with his persistent cough that he went to the doctor again.

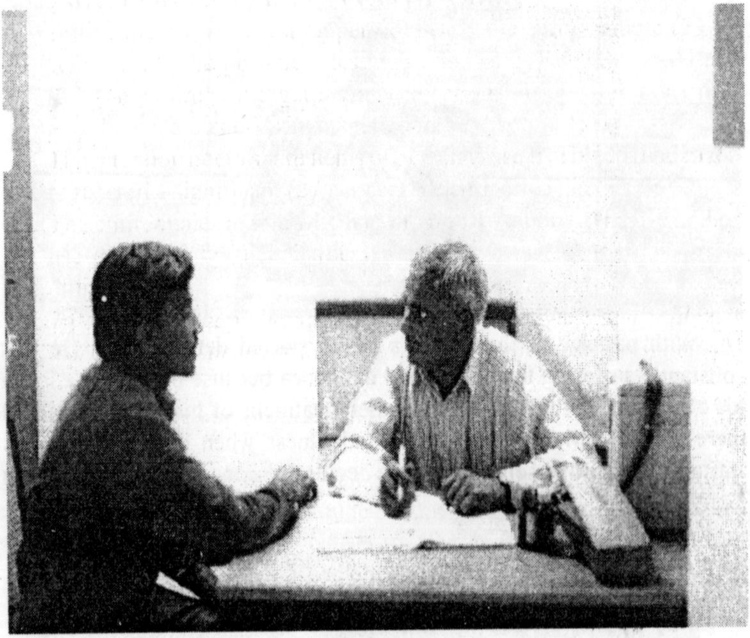

This time the doctor asked him some personal and intimate questions while trying to diagnose his ailment. When the doctor convinced Irfan that without complete knowledge of his habits and behaviour he would not be able to treat him, Irfan confided in him about his extra-marital sexual contacts with various commerical sex workers. After listening to Irfan doctor expressing his concern said "You may be HIV positive." Irfan unknowingly asked "HIV positive? Doctor what is that?" Then the doctor elaborately explained to Irfan "HIV is a very small disease causing virus which enters into our body and after a few years causes the fatal disease called AIDS. Irfan again enquired, "But doctor how does this HIV enter into our body?"

Modes of HIV Transmission in Our Body

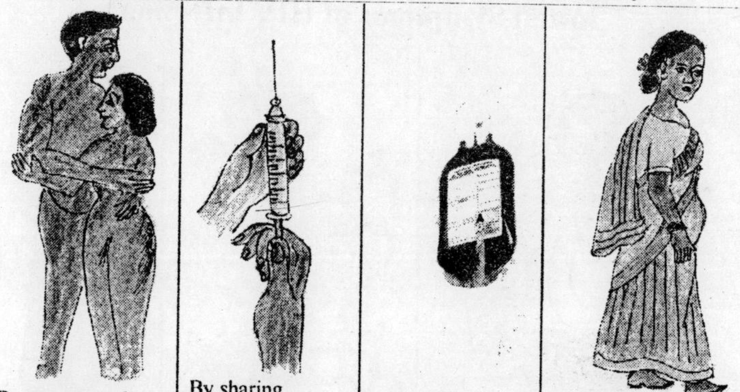

By unprotected sexual contact with an infected partner | By sharing contaminated needle and syringe | By Transfusion with HIV infected Blood | From HIV Infected mother to her child

The doctor while showing him a few pictures explained "There are four known ways of HIV transmission in our body. They are –

(1) By having unprotected sexual contact with a HIV positive partner.

(2) By using HIV contaminated needles and syringes for injecting purposes.

(3) By transfusion with HIV infected blood.

(4) And lastly, mother to child transmission, i.e., a HIV positive mother can pass on the infection to her child before, during or after childbirth."

The doctor explained to Irfan how HIV after entering into a body slowly but steadily kills the body's defense mechanism thereby decreasing its immunity to various infections. Ultimately, when the body's immunity is completely destroyed it falls prey to a host of infections which is known as *Acquired Immune Deficiency Syndrome* commonly known as AIDS.

Initial Symptoms of HIV Infection

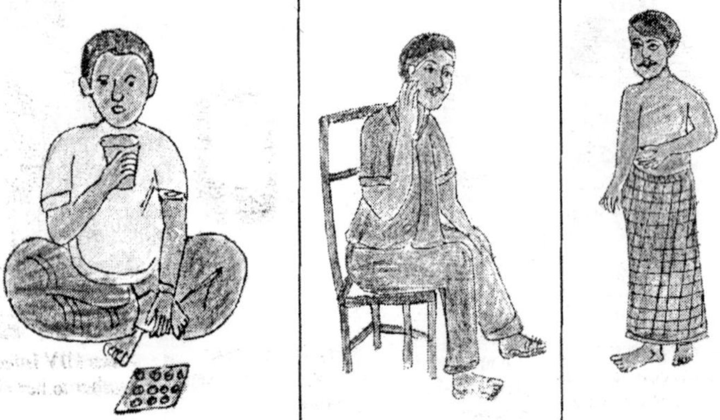

Fever | Headache | Bodyache

Irfan was surprised to hear about a disease which he had earlier not heard about. He further enquired "doctor. what are the symptoms of this disease?" The doctor responded, "After initial infection with HIV the person develops symptoms like flu in which he may suffer from fever, headache and bodyache. But after a few days these symptoms disappear and the HIV infected person looks normal. A HIV infected person can lead an asymptomatic life for 3 to 12 years depending upon his nutritional status and life style. But, during this asymptomatic phase although the HIV positive person may appear to be healthy yet, he can transmit the virus to others by indulging in unprotected sexual contact, by sharing his contaminated needles and syringes, by donating HIV infectef blood, and also a HIV positive mother can transmit the virus to her child before/during childbirth via blood transmission mode and after child birth through breast feeding. With passage of time, as the disease progress so do the symptoms elevate."

Initial Symptoms of AIDS

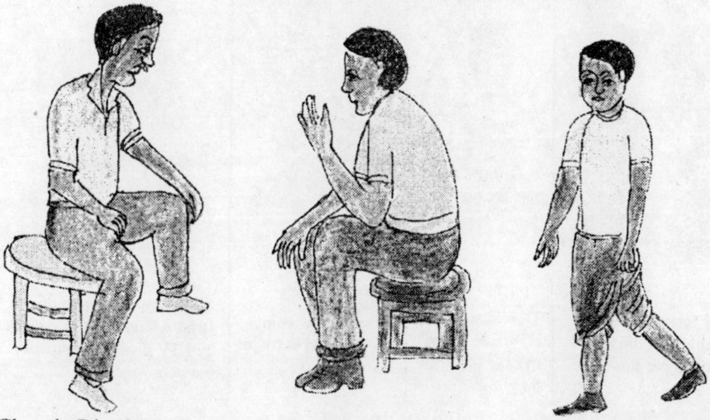

Chronic Diarrhoea — Long Term Fever — Weight loss, more than 10% of the body weight

The doctor further explained "The initial symptoms of AIDS are –

1. Chronic diarrhoea lasting for more than 1 month.
2. Long-term fever
3. Weight loss, i.e., more than 10 per cent of the entire body weight in a month.

As the disease progresses the person falls prey to a host of infections like T.B., Pneumonia, Lymphadenopathy, Oral thrush and Sarcoma. The body is unable to defend itself against these diseases due to completely destroyed immunity as a result of the HIV infection, and the person dies due to these opportunistic infections.

Ways of HIV Prevention

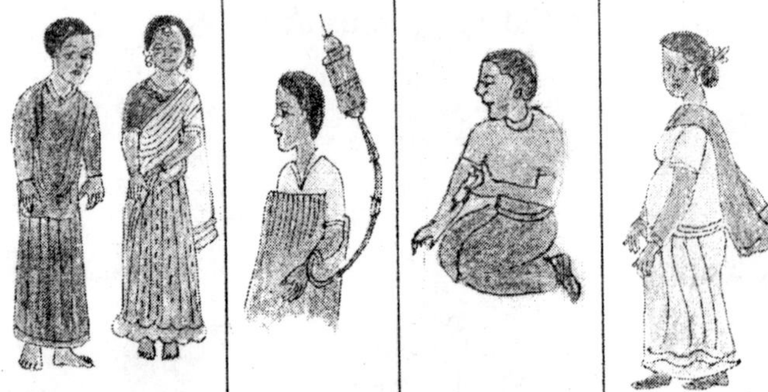

By having Sex with one uninfected sexual partner	Transfusion with HIV free blood in case the need be	Using disposable needles and syringes for injecting	Regular check up and strict adherence to treatment by HIV positive pregnant women

After hearing all this Irfan became doubtful and said "doctor, how can a person be tested for HIV?" The doctor replied that a blood test could reveal the HIV status of an individual. Irfan again questioned "Is there a cure for AIDS?" The doctor thought for a while and replied, – "No, unfortunately till date there is no cure for AIDS. But yet, one can protect oneself from acquiring this disease by adopting safe behaviour and practices. The simple ways by which HIV prevention is possible are –

1. By having sex with one faithful (steady) sexual partner. In case your partner is casual, HIV positive or you have multiple sexual partners then you should always practice safe sex by using a condom.
2. In case a blood transfusion is required one should always ensure that the blood is certified to be HIV free. For this one should always insist on procuring blood from a licenced blood bank.
3. When there is a need to be injected a person should always ensure that a disposable needle and syringe is being used for the purpose. In case of an emergency if a new needle and syringe are not available and a person has to use a previously used needle and syringe then they should be sterilized by placing them in boiling water for atleast 20 minutes.
4. Every HIV positive pregnant women should go to a hospital and put herself under treatment, so as to prevent mother to child transmission.

Symptoms of Sexually Transmitted Diseases

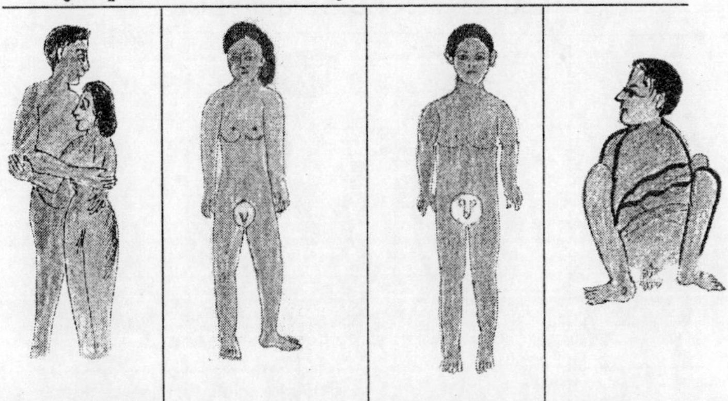

S.T.D. are caused by unprotected sexual contact with an infected partner	Itching, Blisters and Sores in private parts of body	Unusual discharge from private parts of body	Burning Sensation while urinating

The doctor further informed Irfan that presence of sexually transmitted infections could also enhance HIV transmission. Irfan was surprised and enquired "What are sexually transmitted infections?" The doctor replied "Sexually transmitted infections are caused by unprotected sexual contact with an infected partner. One should never be careless about these and get them treated as soon as possible. Irfan anxiously asked "But doctor how can a person know if he is suffering from a sexually transmitted infection? I mean that what are the symptoms of these infections?"

The doctor explained "sexually transmitted infections, manifest themselves in the form of itching, sores or unusual discharge from private body parts, Lower abdominal pain or pain while urinating could also be symptoms of sexually transmitted infection.

Modes of S.T.D. Transmission

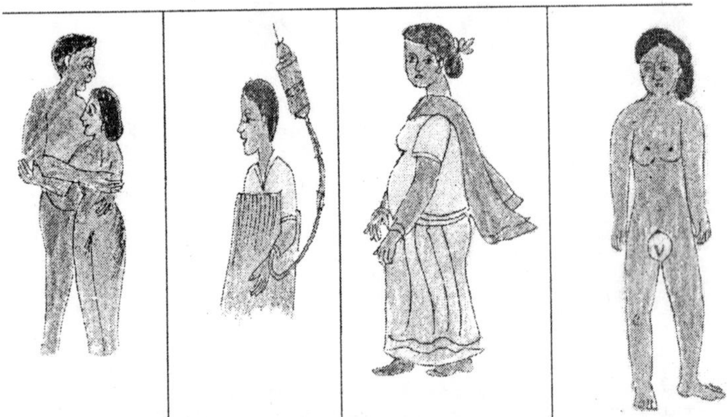

By sexual contact with an infected partner	By Transfusion with blood from an S.T.D. infected person	From S.T.D. infected pragnant women to her unborn child.	S.T.D. enhance the risk of HIV transmission

On hearing this Irfan said, "Yes, Doctor. Now I realise, you are talking about the problem that is caused due to excessive heat in the body". The doctor smiled a little and said "Yes, sometimes people consider sexually transmitted infections as a problem of excessive heat in the body. But this is not true. These infections are not caused by eating hot things or by excessive body heat. These are mere myths sexually transmitted infections are caused only by having unprotected sexual contact with an infected partner, by transfusion with infected blood or from an infected pregnant women to her unborn child before or during birth." The doctor further warned "Sexually transmitted infections cannot only cause congenital defects in an unborn child but also lead to still birth. Moreover the risk of HIV transmission is enhanced because of sores and broken lining around the genitals. That is why it is very important to get timely treatment for sexually transmitted diseases from a specialist."

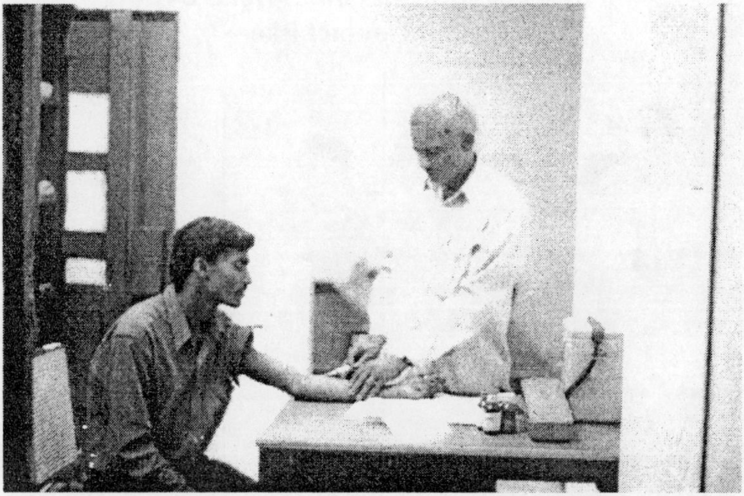

Now Irfan started introspecting. He wished he had not treated sexually transmitted infection as a disease caused due to excessive body heat and got himself treated from a STD specialist. The doctor was quick to grasp the dilemma that Irfan was going through. He supportingly said, "Fine, what has happened, has happened. But now it is very important that you go through a blood test to get your illness diagnosed." Irfan was very tense and nervous. "But doctor you said that till date there is no cure for AIDS so what is the purpose of getting HIV tested now?"

Some of the audience said that Irfan should get himself tested for HIV while a few also opined that he should not be doing so. Everybody tried to justify his/her answer with a reason. Let's see what Irfan did?

The doctor could very well understand what Irfan was going through. He while trying to convince Irfan said "Yes, it is true that as of now there is no cure for HIV/AIDS but also it is true that if HIV related opportunistic infections are treated in time then a HIV positive person can live a asymptomatic healthy life for long years just like any other normal being." On hearing this Irfan felt a little relieved and said "Fine doctor, if this is so then you can take my blood sample for HIV testing."

HIV/AIDS Does not Spread by Casual Contact like –

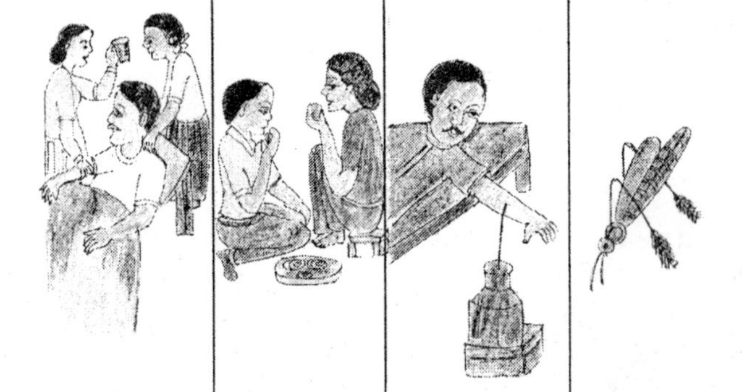

Touching an HIV/AIDS patient	Sharing utensils with HIV/AIDS infected person	By donating blood	Through mosquito or any other insect bite

After some days when Irfan went to collect his blood report he was shocked to learn what he had been unwantingly expecting. The doctor confirmed that he was HIV positive. Irfan was quite nervous and depressed. He sat down and slowly remarked "Doctor, now nobody would like to sit or come in contact with me. My friends have told me that this is a contagious disease and is spread by mere contact."

The doctor contradicted, "No, this is not true. HIV/AIDS does not spread by casual contact. The disease is not acquired by sitting next to HIV positive person or by touching him. Similarly sharing food or utensils with a HIV positive individual does not transmit the virus." The doctor while showing him a few pictures clarified "Look Irfan, HIV is not acquired by –

1. Touching HIV positive person.
2. Sitting, playing or working with a HIV positive individual.
3. Sharing utensils or eating food cooked by a HIV positive person.
4. Donating blood.
5. Mosquito or any other insect bite.

The doctor again emphasized "Irfan, always remember that HIV/AIDS is not a contagious disease. It is acquired only after coming in contact with HIV infected blood or other body fluids. Therefore, we should never discriminate against a HIV positive person rather that person should be treated with love and compassion as any other normal human being. Being HIV positive does not mean that the person is not entitled to basic human rights. So why do we indulge in irrational discrimination of such people?"

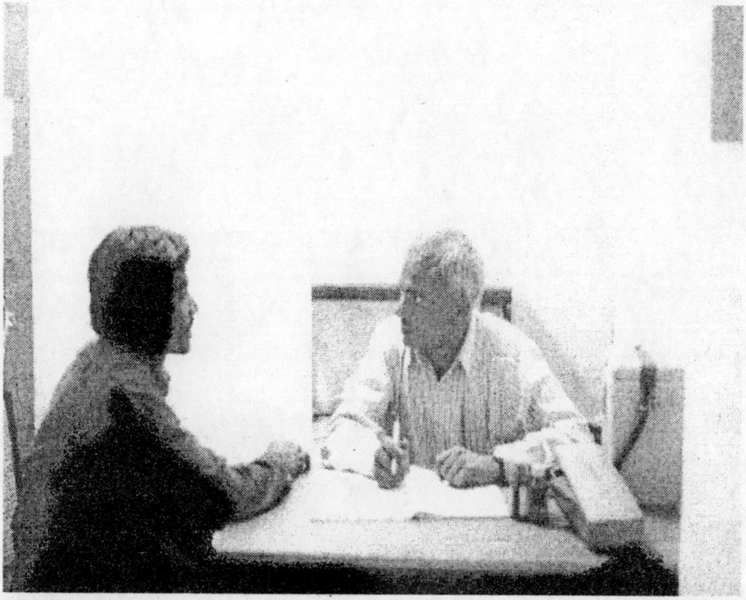

Irfan was quiet for some time. Suddenly he broke his silence and asked "But doctor, how will I tell my wife and family about all this? Moreover I am at a loss to understand that whether I should be telling them all this or not. What do I do doctor?"

At this point, we would again like to ask the audience if they could help Irfan in finding a solution to his problem? Do you all think that Irfan should reveal his HIV status to his family especially his wife? OK. Some of your said "he should." while a few maintained that he should not. Let's see what decision the hero of our story Irfan takes?

The doctor while boosting Irfan's morale said, "Irfan there is still time to correct your mistake. You can still lead a healthy life for long. The only pre-requisite to this a little protection." "What do you mean by this, doctor? Can I still lead a normal life and work like any other uninfected individual?" Irfan asked. The doctor promptly nodded and said, "Yes. It is very much possible. You only need some awareness.

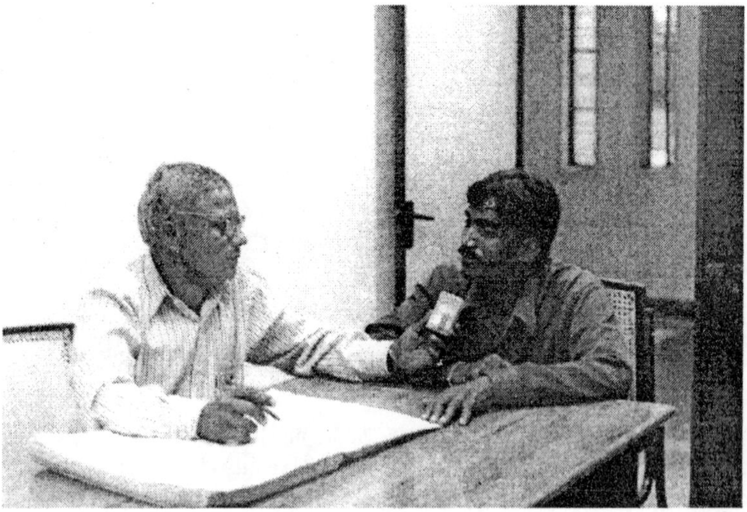

Irfan quickly responded – "Then please do not delay any more and generate that kind of awareness so that I am able to lead a happy life with my family once again." The doctor advised, "Irfan, first of all you have to win over the trust of your wife and tell her that you are HIV positive. After that you should get her tested, so that her HIV status may be known. Luckily, in case she is till not HIV infected then you have to always practice safe behaviour with her.This means you should always use a condom while having sex with her so that she does not acquire the virus from you."

Ways of Boosting Body's Immunity to Fight HIV/AIDS

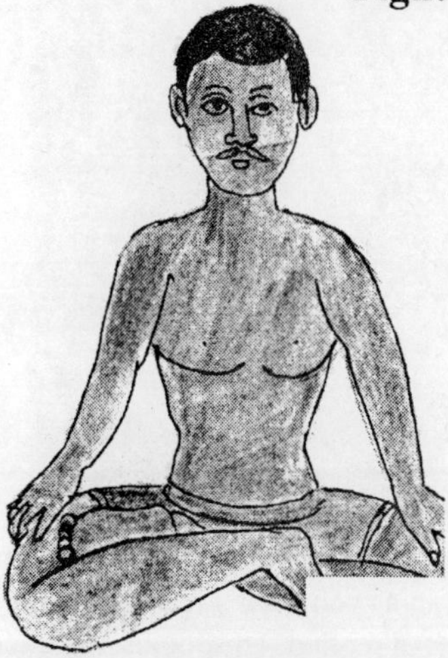

Regular Exercise

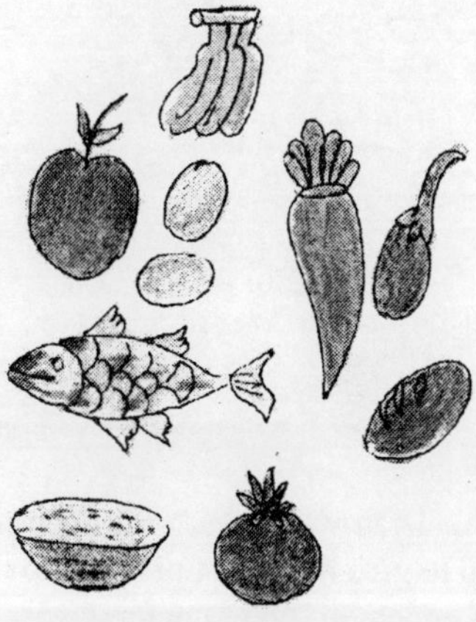

Nutritious Food

The doctor further advised "Irfan from now on you have to regularly exercise everyday and eat nutritious food so as to boost your body's immune system. People sometimes tend to ignore these important aspects but it is very true that we are what we eat. So to maintain a healthy body it is very important to eat nutritious food. I hope you will pay attention to what all I have said. And yes, do not hesitate to come to me whenever you need my advise."

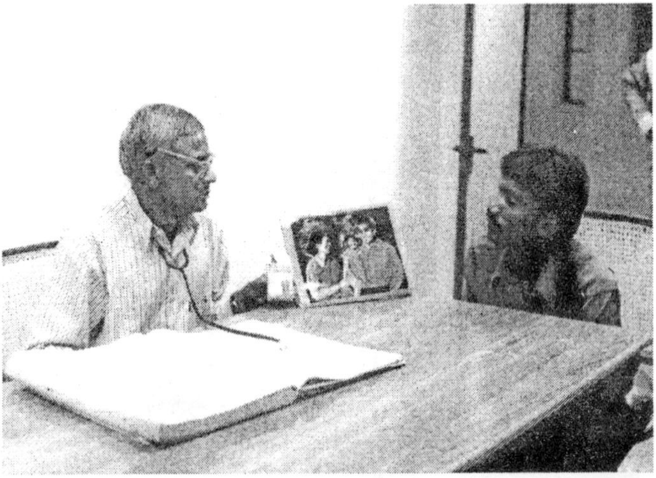

Irfan was about to leave after saying goodbye when the doctor got up to give him a last piece of advise "Irfan as you leave I have something to conclude." "Yes doctor. Please say." Irfan replied. The doctor remarked "Always remember that you should have sexual relationship with one faithful (steady) sexual partner and in case you ever think about having casual sex then you should always have safe sex, i.e., always use a condom."

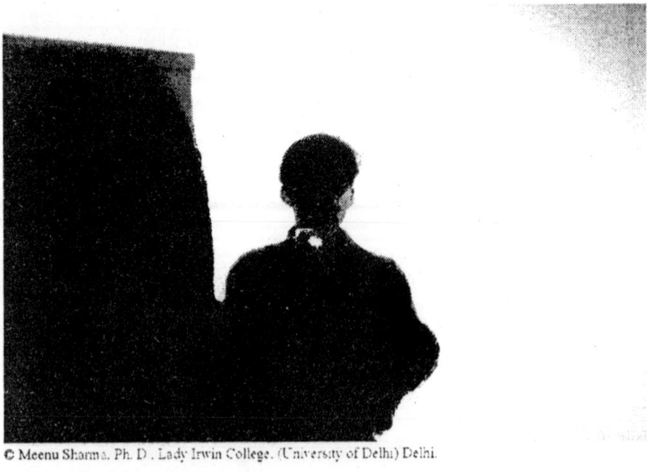

Irfan nodded in consent and said "Yes doctor, now I have fully understood. From today the motto of my life would be '*Adopt safe behaviour to keep AIDS at bay*'."

Annexure II

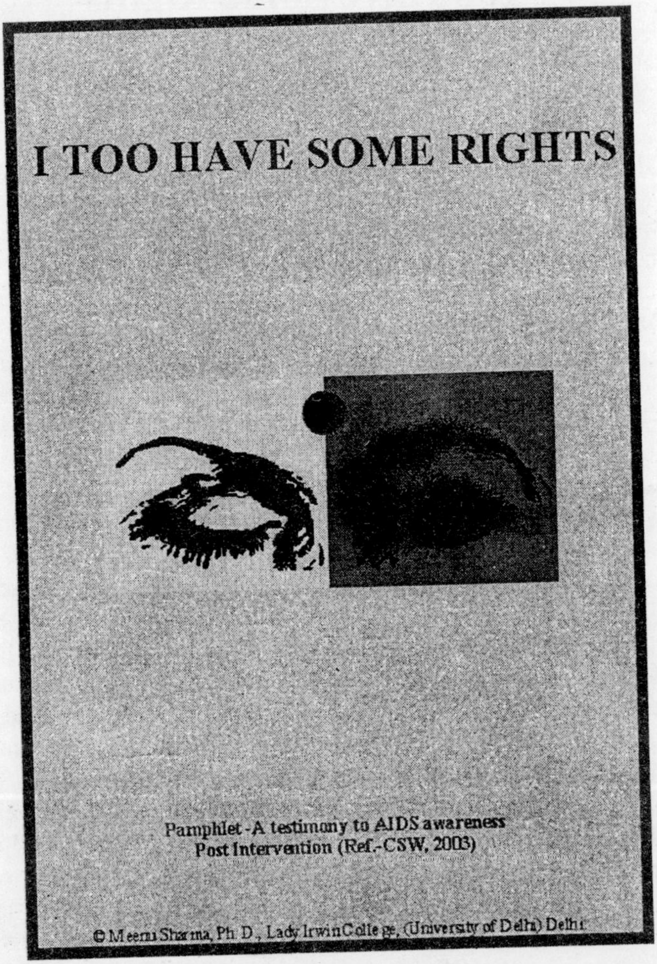
I TOO HAVE SOME RIGHTS
Pamphlet -A testimony to AIDS awareness
Post Intervention (Ref.-CSW, 2003)
© Meenu Sharma, Ph. D., Lady Irwin College, (University of Delhi) Delhi

I Too Have Some Rights

I am a commercial sex worker and am 30 years old. I have been in sex-trade for nearly 10 years. In these long years I have seen and learnt a lot. Now I have come to realize that every worker has some rights irrespective of the kind of work. I too have some rights — like protecting myself and my children from every danger and disease alike. I have heard a lot about AIDS and now I fully understand that the only way to protect oneself from this disease by practising safe behaviour. By safe behaviour I means using a condom for each and every sexual transactions with a customer.

Earlier I used to think that getting a shot could protect me from AIDS but now I know that till date there is no cure for AIDS. That is why if a customer asks me to have unprotected sex I practice my right to say "no". I have started realising that I owe responsibility towards my children and the society too.

Awareness regarding some facts like – Sexually Transmitted Diseases (STD) are not caused by excessive heat in the body but due to unsafe sex and that one should abstain from having sex while suffering from STD has made me a lot more alert. Now, whenever I have pain in the lower abdomen I take medicine from a doctor immediately because I know this could be a symptom of a STD. We should not be careless about any of our ailments as this can be fatal.

Now I am also aware about the right method of using as well as disposing a condom. Sometimes we tend to ignore such tasks but I now realise how important it is to practise things in a proper manner. After gaining awareness about all these things I have become all the more confident. Today, I really feel empowered to take my own decisions and this is all because of AIDS awareness. In the end, I would like to convey to my fellow sisters that "Protection sustains life and life means happiness".

Annexure III

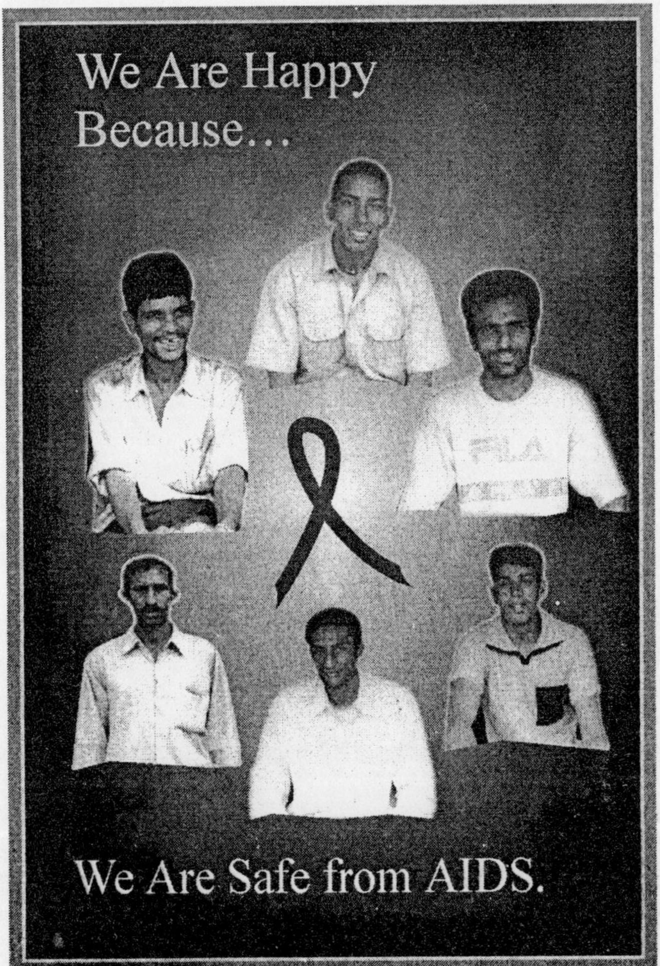

Poster* - *A result of intervention amongst the Truck drivers (Ref.- Truck drivers. 2003)

Bibliography

1. Adrien, A., Godin, G., Cappon, P., Manson-Singer, S., Maticka-Tyndale, E., & Willms, D. Many Voices; HIV/AIDS In The Context of Culture – A National Study. Presented at Eleventh International Conference on AIDS, Vancouver, Canada; 1996. Abstract MoD 1690, Vol. 1, p. 172.
2. Aggarwal, O., & Sharma, A. (1997). AIDS – An Innovative Approach in IEC. HIV/AIDS Research in India. NACO, New Delhi. pp. 779-80.
3. Ahmad, A. (1996). Level of Awareness Among Commercial Sex Workers on AIDS and STD: An Empirical Study. HIV/AIDS Research in India. NACO, 1997, New Delhi. p. 278-79.
4. Ahmed, S. (1997). Truck Drivers as a Vulnerable Group in North East India. HIV/AIDS Research in India. NACO, New Delhi. p. 497.
5. aids/europeer.htm. Department of Community Medicine, Malmo, Sweden.
6. Alam, S., Roy, Biswajit, & Islam. Population Assessment on Truckers on STD/HIV/AIDS. Presented at Eleventh International Conference on AIDS, Vancouver, Canada; 1996. Abstract MoD 1736, Vol. 1, p. 181.
7. Allen, J. Fighting the Tide: Creating a Community Based Response to Women and HIV/AIDS in the Maritimes. Presented at Eleventh International Conference on AIDS, Vancouver, Canada; 1996. Abstract TuD 2733, Vol. 1, p. 390.
8. Allen, S., Tice, J., Vande, P. Effect of Serotesting with Counselling on Condom Use and Seroconversion among HIV Discordant Couples in Africa. In Journal of American Medical Association. HIV/AIDS Patient Education, May 8, 1998. University of California.
9. Almeida, V. D., Parker, R., Terto, V., Galvio, J., & Fernandez, M. Cabaret Prevencao: Expressionist Theater and AIDS Prevention in Rio De Janeiro, Brazil. Presented at Eleventh International Conference on AIDS, Vancouver, Canada; 1996. Abstract TuD 2848, Vol. 1, p. 405.

10. Annan, K. (2004). Global Media AIDS Initiative. *Times of India*, January 16, 2004, New Delhi.
11. APAC-VHS. (2000). High Risk Behaviour Surveillance Survey in Tamil Nadu. AIDS Prevention and Control Project-Voluntary Health Services, Chennai, India, p. 39.
12. Ayala, R.G., Martinez, M., & Dulaney, A. AIDS Prevention and Care in Latin America: A Participatory Investigation. Presented at Eleventh International Conference on AIDS, Vancouver, Canada; 1996. Abstract TuD 2843, Vol. 1, p. 405.
13. Bagasra, O., Lichner, W. (1993). Alcohol intake increases HIV type 1 replication in human peripheral blood. In R. Bansal. Truck Drivers and risk of STD including HIV. HIV/AIDS Research In India. NACO, 1997, New Delhi. pp. 488-90.
14. Balaganesh, G., Chandrasekar, V., Sai, T., & Babu, V. (1994). Survey on Public Awareness on AIDS in a Rural South Indian Community. Indian Journal Community Research, Vol. XIX, No. I. Reproduced in HIV/AIDS Research in India. NACO, 1997, New Delhi. pp. 119-22.
15. Baldo, et al. (1993). Does Sex Education lead to Earlier Sexual Activity in Youth. In R. Mathai, W. Michael, W. Ross, & S. Hira, Concomitants of HIV/STD Risk Behaviour and Intention to Engage in Risk Behaviours in Adolescents in India. HIV/AIDS Research in India. NACO, 1997, New Delhi, pp. 195-60.
16. Bansal, R. (1994). HIV/AIDS and Barber Shop. Indian Medical Gazette, C XX, VIII (I). Reproduced in HIV/AIDS Research in India. NACO, 1997, New Delhi, pp. 261-62.
17. Bansal, R. (1995). Truck drivers and Risk of STDs including HIV. Indian Journal of Community Medicine. Vol. XX. Nos. 1-4. Reproduced in HIV/AIDS Research in India. NACO, New Delhi, pp. 488-90.
18. Bansal, R., & Arya, R. (1993). Tattooing Practices in Bhadbhut Pilgrimage and Risk of Transmission of Infections. Medicine and Surgery. November – December, 1993. Reproduced in HIV/AIDS Research in India. NACO, 1997, New Delhi, pp. 509-11.
19. Bansal, R., Srivastava, R., & Sexena, D. (1994). An Exploratory KABP Study of AIDS in Indigenous Medical Practitioners and RMPs in Central India. Ind, J, Dermatol Venereol Leprol 1994, 60. Reproduced in HIV/AIDS Research in India. NACO, 1997, New Delhi, pp. 154-56.
20. Bascunan, S., & Ana, C. AIDS Prevention in Heterosexual Women with Stable Partners. Presented at Eleventh International Conference

on AIDS, Vancouver, Canada; 1996. Abstract TuC 2450, Vol. 1, p. 342.

21. Bee, H. (1995). The Developing Child. Harper Collins Publishers, New York.
22. Benjamin, A., & Zachairah, P. (1997). KABP Study on Prevention of AIDS among Health Professionals. HIV/AIDS Research in India. NACO, New Delhi, pp. 294-98.
23. Benjamin, J.A., Engel, D., & De Buysscher, R. AIDS Prevention Amid Chaos: The Case of Rwandan Refugees in Tanzania. Presented at Eleventh International Conference on AIDS, Vancouver, Canada; 1996. Abstract TuD 241, Vol. 1, p. 255.
24. Bertinato, L., Poli, S., Mirandola, M., Greco, D., Serain, I. Lessons Learnt in Five Years National HIV Prevention Strategy in School: The Italian Experience. Presented at Eleventh International Conference on AIDS, Vancouver, Canada; 1996. Abstract TuD 2797, Vol. 1, p. 399.
25. Betancourt & Lopez, (1993) and Cole, (1992). In Helen Bee. The Developing Child. Harper Collins College Publishers, 1995, New York.
26. Bharat, S. (1996). Facing The Challenge: Household and Community Response to HIV/AIDS in Mumbai, India. HIV/AIDS Research in India. NACO, 1997, New Delhi, pp. 372-75.
27. Bharat, S. (1995). Female Socialization for Reproductive Role: Implications for HIV/AIDS Prevention. In R. Mathai, W. Michael, W. Ross, & S. Hira. Concomitants of HIV/STD Risk Behaviour and Intention to Engage in Risk Behaviours in Adolescents in India. HIV/AIDS Research in India. NACO, 1997, New Delhi, pp. 195-207.
28. Bhave G., Lindan, P., Christina, E.S.H., Desai, S., Wagle, U., Tripathi, P.S., & Mandel, S.J. (1995). Impact of an Intervention on HIV, Sexually Transmitted Diseases, and Condom Use Among Sex Workers in Bombay, India. HIV/AIDS Research in India. NACO, 1997, New Delhi, pp. 781-92.
29. Bianco, M., ReMaria, I., Pagani, L. Women's Prevention: A Dilemma in Developing Countries. Presented at Eleventh International Conference on AIDS, Vancouver, Canada; 1996. Abstract TuD 353, Vol. 1, p. 258.
30. Bora, P., & Gilada, I. (1997). Religious Festivities and AIDS Awareness. CARC Calling. Reproduced in HIV/AIDS Research in India. NACO, New Delhi, pp. 134-36.
31. Brashers, D., Neigig, J., Hass, S., & McDonald, M. The Role of HIV/AIDS Patient Activism in Healthcare Decision Making. Presented

at Eleventh International Conference on AIDS, Vancouver, Canada; 1996. Abstract TuD 2949, Vol. 1, p. 420.

32. Bronfman, P.M., & Rubin-Kurtzman, J. Two Borders, One Country: Sexual Behaviour of Migrants and HIV Infection Risk Practices at Mexico's Southern and Northern Borders. Presented at Eleventh International Conference on AIDS, Vancouver, Canada; 1996. Abstract TuD 2904, Vol. 1, p. 414.

33. Brookman, J. Client-Centered Counselling Utilizing a Harm Reduction Approach for Populations Resistant to Behavioural Change. Presented at Eleventh International Conference on AIDS, Vancouver, Canada; 1996. Abstract MoD 1757, Vol. 1, p. 184.

34. Brooks-Gun & Paikoff. Sex is a Gamble, Kissing is a Game. New York: Oxford Press. In R. Mathai, W. Michael, W. Ross, & S. Hira. Concomitants of HIV/STD Risk Behaviour and Intention to Engage in Risk Behaviours in Adolescents in India. HIV/AIDS Research in India. NACO, 1997, New Delhi, pp. 195-82.

35. Bullock, S.L., Myers T., Calzavara, L.M., Cockerill, R., Marshall, V.W., & Burchell, A. Unprotected Intercourse and the Meanings Ascribed to Sex by Aboriginal People Living on Reserve in Ontario, Canada. Presented at Eleventh International Conference on AIDS, Vancouver, Canada; 1996. Abstract MoD 483, Vol. 1, p. 50.

36. Buysse, A., Van Renterghem, H., Drieghe, L., & Wouters, R. Super Sex Strategies Among Belgian U.N. Blue Helmets on a Peace Keeping Mission in a High HIV/AIDS Prevalence Area. Presented at Eleventh International Conference on AIDS, Vancouver, Canada; 1996. Abstract TuC 2616, Vol. 1, p. 371.

37. Campbell, I.D., & Rader, A.D. A Continuum of Confidentiality Linking the Continuum of Care and Prevention of HIV/AIDS. Presented at Eleventh International Conference on AIDS, Vancouver, Canada; 1996. Abstract TuD 2929, Vol. 1, p. 417.

38. Campos-Lopez, P. I., Martinez-Lopez, J., Diaz-Camarena, A., Avalos-Huizar, P., Lopez-Marquez, F.C., Sierra-Quevedo, J., & Vazquez-Valls, E. Developing HIV/AIDS Education and Training Program to Target Groups From Jalisco, Mexico. Presented at Eleventh International Conference on AIDS, Vancouver, Canada; 1996. Abstract MoC 1600, Vol. 1, p. 158.

39. Carneiro, P., Boer, A., & Santos, S. Seductive Images: A Life-Oriented Campaign for AIDS Prevention. Presented at Eleventh International Conference on AIDS, Vancouver, Canada; 1996. Abstract MoD 1813, Vol. 1, p. 192.

40. Castaneda, X., Allen, B., & Castaneda, I. Migration, Virginity and Sexual Initiation: Factors Associated with STD/AIDS Risk Perception Among Rural Adolescents in Mexico. Presented at Eleventh International Conference on AIDS, Vancouver, Canada; 1996. Abstract TuD 2703, Vol. 1, p. 385.

41. Castillo, J., Moreno, L. Provocative Theater: Innovative Strategy for HIV/AIDS Prevention in the Commercial Sex Industry. Presented at Eleventh International Conference on AIDS, Vancouver, Canada; 1996. Abstract MoD 1855, Vol. 1, p. 199.

42. Castro, J.R., & Fleras, J.B. Identifying the Rights of Women in the Sex Industry: An Approach Towards Advocacy. Presented at Eleventh International Conference on AIDS, Vancouver, Canada; 1996. Abstract TuC 2638, Vol. 1, p. 375.

43. Center of Concern for Child Labour. (1998). In Adolescents in India – a Profile. UNFPA (2000), New Delhi.

44. Chabbra, R. (2003). HIV Infection on the rise in colonies. *Times of India,* September 10, 2003. New Delhi.

45. Chan, R.K.W., Wong, M.L., Lee, J., Koh, D., Wong, C. A Behavioural Intervention Programme to Increase Condom Use Among Sex Workers in Singapore. Presented at Eleventh International Conference on AIDS, Vancouver, Canada; 1996. Abstract MoD 1747, Vol. 1, p. 182.

46. Chandlok, K., Sankaran, P.S., Mathew, G., & Manoharan, S. Developing Comprehensive Intervention Programme for Women in Reproductive Age Group. Presented at Eleventh International Conference on AIDS, Vancouver, Canada; 1996. Abstract TuD 2453, Vol. 1, p. 343.

47. Chatterjee, S. (2001). Preying on Flesh Trade. *Times of India,* August 26, 2001, New Delhi.

48. Chauhan, C. (2003). Government Survey Identifies 400 Paid Sex Hot spots in City. *Hindustan Times*, August 6, 2003, New Delhi.

49. Chhabra, R. (2003). Condomisation of Society. *Hindustan Times,* January 20, 2003, New Delhi.

50. Chipo, M. What Makes Programme Impact Last. Presented at Eleventh International Conference on AIDS, Vancouver, Canada; 1996. Abstract TuD 2937, Vol. 1, p. 418.

51. Clarke, A., & Stewart. (1987). *Child Development : Infancy Through Adolescence*. John Wiley and Sons, Inc. U.S.A.

52. Coll-Seck, A.M., Diop-Ly, F., Mbengue, C.S.A., & Sall, L.F. Socio-Economic Factors of the HIV/AIDS Epidemic in Senegal. Presented

at Eleventh International Conference on AIDS, Vancouver, Canada; 1996. Abstract MoD 1883, Vol. 1, p. 203.

53. Dahl, D.W., Gorn, G. J., & Weinberg, C.B. Purchase and Availability of Condoms: A Social Marketing Experiment. Presented at Eleventh International Conference on AIDS, Vancouver, Canada; 1996. Abstract TuD 2875, Vol. 1, p. 409.

54. Dawson, C. J., Alstead, M., Hartfield, K., Goldbaum, G., & Campsmith, M. "4 Out of 4 Persons Surveyed Prefer Condoms over Herpes!!!": A Mass Media Campaign Targeting Sexually Active Adolescents. Presented at Eleventh International Conference on AIDS, Vancouver, Canada; 1996. Abstract MoD 1830, Vol. 1, p. 195.

55. De Wit, J. The Epidemic of HIV Among Young Gay Men. Presented at Eleventh International Conference on AIDS, Vancouver, Canada; 1996. Abstract Mo.03, Vol. 1, p. 2.

56. Dlamini-Kapenda, W. Traditional and Cultural Practices That Promote The Spread of HIV Infection. Presented at Eleventh International Conference on AIDS, Vancouver, Canada; 1996. Abstract MoD 1874, Vol. 1, p. 201.

57. Dodds, J. V., & Braidele, S. Macro Vs Micro: Developing A Provincial Coalition to Address the Macro Issues Around HIV/AIDS. Presented at Eleventh International Conference On AIDS, Vancouver, Canada; 1996. Abstract TuD 2922, Vol. 1, p. 416.

58. Dortzbach, D., Njorge, L., Kiiti, N., Robinson, P., Amalemba, W., & Mallet, S. Marshalling the Influence of Church Leaders in AIDS Prevention and Counselling: Lessons Learned From Kenya. Presented at Eleventh International Conference on AIDS, Vancouver, Canada; 1996. Abstract TuD 460, Vol. 1, p. 260.

59. Drew, R. Spirituality–A Key Issue for HIV/AIDS Programmes. Presented at Eleventh International Conference on AIDS, Vancouver, Canada; 1996. Abstract TuD 2840, Vol. 1, p. 404.

60. DuBois, & Marcel, J. Examining the Pros and Cons of Spirituality on Canada's Aboriginal People Living with HIV/AIDS. Presented at Eleventh International Conference on AIDS, Vancouver, Canada; 1996. Abstract MoD 1898, Vol. 1, p. 205.

61. Edward, W. Minium, Bruce, M. King, Gordon Bear. Statistical Reasoning in Psychology and Education. 3rd Edition, 1993. John Wiley & Sons, Inc.

62. Eldridge, G., Lawrence, J., Little, C., Shelby, M., Service, J., & Singh, J. Evaluation of an HIV Risk Reduction Intervention for Women in Inpatient Drug Treatment. Presented at Eleventh International

Conference on AIDS, Vancouver, Canada; 1996. Abstract MoD 1771, Vol. 1, p. 186.

63. Fabian, A M., Roca de Torres, I., & Rodriguez, O. Women Living With HIV In Puerto Rico: Impact of HIV on the Lives of a Group of Hispanic Women. Presented at Eleventh International Conference on AIDS, Vancouver, Canada; 1996. Abstract TuD 2751, Vol. 1, p. 392.

64. Fernandez, E., Ramirez, A.G., & Villarreal, R. Sexual Risk Behaviours Among Latinos : A Community– Based Study Across the United States. Presented at Eleventh International Conference On AIDS, Vancouver, Canada; 1996. Abstract TuC 2665, Vol. 1, p. 380.

65. Fishbein, M., & Johnson, W.D. The AIDS Community Demonstration Projects (ACDP): A Successful Multi-Site Community-Level Behavioural Intervention. Presented at Eleventh International Conference on AIDS, Vancouver, Canada; 1996. Abstract MoD 580, Vol. 1, p. 52.

66. Frew, R.L. Theological and Scriptural HIV/AIDS Training for Congregations, Local Communities and ASOS. Presented at Eleventh International Conference on AIDS, Vancouver, Canada; 1996. Abstract TuD 2839, Vol. 1, p. 404.

67. Gardner, K., Nikitina, M., & Karimova, L. Building a National Sexual Health Coalition in Russia: From Community Activism to Policy. Presented at Eleventh International Conference on AIDS, Vancouver, Canada; 1996. Abstract TuD 486, Vol. 1, p. 263.

68. Gates, B. (2002). Act Decisively Now – India Can Avert an AIDS Tragedy, *Times of India*, November 11, 2002. New Delhi.

69. Gates, B. (November 12, 2002). Aids for AIDS. *Times of India*, November12, 2002. New Delhi.

70. Ghosh, S., Chowdhury, S., & Gill, J.S. (1997). Knowledge of HIV/AIDS/STD and High Risk Sexual Practices in Two Slums in South Delhi. HIV/AIDS Research in India. NACO, 1997, New Delhi, pp. 123-25.

71. Gilliam, G A., Brown, M., Aymer, F., O'Neill, C., Collins, J. Designing Culturally Appropriate Theory-Based Behavioural Interventions: The Antigua Schools Project. Presented at Eleventh International Conference on AIDS, Vancouver, Canada; 1996. Abstract TuD 2860, Vol. 1, p. 407.

72. Gillies, P. A., James, N., Slack, R., & Johnson, S. Effective Community Development for HIV Prevention and Sexual Health Promotion: POW.

Presented at Eleventh International Conference on AIDS, Vancouver, Canada; 1996. Abstract TuD 2930, Vol. 1, p. 417.

73. Goyal, R.C., Kukarni, A.T., & Somasundaram, K.V. (1994). AIDS Awareness Among Rural Community – A Study. Swasth Hind XVIII: (11-12). Reproduced in HIV/AIDS Research in India. NACO, 1997, New Delhi, pp. 116-18.

74. Gray, L.A., House, R.M., Devadas, R.P., Vijayalakshmi, O., & Kamalanathan, G. Knowledge, Attitudes, and Beliefs About HIV/AIDS Among Women Students at an Indian University. Presented at Eleventh International Conferenceo on AIDS, Vancouver, Canada; 1996. Abstract TuD 2742, Vol. 1, p. 391.

75. Grinard, B., & Cato, M. PSI Haiti Social Marketing STD/AIDS Prevention During High Risk Carnival Period. Presented at Eleventh International Conference on AIDS, Vancouver, Canada; 1996. Abstract TuD 2893, Vol. 1, p. 412.

76. Guyer, J., & Wooti, S. The Health Promotion Center: A Home Based Care. Model for Supporting People Living with HIV/AIDS in Thailand. Presented at Eleventh International Conference on AIDS, Vancouver, Canada; 1996. Abstract MoD 234, Vol. 1, p. 44.

77. Halloran, J.P., Ross, M., & Huffrman, L. Training PLWHIV for Involvement in Community Planning Processes: Project Leap (Learning, Empowerment, Advocacy, Participation). Presented at Eleventh International Conference on AIDS, Vancouver, Canada; 1996. Abstract TuC 234, Vol. 1, p. 255.

78. Herkommer, H., Lenuweit, B., Staszewski, S., & Stille, W.J. Epidemiological and Psychosocial Problems of Immigrants With HIV and AIDS. Presented at Eleventh International Conference on AIDS, Vancouver, Canada; 1996. Abstract TuC 2677, Vol. 1, p. 381.

79. *Hindustan Times,* September 11, 2001. No more Licenses Needed for Plying Cycle Rickshaws. *Hindustan Times*, New Delhi.

80. *Hindustan Times*, July 10, 2003. AIDS victim stoned to death in Andhra Pradesh. *Hindustan Times*, New Delhi.

81. *Hindustan Times,* (November 8, 2003). 75 per cent Jabs in Third World-used. London. *Hindustan Times,* New Delhi.

82. Honigsbaum, N., & Neil, O. The UN Convention on the Rights of the Child and Children Affected by HIV. Presented at Eleventh International Conference on AIDS, Vancouver, Canada; 1996. Abstract TuD 462, Vol. 1, p. 260.

83. Human Development Report. (2003). Wonder years in South Asia. *Times of India,* December 12, 2003, New Delhi.

84. ICMR. (1996). Turning Point in HIV/AIDS Research: Vision of Hope. ICMR Bulletin. Vol. 26, No. 12. Reproduced in HIV/AIDS Research in India. NACO, 1997, New Delhi, pp. 7-17.

85. India Abroad. (June-July, 2002). Joining India in the Fight Against AIDS. India Abroad, U.S.A.

86. *Indian Express*, April 4, 2002. Delhi Government Spends Crores on AIDS Awareness, Few Seem to be Learning. *Indian Express*, New Delhi.

87. *Indian Express*, December 9, 2003. AIDS – New Delhi at High Risk. *Indian Express*, New Delhi.

88. Jahoda, M., Deutsch, M., & Cook, S.W. (1955). Research Methods in Social Relations. The Dryden Press, Inc. New York.

89. Jain, K. (2001). Concern over Drug Resistant HIV Strains. *Times of India*, Undated. New Delhi.

90. Jain, K. (2002). Blood Banks Can Tell Donors HIV Status. *Times of India*, December 2, 2002. New Delhi.

91. JAMA. (1998). AIDS and Public Policy Journal. University Publishing Group. Vol. 13, No. 2.

92. Jayadekar, S., Pratinidhi, A., & Rodrigues. (1997). HIV Seropositivity in Truck Drivers. HIV/AIDS Research in India. NACO, New Delhi. pp. 491-92.

93. Jayaseelan, J. An HIV/AIDS Organization of Communities – Emphasizing Community Building, Consultation and Evaluation. Presented at Eleventh International Conference on AIDS, Vancouver, Canada; 1996. Abstract TuD 481, Vol. 1, p. 262.

94. Jemmott, L.S. Effective HIV/AIDS Prevention Interventions for Adolescents And Women: Results of a Decade of Research. Presented at Eleventh International Conference on AIDS, Vancouver, Canada; 1996. Abstract MoD 1779, Vol. 1, p. 187.

95. Josefina, G., & Tayag, D.P.A. Value Formation Among Male and Female Sex Workers: An Intervention Scheme for Behaviour Modification. Presented at Eleventh International Conference on AIDS, Vancouver, Canada; 1996. Abstract MoD 1851, Vol. 1, p. 198.

96. Julia, R., & Baume, C. When You Can't Be A Fly on the Wall: Improving Measures of Reported Risk Behaviour. Presented at Eleventh International Conference on AIDS, Vancouver, Canada; 1996. Abstract MoD 1859, Vol. 1, p. 200.

97. Kagimu, M., Walakira, Y., Nakyanjo, N., & Marum, E. The Effect of AIDS Education on Sexual Behaviour Among Women in the Muslim Community in Uganda. Presented at Eleventh International

Conference on AIDS, Vancouver, Canada; 1996. Abstract TuD 2837, Vol. 1, p. 404.

98. Kashyap, S. (2003). AIDS Victims Unite Against Discrimination. *Times of India,* October 20, 2002, New Delhi.

99. Kelly, J., Murphy, et al. The Effects of HIV/AIDS Intervention Groups for High-Risk Women in Urban Clinics. In *Journal of American Medical Association.* HIV/AIDS Patient Education, May 1998. University of California.

100. Kemmegne, J., Touko, A., & Kamta, C. Obstacles due to Religion and Traditional Medicine in the Prevention of HIV/AIDS in Cameroon. Presented at Eleventh International Conference on AIDS, Vancouver, Canada; 1996. Abstract TuD 2831, Vol. 1, p. 403.

101. Khan, M., & Sharma, A. (1997). Psycho-social Aspects of STD and HIV Infection Amongst Commercial Sex Workers in Delhi. HIV/AIDS Research In India. NACO, New Delhi, pp. 469-72.

102. Kiran, A., & Sharma, A. (1997). Psychosocial Aspects of STD and HIV Infection amongst CSWs in Delhi. HIV/AIDS Research In India. NACO, New Delhi, pp. 469-72.

103. Kirby, D. (1992). School Based Prevention Programmes. In R. Mathai, W. Michael, W. Ross, & S. Hira. Concomitants of HIV/STD Risk Behaviour and Intention to Engage in Risk Behaviours in Adolescents in India. HIV/AIDS Research in India. NACO, 1997, New Delhi, pp. 195-07.

104. Koester, S., Anderson, K., & Hoffer, L. Drug Sharing: Implication for HIV Prevention. Presented at Eleventh International Conference on AIDS, Vancouver, Canada; 1996. Abstract TuC 2553, Vol. 1, p. 360.

105. Koo, Henry, & Tang, D. Action Now! Asian Communities for Two Initiatives with One Need Now! A Model that Addresses Cultural Determinant Factors in the Larger Social Context of Community. Presented at Eleventh International Conference on AIDS, Vancouver, Canada; 1996. Abstract TuD 2923, Vol. 1, p. 416.

106. Krizansky, J., Lunin, I., Filimonov, S., & Vladimir. Sexual Prejudices of General Population in Russia. Presented at Eleventh International Conference on AIDS, Vancouver, Canada; 1996. Abstract TuD 2721, Vol. 1, p. 388.

107. Kumar, D. (1998). AIDS Spectre Haunts Armed Forces. *The Times of India,* (undated), New Delhi.

108. Kurth, A., Keller, S. L., & Getty, C. The Impact of Care Site on HIV Test-Seeking By Women. Presented at Eleventh International Conference on AIDS, Vancouver, Canada; 1996. Abstract TuC 2771, Vol. 1, p. 395.

109. Kutikuppala, S.R., Rao, M.V., Brahman, K.K., Murty, M.V., & Kumar, K. An Epidemiological Study on Sexual Reproductive Health in Promotion of Family Planning/AIDS Prevention in Slums of South India. Presented at Eleventh International Conference on AIDS, Vancouver, Canada; 1996. Abstract MoC 1497, Vol. 1, p. 141.

110. Lelievre, D., & Maison P. C. Art Therapy Support Group Conceived In An Integrative Way: A Global Approach for Reinforcing Self-Esteem of People Living With HIV/AIDS. Presented at Eleventh International Conference on AIDS, Vancouver, Canada; 1996. Abstract TuD 2851, Vol. 1, p. 406.

111. Lewis, Y.P., Young, P., Williams, M.L., & Wild, J. Structure of AIDS Risk For Female Sexual Partners of Injection Drug Users. Presented at Eleventh International Conference on AIDS, Vancouver, Canada; 1996. Abstract TuC 2469, Vol. 1, p. 346.

112. Londero, M.T., & Damond, M.E. Recent Immigrant Hispanics and HIV/AIDS Preventive Education: Program and Impact Evaluation That Work. Presented at Eleventh International Conference on AIDS, Vancouver, Canada; 1996. Abstract MoD 1799, Vol. 1, p. 191.

113. Mahler, H.M., & Flanagan. Afraid To Use Fear? Observations and Recommendation from Africa, Asia and Latin America. Presented at Eleventh International Conference on AIDS, Vancouver, Canada; 1996. Abstract TuD 2916, Vol. 1, p. 415.

114. Mahler, H.R., Flanagan, D., & Hassig, S.E. Emma Says and The Fleet of Hope: The Appeal of Global Messages and Icons. Presented at Eleventh International Conference on AIDS, Vancouver, Canada; 1996. Abstract TuD 2862, Vol. 1, p. 407.

115. Mane, P., & Maitra, S. (1992). AIDS Prevention: The Socio-Cultural Context in India. Tata Institute of Social Sciences. In R. Mathai, W. Michael, W. Ross, & S. Hira. Concomitants of HIV/AIDS Risk Behaviour and Intention to Engage in Risk Behaviour in Adolescents in India. NACO, 1997, New Delhi.

116. Manson-Singer, S., Willms, D., Adrien, A., Godin, G., Maticka-Tyndale, E., & Cappon, P. South Asian Immigrants' Risk Factors For HIV Transmission in Vancouver, Canada. Presented at Eleventh International Conference on AIDS, Vancouver, Canada; 1996. Abstract TuD 2901, Vol. 1, p. 413.

117. Martin, C., Love, J., & Stover, D. Reaching and Involving Youth: A Prevention Marketing Approach. Presented at Eleventh International Conference on AIDS, Vancouver, Canada; 1996. Abstract TuD 2881, Vol. 1, p. 410.

118. Martin, J. Transferable Concepts in Community Development Response to HIV/AIDS. Presented at Eleventh International Conference on AIDS, Vancouver, Canada; 1996. Abstract TuD 2934, Vol. 1, p. 418.
119. Mathai, R., Michael, W., Ross, W. & Hira, S. (1997) Concomitants of HIV/STD Risk Behaviour and Intention to Engage in Risk Behaviours in Adolescents in India. HIV/AIDS Research in India. NACO, New Delhi. pp. 195-207.
120. Maticka, T. E., Elkins, D., Rujkarakorn, D., Dole, L., Stam, K., & Haswell, E. Field-Based Programmes for Reduction of Sexual Transmission of HIV in North-East Thailand. Presented at Eleventh International Conference on AIDS, Vancouver, Canada; 1996. Abstract TuC 450, Vol. 1, p. 250.
121. Mc Clure, C. M., Naumovich, W., & Robinson, B. HIV + Peers as Treatment Information Counsellors: Training Program and Service Delivery. Presented at Eleventh International Conference on AIDS, Vancouver, Canada; 1996. Abstract MoD 1785, Vol. 1, p. 188.
122. Mehra, S. (2003). *Times of India*, January 20, 2003, New Delhi.
123. Metsch, L.R., McCoy, C. B., McCoy, H.V., Lai, S., & Correa, R. Influence of Living Arrangements in Predicting Behaviour Change Among Drug Using Women at Risk for HIV Infection. Presented at Eleventh International Conference on AIDS, Vancouver, Canada; 1996. Abstract TuD 2770, Vol. 1, p. 395.
124. Miller, L. C., Murphy, S.T., Clark, L., & Mackie, D. Selling Safer Sex: Do AIDS Messages Fit The Everyday Goals of the High Risk Women? Presented at Eleventh International Conference on AIDS, Vancouver, Canada; 1996. Abstract MoD 1834, Vol. 1, p. 196.
125. Mishra, M. (2003). AIDS a Curse for U.P. Government Hospitals. *Times of India*, August 25, 2003, New Delhi.
126. Mittal, M., Garg, S., Sehgal, K., & Bansal, R. (1995). A Study of KABP Regarding STD and HIV/AIDS Amongst Women of an Urban Slum: Health Issues in Delhi. In HIV/AIDS Research in India. NACO, 1997, New Delhi, pp. 130-33.
127. Morais de Sa, C.A., Sion, F.S., Moura E.M., Oliveira, E.R., Meria – de- Vasconcellos., Borges, M. R. Male Sexual Behavior and Women's Risk for HIV Infection in Rio De Janeiro, Brazil. Presented at Eleventh International Conference on AIDS, Vancouver, Canada; 1996. Abstract TuC 2425, Vol. 1, p. 339.
128. Morrill, A.M., & Ickovics, J. Surviving Abuse and HIV Risk– How Women's Experiences of Abuse Shape their Heterosexual Risk for

HIV. Presented at Eleventh International Conference on AIDS, Vancouver, Canada; 1996. Abstract TuD 134, Vol. 1, p. 254.

129. Muncy, S., Pablo, C., Luwalhati, F., & Gudaca, R. T. "Community Based Approach to the Prevention of HIV/AIDS in Palawan, Philippines". Presented at Eleventh International Conference on AIDS, Vancouver, Canada; 1996. Abstract TuC 2671, Vol. 1, p. 381.

130. Musuamba, N., & Mutombo, T. Education Programme Inviting Women to Use Their Rights for the Preservation of Sexual Relationships Against HIV Infection: The Human Rights Programme. Presented at Eleventh International Conference on AIDS, Vancouver, Canada; 1996. Abstract TuD 356, Vol. 1, p. 258.

131. NACO. (1996 – 2003). Yearly Updates Published on December 1, World AIDS Day. *Times of India,* New Delhi.

132. NACO. (1996). *National AIDS Control Programme – India, Country Scenario: An Update.* NACO, New Delhi.

133. NACO. (2000). *Specialist's Training and Reference Module – 2000.* NACO, New Delhi.

134. NACO. (2001). *National Baseline High Risk And Bridge Population Behavioural Surveillance Survey – 2001, Part – I, Female Commercial Sex Workers and Their Clients.* NACO, New Delhi.

135. NACO. (2002). India responds to AIDS. NACO, New Delhi.

136. NACO. (2003). In K. Jain. AIDS Bomb in India Ticking at a Faster Rate. *Times of India*, July/August, 2003, New Delhi.

137. NACO. (2004). *Hindustan Times*, May 27, 2005, New Delhi.

138. NACO. (April, 2000). AIDS in India. NACO, New Delhi. Vol. 1, No. 2, p. 3.

139. NACO. (December 1, 2001). Resurgent India Meets the AIDS Challenge. In *Times of India*, December 1, 2001, New Delhi.

140. NACO. (December, 2000). Towards an AIDS – Free India. *Times of India*, December 1, 2000, New Delhi.

141. NACO. (July-Sept., 2000). AIDS in India. NACO, New Delhi, Vol. 1, No. 3.

142. NACO. (March, 1994). *High Risk Behaviour Assessment Guide.* NACO, New Delhi.

143. NACO. (Oct. – Dec., 2000). AIDS in India. NACO, New Delhi, Vol. 1, No. 4.

144. Nankunda, A. Factors That Influence Sustained Behaviour Change Among Rural Women in South Western Uganda, in Relation to HIV Prevention. Presented at Eleventh International Conference on AIDS, Vancouver, Canada; 1996. Abstract TuD 2741, Vol. 1, p. 391.

145. Narain, J., & Jha, A. (1997). *NGOs and AIDS – Responding to the Expanding Epidemic.* WHO, New Delhi.
146. Nickson, A., & Kosch, D. Raising Relevance, Not Prevalence: An Example of Improvisational Drama in Gay Community Development and Education. Presented at Eleventh International Conference on AIDS, Vancouver, Canada; 1996. Abstract TuD 2933, Vol. 1, p. 418.
147. Nicolosi, et al. (1994) & Padian, et al. (1995). In NACO. Women and HIV Infection – Including Mother to Child Transmission. *Specialist's Training and Reference Module.* NACO, 2000, New Delhi.
148. Nordenberg, D. F., & Bernstein, C.W. HIV Youth Intervention: A School Based Theatre Performance and Related Intervention Activities. Presented at Eleventh International Conference on AIDS, Vancouver, Canada; 1996. Abstract MoD 244, Vol. 1, p. 45.
149. Nowlan, M., Clayton–Davis, J., Dennie, S., Love, J., & Word, E. Community Planning Process That Fosters Responsibility, Ownership and Commitment: The Nashville Preventing Marketing Initiative. Presented at Eleventh International Conference on AIDS, Vancouver, Canada; 1996. Abstract TuD 2942, Vol. 1, p. 419.
150. O'Neill, Joseph, F., Talmadge, S., Gordon, S., Gerber R., & Sumaya, C. Analysis of the U.S., Public Health Service Programs to Increase Access to Care and Services for Women Living With HIV/AIDS. Presented at Eleventh International Conference on AIDS, Vancouver, Canada; 1996. Abstract TuD 2760, Vol. 1, p. 394.
151. Oetomo, D. Cultural Sensitivity to Gender and Sexual Diversity as a Prerequisite to Effective HIV/AIDS Programme. Presented at Eleventh International Conference on AIDS, Vancouver, Canada; 1996. Abstract TuD 601, Vol. 1, p. 263.
152. Ortiz-Torres, B., Ehrhardt, A., Van Dommelen, E., & River, M.G. Testing A Diffusion-Of Innovation Approach to Encourage HIV Risk Reduction Behaviour Among Latin Women. Presented at Eleventh International Conference on AIDS, Vancouver, Canada; 1996. Abstract TuD 2750, Vol. 1, p. 392.
153. Pachauri, S. (1994). Women's Reproductive Health in India: Research Needs and Priorities. In R. Mathai, W. Michael, W. Ross, & S. Hira. Concomitants of HIV/STD Risk Behaviour and Intention to Engage in Risk Behaviour in Adolescents in India. HIV/AIDS Research in India. NACO, 1997, New Delhi, pp. 195-207.
154. Pandey, V., Bhargava, N., & Tiwari, V. (1989) AIDS Awareness and Knowledge among STD Patients. Swasth Hind, 1989:33 (12). Reproduced in HIV/AIDS Research in India. NACO, 1997, New Delhi, pp. 804-05.

155. Paula, K. The Development of a Cultural Model for Behaviour Change. Presented at Eleventh International Conference on AIDS, Vancouver, Canada; 1996. Abstract TuD 2864, Vol. 1, p. 408.

156. Pinckney, L.D., Hare, M., Rugg, D., & Kennedy, M. Case Study Methods for Evaluation Process of Participatory Social Marketing. Presented at Eleventh International Conference on AIDS, Vancouver, Canada; 1996. Abstract MoC 1606, Vol. 1, p. 159.

157. Pinel, A. Personal Dynamics of Women Who Risk Unprotected Sex With HIV Infected Partners. Presented at Eleventh International Conference on AIDS, Vancouver, Canada; 1996. Abstract MoD 1684, Vol. 1, p. 171.

158. Pott, E., Toppich, J., & Christiansen, G. The Important Role of Audio-visual Media in AIDS Prevention. Presented at Eleventh International Conference on AIDS, Vancouver, Canada; 1996. Abstract MoD 1820, Vol. 1, p. 194.

159. Pran, N. (undated). Sex Workers Need Help. *Hindustan Times*. New Delhi.

160. Radford, J., King, A., & Warren, W. Street Youth and AIDS. Ontario: Kingston, 1989. In R. Bansal. Truck Drivers and Risk of STD Including HIV. HIV/AIDS Research in India. NACO, 1997, New Delhi, pp. 488-90.

161. Ramakrishnaiah, Y., Lakshmi, N., Gururaj, A., Srinivasula, M., & Veerappa, M. (1991). Clinical and Serological Profile of Hotel Workers in Tirupati. Reproduced in HIV/AIDS Research in India. NACO, 1997, New Delhi, pp. 452-53.

162. Ravelo, N., Herndez, R., Williams, N. Kalinga, A., & Cavite. The Influence of Customers and Employers on Condom Use Among Sex Workers in the Philippines. Presented at Eleventh International Conference on AIDS, Vancouver, Canada; 1996. Abstract TuC 2670, Vol. 1, p. 380.

163. Rompa, D. J., Kalichaman, S.C., & Kelly, J.A. Age and Ethnicity in Relation to HIV Risk Behavior Levels in a Diverse Community Sample of Men Who Have Sex with Men. Presented at Eleventh International Conference on AIDS, Vancouver, Canada; 1996. Abstract TuC 2406, Vol. 1, p. 336.

164. Rosas Solis, A., Rangel, G., & Diaz, J. Social Factors Of Female Prostitution That Influence on Their Health Condition: HIV and Sexually Transmitted Diseases. The Case of Tijuana, B.C., Mexico. Presented at Eleventh International Conference on AIDS, Vancouver, Canada; 1996. Abstract TuC 2666, Vol. 1, p. 380.

165. Rosensnard, C., & Campbell, T.A. Review of Sexual Behaviour Change Studies From Sub-Saharan Africa: What Lessons Can We Learn For The Future. Presented at Eleventh International Conference on AIDS, Vancouver, Canada; 1996. Abstract MoD 1831, Vol. 1, p. 196.

166. Roy, P., & Chowdhury, S. (1997). Knowledge and Attitude Regarding HIV/AIDS of General Medical Practitioners from Delhi. HIV/AIDS Research in India. NACO, New Delhi, pp. 148-50.

167. Roy, S., Aggarwal, O.P., Gupta, P. & Ramchandran, V.G. (1997). HIV Seropositivity Among Truck Drivers Plying Through the Eastern Border of Delhi. HIV/AIDS Research in India. NACO, 1997, New Delhi, p. 493.

168. Rudelic-Fernandez, D., Bajos, N., Lert, F., Ducot, B., & Sipra, A. Towards a New Model for Public Awareness Campaigns: The Role of Fiction in Supporting Identification and Social Interaction. Presented at Eleventh International Conference on AIDS, Vancouver, Canada; 1996. Abstract MoD 1832, Vol. 1, p. 196.

169. Rugg, D.L., Nowak, G., Westover, B., Monterroso, M., Pinckney, L., Kennedy M., & Shepherd, M. Evaluating the Contributions of Social Marketing to HIV Prevention in Five U.S. Communities. Presented at Eleventh International Conference on AIDS, Vancouver, Canada; 1996. Abstract TuD 2880, Vol. 1, p. 410.

170. Ruiz, BA., Magis, R.C., Ortiz, M. R., Bronfman, M. del Rio C. The Uses of Attitudes Assessment in Research About AIDS in Mexico. Presented at Eleventh International Conference on AIDS, Vancouver, Canada; 1996. Abstract MoD 1869, Vol. 1, p. 201.

171. Sarman, S., & Niti, S. Human Immunodeficiency Virus Reaches Small Villages in Rural India. Presented at Eleventh International Conference on AIDS, Vancouver, Canada; 1996. Abstract MoC 4554, Vol. 1, p. 40.

172. Schechter, C., Lee, A., Zucker, D., Stover, D., Puryer, M., Rowland, S., & Puryear, M. Enhancing Collaboration Between Community – Based Organizations, Behavioural Research, and Social Marketers in Developing HIV Prevention Programmes for Youth: The Prevention Marketing Initiative (PMI). Presented at Eleventh International Conference on AIDS, Vancouver, Canada; 1996. Abstract TuD 2886, Vol. 1, p. 411.

173. Sehgal, P. N., & Singh, K. (1997). KABP Study related to AIDS in Manipur State, India and Intervention. HIV/AIDS Research in India. NACO, New Delhi, pp. 137-40.

174. Sehgal, P.N. (1997). KABP Study Related to AIDS in Tamil Nadu State, India and Intervention Strategies. HIV/AIDS Research in India. NACO, New Delhi, pp. 141-47.

175. Seth, M., & Capila, A. (1998). In Vasuja, S. Towards Better Health and Hygiene: An Intervention in S.O. S. Children's Villages, Unpublished Master's Dissertation (1999). University of Delhi, Delhi.

176. Sethi, G., & Lal, S. High Risk Behaviour Study in 35 Cities. Presented at Eleventh International Conference on AIDS, Vancouver, Canada; 1996. Abstract MoD 1697, Vol. 1, p. 174.

177. Shain, R., Piper, J., Newton, E., Perdue, S., Ramos, R., Dimmitt, J., Guerra, F., Porto, M. Preventing Sexually Transmitted Disease Among Minority Women: Results of a Controlled Randomized Trial at 12 months' Follow-Up. Presented at Eleventh International Conference on AIDS, Vancouver, Canada; 1996. Abstract MoD 1773, Vol. 1, p. 187.

178. Shanmuganandan, S., & Maniyosai, R. Geographic Distributions And Patterns of Spatial Diffusion of AIDS Epidemic In Tamil Nadu, India. Presented at Eleventh International Conference on AIDS, Vancouver, Canada; 1996. Abstract MoC 1498, Vol. 1, p. 141.

179. Sharma, A., Sehgal, V., Kant, S., & Chawla, S. (1994). Knowledge, Attitude Survey of Rural Adolescents. International Conference on AIDS. In R. Mathai, W. Michael, W. Ross, & S. Hira. Concomitants of HIV/AIDS Risk Behaviour and Intention to Engage in Risk Behaviour in Adolescents in India. NACO, 1997, New Delhi, pp. 195-207.

180. Sharma, N. (2001). For Free AIDS Treatment, Go to Jail. *Times of India*, August 8, 2001, New Delhi.

181. Sharma, S. (2003). Free Drugs for HIV Positive Kids, Mothers. *Hindustan Times*, November 13, 2003, New Delhi.

182. Shreedhar, J. (2002). A Bitter Pill – Coping with New Strains of HIV. *Times of India*, August 2, 2002, New Delhi.

183. Shubhandha, S., Jayadekar, A. P., Sanjay, S.M., & Rodrigues. (1997). HIV Seropostivity in Truck Drivers. HIV/AIDS Research in India. NACO, New Delhi. pp. 491-92.

184. Siegel, L. (1986). Relationship to Alcohol and Other Drugs Journal of Substance Abuse Treatment. In R.K. Bansal. HIV/AIDS Research in India. NACO, 1997, New Delhi, pp. 494-96.

185. Sikos, G. Risk Concepts and Sexual Protection in the Imagery and Customs. Presented at Eleventh International Conference on AIDS, Vancouver, Canada; 1996. Abstract MoD 1780, Vol. 1, p. 188.

186. Silva, J. L., Nakata, A.K., Figueiredo, C.R., Andrade, L.F., Passador, L. H. STD/AIDS Prevention Among Female Prostitutes in Sao Paulo State. Presented at Eleventh International Conference on AIDS, Vancouver, Canada; 1996. Abstract Tuc 2622, Vol. 1, p. 372.

187. Sin, E. Asian Volunteer Coordination and Training Modules. Presented at Eleventh International Conference on AIDS, Vancouver, Canada; 1996. Abstract TuD 2850, Vol. 1, p. 405.

188. Singh, B., Bedi, Y., Singh, S., & Sehgal, S. (1994). AIDS awareness among Truck Drivers in Punjab. Ann Natl Acad Med Sci (India). Reproduced in HIV/AIDS Research In India. NACO, 1997, New Delhi, pp. 263-72.

189. Skinner, S., Ruiz, J., & Stempliuk, V. Youth Divided: HIV Prevention in a Brazilian Inner City Community. Presented at Eleventh International Conference on AIDS, Vancouver, Canada; 1996. Abstract TuD 2940, Vol. 1, p. 419.

190. Span. (2001). The Quiet AIDS Crisis. Sept./Oct. New Delhi.

191. Srivastava, R. (2003). Bill for Treating AIDS Patients. *Times of India*, January 14, 2003, New Delhi.

192. Stayanoff, S.R., Weber M.D., Ford, W.L., Kerndt, P.R., Sexual Behaviors and Non-injection Drug Use Among Young Men, 15-22 Years of Age Who Have Sex with Men: Young Men's Survey. Presented at Eleventh International Conference on AIDS, Vancouver, Canada; 1996. Abstract TuC 2411, Vol. 1, p. 337.

193. Stokes, D., & Mestman, B. (1996). SPV- 30: An Activist Initiated Informal Study to Collect Data to determine the Efficacy of a Natural Alternative Therapy For HIV/AIDS. Presented at Eleventh International Conference on AIDS, Vancouver, Canada; 1996. Abstract TuD 2946, Vol. 1, p. 420.

194. Stratford, D., & Ellerbrock, T. Social Organization of Sexual Behaviour and its Relation to HIV Risk and Transmission in a Rural Community in the South Eastern United States. Presented at Eleventh International Conference On AIDS, Vancouver, Canada; 1996. Abstract TuD 2712, Vol. 1, p. 386.

195. Strathdee Steffanie, A., Patric, D. M. Archibald, C., Ofner, M., Craib, K.P., Cornelisse, P., Eades, G., Schechter, M., Rekart, M., & O'Shughnessy, M. Social Determinants Predict Needle Sharing Behaviour Among Injection Drug Users in Vancouver. Presented at Eleventh International Conference on AIDS, Vancouver, Canada; 1996. Abstract MoD 363, Vol. 1, p. 48.

196. Susan, M., Shepherd, M., Bhattacharya, K., Rosenbaum, J., Baume, C., & Weiss. L. Use of a Theory-Based Semi-Structured Elicitation Questionnaire to Explore Determinants of Consist Condom Use. Presented at Eleventh International Conference on AIDS, Vancouver, Canada; 1996. Abstract MoD 1727, Vol. 1, p. 179.

197. *The Week.* (2000). Shadows of the Dead. December 10, 2000. Vol. 18, No.52, pp. 15-17.

198. Thorens, J. J. Eurocaso/Positive Action Twinning Process of Structured Skill Exchange. Presented at Eleventh International Conference on AIDS, Vancouver, Canada; 1996. Abstract TuD 2879, Vol. 1, p. 410.

199. Tikoo, M., Bollman, S., & Bergen, M. (1995). Knowledge Level of Youth in India regarding Human Sexuality and AIDS. Journal of Sex and Marital Therapy. Reproduced in HIV/AIDS Research In India. NACO, 1997, New Delhi, pp. 208-12.

200. *Times of India*. (2001). Rescued Minors May Have Been Given Estrogen. *Times of India*, June, 2001, New Delhi.

201. *Times of India.* (August 26, 2003). Our Future is Sealed. *Times of India,* New Delhi.

202. *Times of India*. (December 1, 2001). AIDS Spread in India, *Times of India*, New Delhi.

203. *Times of India*. (December 12, 2003). Human Development Report. New Delhi.

204. *Times of India*. (December 2, 2003). India to Supply Free Drugs to AIDS Patients. *Times of India*, New Delhi.

205. *Times of India.* (January 4, 2002). Capital has 646 cases of full-blown AIDS. *Times of India,* New Delhi.

206. *Times of India*. (July 18, 2003). Schools deny admission to HIV positive. *Times of India*, New Delhi.

207. *Times of India*. (July 28, 2003). Don't Rob Education to Pay for AIDS. *Times of India*, New Delhi.

208. *Times of India.* (July 4, 2003). AIDS Awareness Dismal. *Times of India,* New Delhi.

209. *Times of India.* (June, 2001). UN Special Session on HIV/AIDS. *Times of India,* June, 2001. New Delhi.

210. *Times of India.* (September 22, 2003). Huge Response to DT Articles. *Times of India,* New Delhi.

211. TNN. (2001). 38 Minor Girls Rescued from Brothel Owners. *Times of India,* June, 2001, New Delhi.

212. Toppich, J., Christiansen, G., & Pott, E. Effectiveness of the First 10 Years of the National AIDS Prevention Campaign in Germany. Presented at Eleventh International Conference on AIDS, Vancouver, Canada; 1996. Abstract MoD 1819, Vol. 1, p. 193.

213. UNAIDS. (1999). Listen, Learn and Live! 1999 World AIDS Campaign with Children and Young People. UNAIDS, Geneva.

214. UNAIDS. (2003). Progress Report on the Global Response to the HIV/AIDS Epidemic, 2003. UNAIDS, Geneva.

215. UNAIDS. (September, 1999). From Principle to Practice. UNAIDS, Geneva.

216. UNAIDS/WHO. (December, 1998). AIDS Epidemic Update: December 1998. UNAIDS, Geneva.

217. UNAIDS/WHO. (December, 1999). AIDS Epidemic Update: December 1999. UNAIDS, Geneva.

218. UNAIDS/WHO. (December, 2000). AIDS Epidemic Update: December 2000. UNAIDS, Geneva.

219. UNAIDS/WHO. (December, 2001). AIDS Epidemic Update: December 2001. UNAIDS, Geneva.

220. UNAIDS/WHO. (December, 2003). AIDS Epidemic Update: December 2003. UNAIDS, Geneva.

221. UNAIDS/WHO. (December, 2003).AIDS Epidemic Update: December 2004. UNAIDS, Geneva.

222. UNAIDS/WHO. (June 1998). Report on the Global HIV/AIDS Epidemic. UNAIDS, Geneva.

223. UNFPA. (September, 2000). Adolescents in India – A Profile. New Delhi.

224. UNICEF (December 12, 2003). Wonder years in South Asia. *Times of India*, New Delhi.

225. USAID. (1997). In NACO. Women and HIV Infection. *Specialist's Training and Reference Module,* NACO, 2000, New Delhi.

226. Velyvis, K.A., Onyango, P., Hasselblad, W., Ndaiye, F. & Lawson, A. Market Women in Senegals: Realities, Risks, and Appropriate Interventions. Presented at Eleventh International Conference on AIDS, Vancouver, Canada; 1996. Abstract TuD 2765, Vol. 1, p. 394.

227. Wadhwa, S., Wahab, S., Gupta, S., & Deshmukh, S. (1997). Knowledge and Attitude of Secondary Students Towards HIV/AIDS. HIV/AIDS Research in India. NACO, New Delhi. pp. 184-88.

228. Wanjpe, A., & Akarte, S. (1997). Knowledge Attitude and Practices – Study of Barbers about HIV Transmission in Bombay. HIV/AIDS Research in India. NACO, New Delhi. pp. 258-60.

229. Warren, P. Participatory Research With Adolescents to Develop Appropriate Media Products for HIV, STD and Pregnancy Prevention. Presented at Eleventh International Conference on AIDS, Vancouver, Canada; 1996. Abstract TuD 2899, Vol. 1, p. 413.

230. Weinrich, J., Atkinson, J. H., & Grant, I., Buried Pleasures: Childhood Family and Environment Predicts Preferences for Certain Safe and Unsafe Sexual Acts. Presented at Eleventh International Conference on AIDS, Vancouver, Canada; 1996. Abstract TuD 2714, Vol. 1, p. 387.

231. Westover, B., Nowa, G., Rugg, D., Kasprzyk, & Mitchell, K. Designing Evaluations of Community-Level HIV Prevention Plans. Presented at Eleventh International Conference On AIDS, Vancouver, Canada; 1996. Abstract MoD 1801, Vol. 1, p. 191.

232. WHO. (1997). *AIDS No Time for Complacency.* New Delhi.

233. WHO. (1998). World AIDS day – Force for Change, World AIDS Campaign with Young People. WHO, New Delhi.

234. WHO. (1999). AIDS The Challenge. New Delhi.

235. WHO. (January – April, 2000). AIDS Watch. Vol. 5, No. 1, New Delhi.

236. WHO. (November, 1998). AIDS Watch. Vol. 3, No. 4, New Delhi.

237. Wolf, R.C., & DeJong, W. Enough Already: Re-evaluating The Future of the U.S. Government's AIDS Awareness Campaign. Presented at Eleventh International Conference on AIDS, Vancouver, Canada; 1996. Abstract MoD 1828, Vol. 1, p. 195.

238. Woody, G. E., Metzger, D., Marmor, M., Gross, M., McKirman, D., Koblin, B., & Donnel, D. Substance use and risky behaviour among men having sex with men. Presented at Eleventh International Conference on AIDS, Vancouver, Canada; 1996. Abstract TuC 2414, Vol. 1, p. 337.

239. www.excite.com. (November 26, 2001). Home Page, News.

240. www.unaids.org. (1999). Listen, Learn and Live! Challenges for Latin America and the Carribean. UNAIDS, Geneva.

241. www.unaids.org. (June, 1998). Report on the global HIV/AIDS epidemic. UNAIDS, Geneva.

242. www.unaids.org. (September, 1998). UNAIDS, Geneva.

243. Yameogo, V., Watts, S., Devine, J. The Female Minstrels of Bobo-Dioulasso, Use of Traditional Channel for AIDS IEC. Presented at Eleventh International Conference on AIDS, Vancouver, Canada; 1996. Abstract MoD 246, Vol. 1, p. 46.

Index